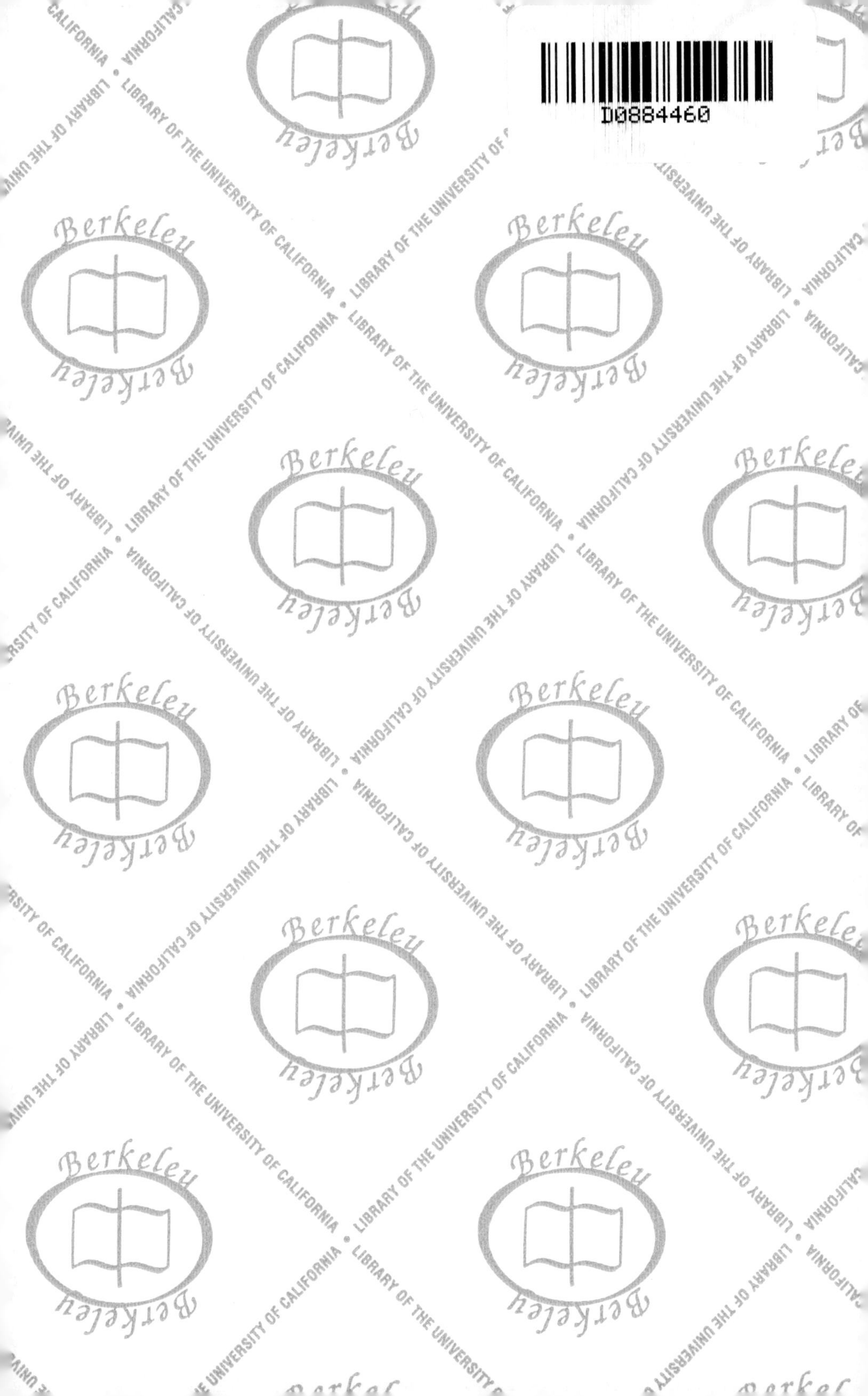

Color Atlas & Synopsis of Clinical Ophthalmology

WILLS EYE HOSPITAL

OCULOPLASTICS

COLOR ATLAS AND SYNOPSIS OF CLINICAL OPHTHALMOLOGY SERIES

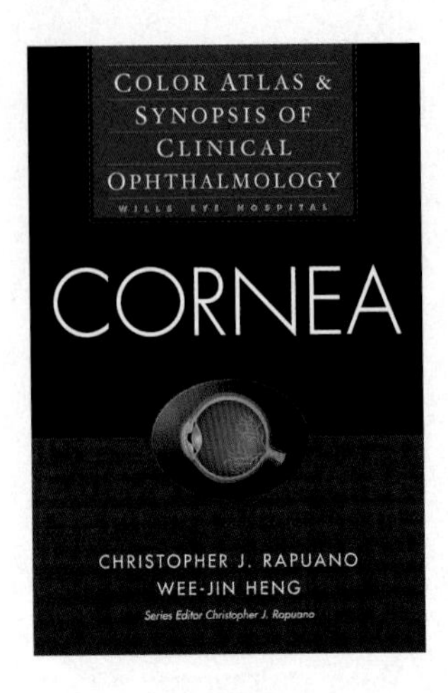

CORNEA
Christopher J. Rapuano, MD
Wee-Jin Heng, MD
0-07-137589-9

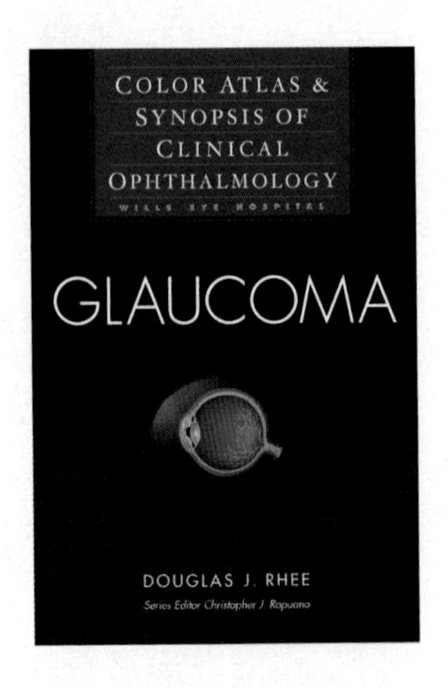

GLAUCOMA
Douglas J. Rhee, MD
0-07-137597-X

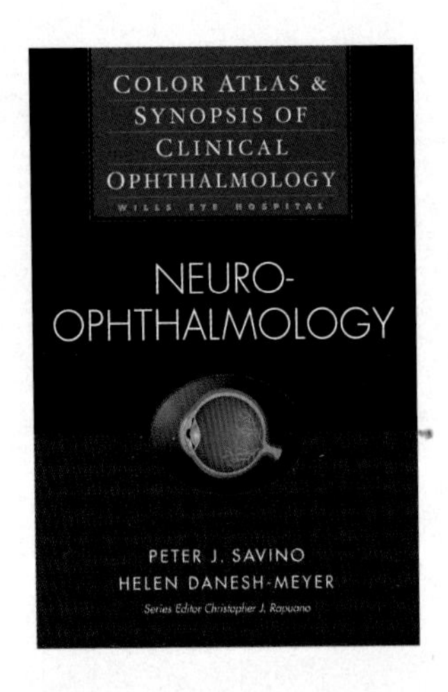

NEUROOPHTHALMOLOGY
Peter J. Savino, MD
Helen Danesh-Meyer, MD
0-07-137595-3

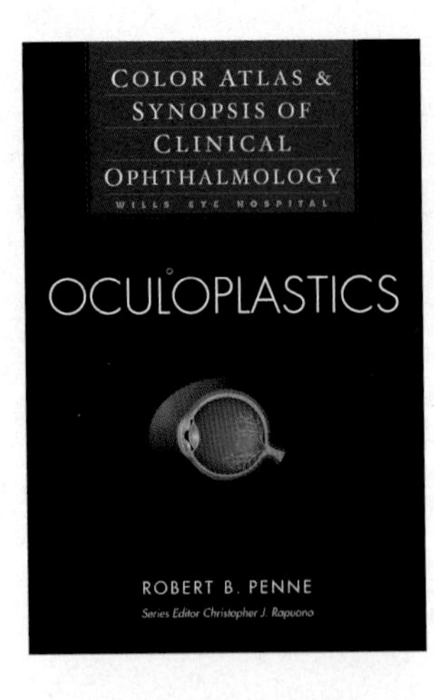

OCULOPLASTICS
Robert B. Penne, MD
0-07-137594-5

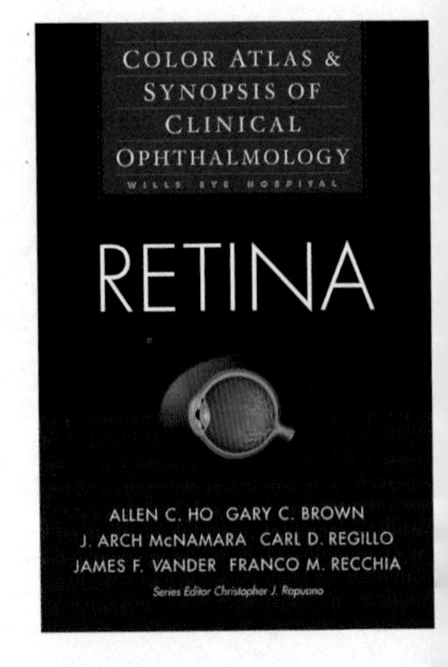

RETINA
Allen C. Ho, MD
Gary C. Brown, MD
J. Arch McNamara, MD
Franco M. Recchia, MD
Carl D. Regillo, MD
James F. Vander, MD
0-07-137596-1

Color Atlas & Synopsis of Clinical Ophthalmology

Wills Eye Hospital

Oculoplastics

Robert B. Penne, MD
Co-Director of the Oculoplastics Service
Wills Eye Hospital
Philadelphia, Pennsylvania

McGraw-Hill
Medical Publishing Division

New York Chicago San Francisco Lisbon London
Madrid Mexico City Milan New Delhi San Juan Seoul
Singapore Sydney Toronto

McGraw-Hill

A Division of The McGraw-Hill Companies

Oculoplastics: Color Atlas and Synopsis of Clinical Ophthalmology

1234567890 IMA IMA 098765432

ISBN 0-07-137594-5

This book was set in Times Roman by TechBooks.
The editors were Darlene Cooke, Susan Noujaim, and Karen Davis.
The production supervisor was Richard Ruzycka.
The book designer was Marsha Cohen.
The cover designer was Mary Belibasakis.
The index was prepared by Editorial Services, Maria Coughlin.
Imago, Singapore, was printer and binder.

This book is printed on acid-free paper.

Library of Congress Cataloging-in-Publication Data

Penne, Robert.
Oculoplastics : color atlas and synopsis of clinical ophthalmology / Robert Penne.
p. ; cm.—(Color atlas and synopsis of clinical ophthalmology series)
Includes bibliographical references and index.
ISBN 0-07-137594-5
1. Ophthalmic plastic surgery—Atlases. 2. Ophthalmic plastic surgery—Handbooks, manuals, etc. I. Title. II. Series.
[DNLM: 1. Ophthalmologic Surgical Procedures—Atlases. 2. Eye Diseases—surgery—Atlases. 3. Reconstructive Surgical Procedures—Atlases. WW 17 P412o 2003]
RE87 .P46 2003
617.7′1—dc21 2002075359

To Devany, Daniel, and Mara

the source of pride and balance in my life

NOTICE

CONTENTS

ABOUT THE SERIES

The beauty of the atlas/synopsis concept is the powerful combination of illustrative photographs and a summary approach to the text. Ophthalmology is a very visual discipline which lends itself nicely to clinical photographs. While the five ophthalmic subspecialties in this series, Cornea, Retina, Glaucoma, Oculoplastics, and Neuroophthalmology, employ varying levels of visual recognition, a relatively standard format for the text is used for all volumes.

The goal of the series is to provide an up-to-date clinical overview of the major areas of ophthalmology for students, residents, and practitioners in all the healthcare professions. The abundance of large, excellent quality photographs and concise, outline-form text will help achieve that objective.

Christopher J. Rapuano, MD.
Series Editor

PREFACE

Oculoplastics: Color Atlas & Synopsis of Clinical Ophthalmology is aimed at assisting physicians (ophthalmologists and nonophthalmologists) in recognizing most common oculoplastic conditions. Many oculoplastic conditions can be diagnosed on simple visual examination which makes this atlas an ideal resource to have in emergency rooms and in the office. This atlas provides a solid basis of photographic and descriptive information to diagnose oculoplastic conditions. Once these conditions are recognized, the text describes other tests that may be needed and the differential diagnoses that should be considered. The management options for these conditions are also described.

ACKNOWLEDGMENTS

Special thank to my colleagues who provided assistance: Edward Bedrossian, MD; Jurij Bilyk, MD; Richard Hertle, MD; and Mary A Stefanyszyn, MD. Thank you to Chris Rapuano, MD, who went well beyond his duties as editor in his assistance at every stage of creation of this atlas.

Color Atlas & Synopsis of Clinical Ophthalmology

Wills Eye Hospital

Oculoplastics

Section I

EYELIDS

Chapter 1

BENIGN EYELID LESIONS

PAPILLOMA

A papilloma is a common benign, often asymptomatic, skin lesion that occurs most commonly in the intertriginous areas (axillae, inframammary, and groin) but is also commonly seen on the neck and eyelids. These are often numerous on the eyelids when present and the number tends to increase with age.
Synonyms: skin tag, acrochordon.

Epidemiology and Etiology

Age More common in middle-aged and elderly people.

Gender More common in females.

Etiology Unknown.

History

Most commonly asymptomatic but may become tender after trauma. With time, lesions may become crusted or hemorrhagic.

Examination

Lesions are soft; skin-colored, tan, or brown; round or oval, pedunculated papillomas (Fig. 1-1A to C). The lesion is often constricted at the base. Size ranges from less than 1 mm to 10 mm.

Special Considerations

May grow or become more numerous during pregnancy. More common in obese patients.

Differential Diagnosis

- Pedunculated seborrheic keratosis
- Dermal nevus
- Solitary neurofibroma
- Molluscum contagiosum.
- Conjunctival papillomas (Fig. 1-1B) can appear on the eyelid margin but have a different appearance and the base of the lesion is from the conjunctival surface.

Treatment

Excision by simply snipping the lesion at the base.

Prognosis

Excellent. Patients may develop other papillomas with time.

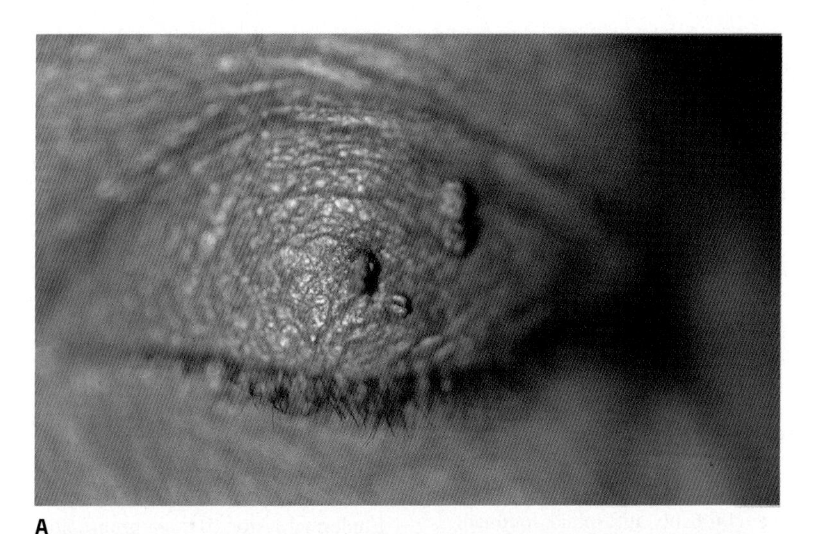

A

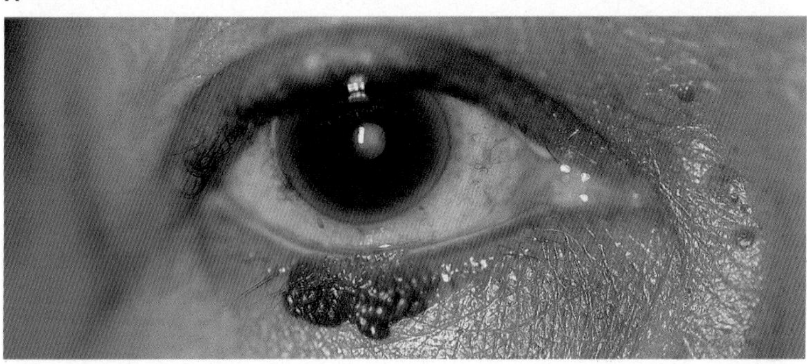

B

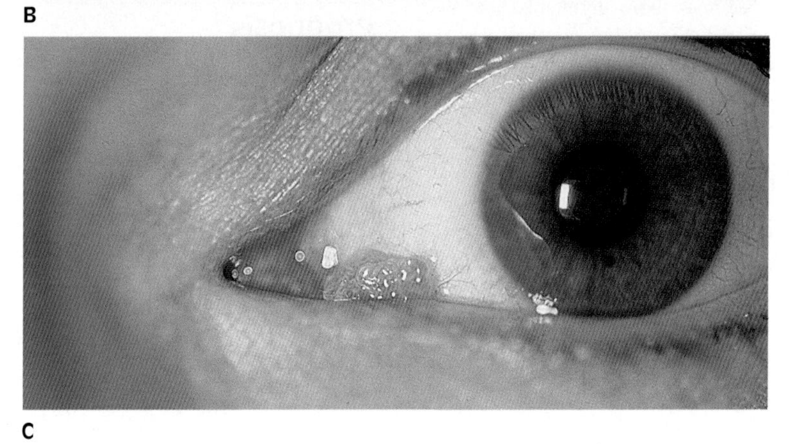

C

Figure 1-1 Papilloma **A.** *Multiple small papillomas of the upper eyelid.* **B.** *Larger papilloma of the right lower eyelid.* **Conjunctival papilloma** **C.** *Papillomatous lesions may grow from the conjunctival surface and protrude onto the eyelid margin. These papillomas are flesh colored and more friable than cutaneous papillomas. Conjunctival papillomas can be associated with a viral origin.*

SEBORRHEIC KERATOSIS

The seborrheic keratosis is one of the most common benign epithelial tumors. These lesions are hereditary, are rarely seen before the age of 30 years, and will continue to increase over a lifetime. Some patients will only have a few and others can have hundreds over their body.

Epidemiology and Etiology

Age More common as patients age. Rare before age 30 years.

Gender More common and more extensive in males.

Etiology Unknown.

Inheritance Probably autosomal dominant.

History

Lesions are often present for months to years and are often asymptomatic. They are most common on the face, trunk, and upper extremities.

Examination

Lesion starts as a flat, light tan lesion. With time, the lesion becomes more pigmented and will become elevated (Fig. 1-2A). As they age, the lesion's surface becomes "warty" (Fig. 1-2B). Lesions vary in size from 1 mm to 6 cm.

Special Considerations

Most common on lower lids.

Differential Diagnosis

- Pigmented actinic keratosis
- Verruca vulgaris
- Pigmented basal cell carcinoma

Pathophysiology

Epidermal lesion. Benign proliferation of keratinocytes, melanocytes, and formation of horn cysts.

Treatment

Light electrocautery or cryotherapy will permit the lesion to be easily rubbed or curretted off. The underlying base can then be retreated with cautery.

Prognosis

Excellent with rare recurrence. Patient will often have many lesions and will develop additional lesions over time.

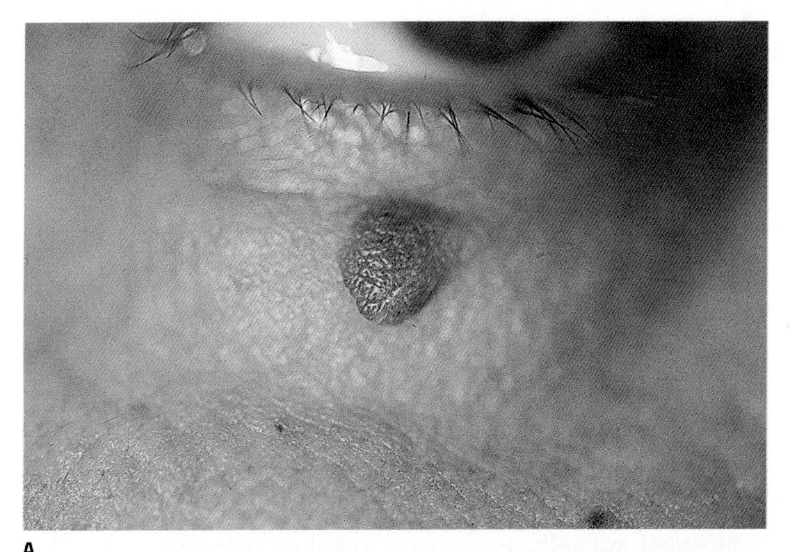

A

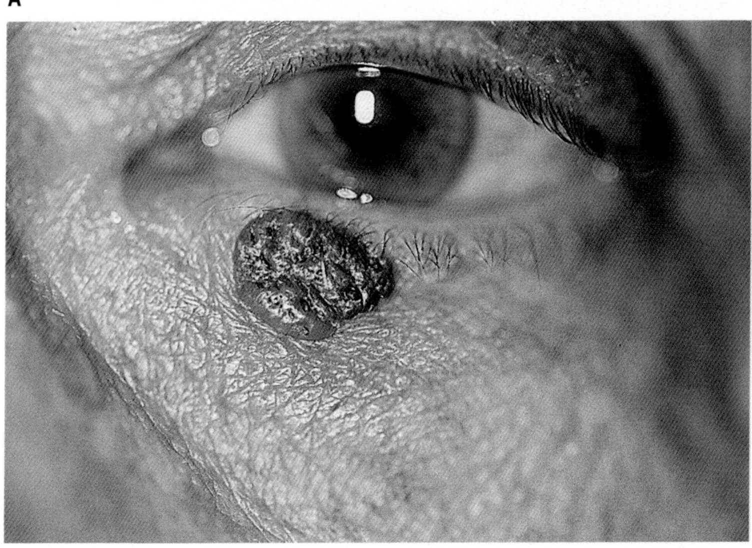

B

Figure 1-2 Seborrheic keratosis **A** *and* **B.** *Seborrheic keratosis are common lesions of the eyelids. They tend to get darker as they have been present longer as seen in* **B.**

CUTANEOUS HORN

Cutaneous horn is a clinically descriptive term for lesions with exuberant hyperkeratosis. The etiology of this hyperkeratosis can be variable and biopsy to determine the cause is required.

Epidemiology and Etiology

Age Older adults.

Gender Equal in males and females.

Etiology Hyperkeratosis associated with a variety of underlying lesions.

History

Lesion may grow slowly or rapidly.

Examination

Raised lesion, often like a stalk, usually white in color. The surface is hyperkeratotic (Fig. 1-3).

Special Considerations

Biopsy of these lesions is required to rule out malignant lesion at the base of the lesion such as basal cell carcinoma or squamous cell carcinoma.

Differential Diagnosis

- This is a descriptive term and not a pathologic, diagnostic term.
- The base of this lesion may be a seborrheic keratosis, verruca vulgaris, basal cell carcinoma, or squamous cell carcinoma.

Laboratory Tests

Pathologic evaluation.

Treatment

Excisional biopsy with pathologic evaluation.

Prognosis

Good.

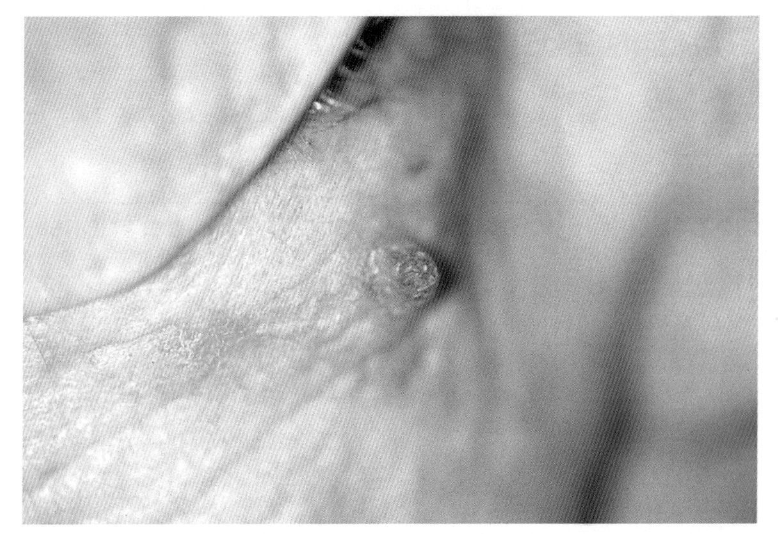

Figure 1-3 Cutaneous horn *A cutaneous horn has a hard, rough surface that is white in color. This lesion is less pointed but some lesions end in a point giving them their name of cutaneous "horn."*

EPIDERMAL INCLUSION CYST

Common white to yellow cyst seen around the eyes and elsewhere on the face. Easily treated with excision.

Epidemiology and Etiology

Age Any.

Gender Equal in males and females.

Etiology Arises spontaneously from the infundibulum of the hair follicle or following traumatic implantation of epidermal tissue into the dermis.

History

May have history of trauma to the area. Usually, lesions grow slowly for a period of time and then remain stable.

Examination

Smooth, round, elevated cyst. The underlying cyst is white and can often be visualized through the thin eyelid skin (Fig. 1-4A and B).

Special Considerations

These cysts may become secondarily infected and cause a cellulitis.

Differential Diagnosis

- Molluscum contagiosum
- Chalazion
- Syringoma

Treatment

Excision; attempt should be made to either excise the entire cyst wall or if left at the base, it should be destroyed with cautery.

Prognosis

Excellent. Recurrence is rare.

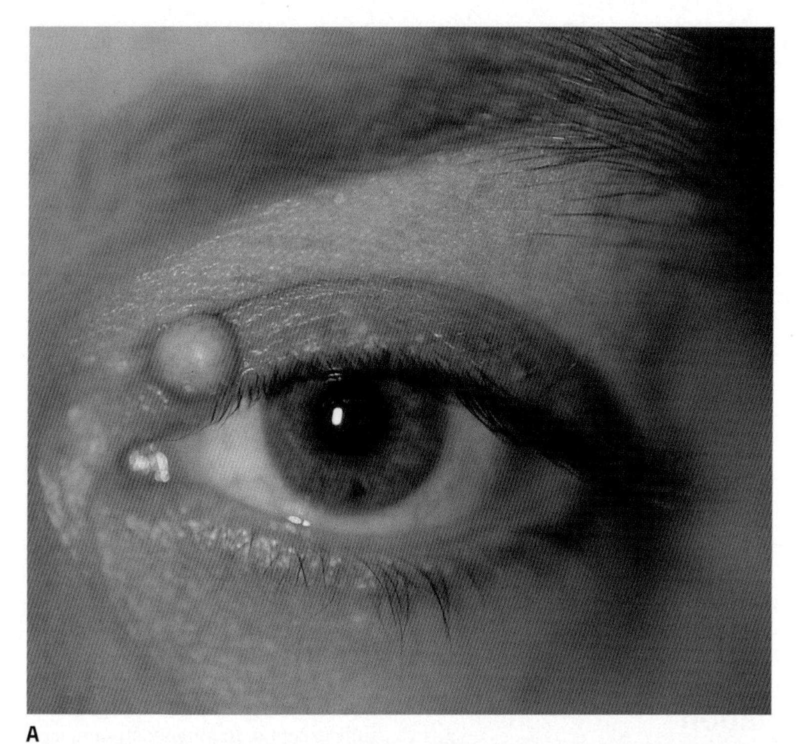

A

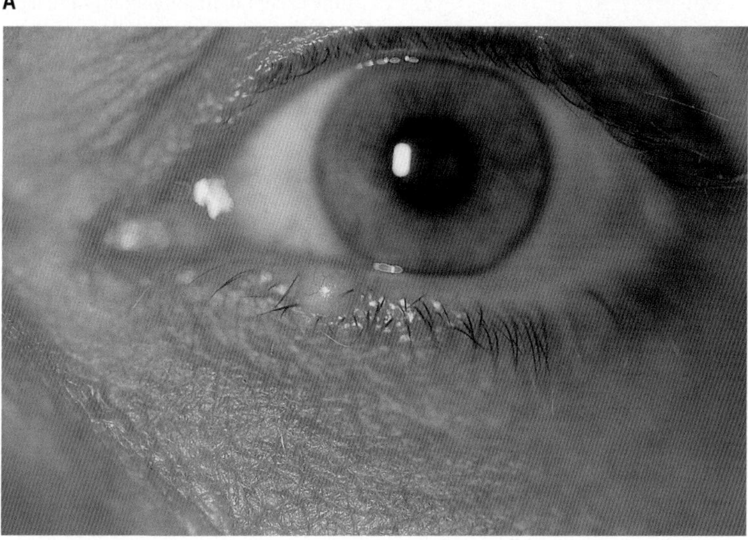

B

Figure 1-4 Inclusion cyst **A.** *Inclusion cyst of the left upper eyelid.* **B.** *A smaller cyst of the left lower lid. Patients with inclusion cysts on the eyelids often seek treatment before they become very large.*

MOLLUSCUM CONTAGIOSUM

Molluscum contagiosum is a self-limited viral infection characterized by skin-colored papules that are often umbilicated in the center. In immunocompromised individuals, this may not be self-limited and can lead to large cosmetically disfiguring lesions. If these lesions are located on the eyelid margin, they may cause a follicular conjunctivitis.

Epidemiology and Etiology

Age Children and young adults.

Gender Males more common than females.

Etiology Viral lesions spread by skin-to-skin contact.

History

Spontaneously occurring lesions. Known contact with other person with lesions is not usual.

Examination

Single or multiple small 1- to 2-mm papules (Fig. 1-5A and B). Rarely, these lesions can become larger. They are pearly white or skin colored with a central keratin plug that gives them their central umbilication.

Special Considerations

If these lesions are located on the eyelid margin, they may cause a mild to severe, chronic follicular conjunctivitis. In immunocompromised patients, this viral infection may not be self-limited and can lead to large, cosmetically disfiguring lesions, especially on the face.

Differential Diagnosis

- Epidermal inclusion cyst
- Syringoma
- Keratoacanthoma

Laboratory Tests

Direct microscopy of the keratin plug with Giemsa stain shows "molluscum bodies."

Treatment

These lesions will regress spontaneously over time except in immunocompromised patients. If removal is desired, small lesions can be frozen or the core can be treated with electrodesiccation. Curettage or direct excision is also effective.

Prognosis

Good in healthy people. The chance of infecting other people is low when the lesions are present but infected patients should avoid skin-to-skin contact.

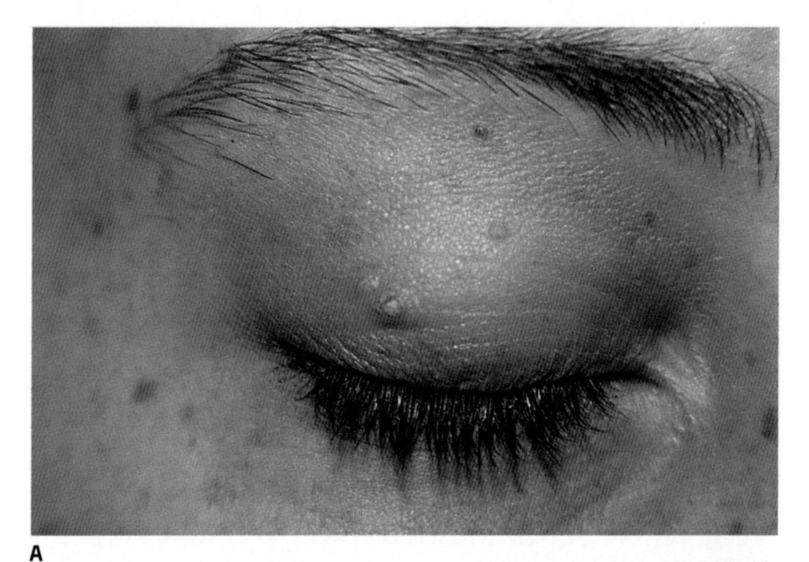

A

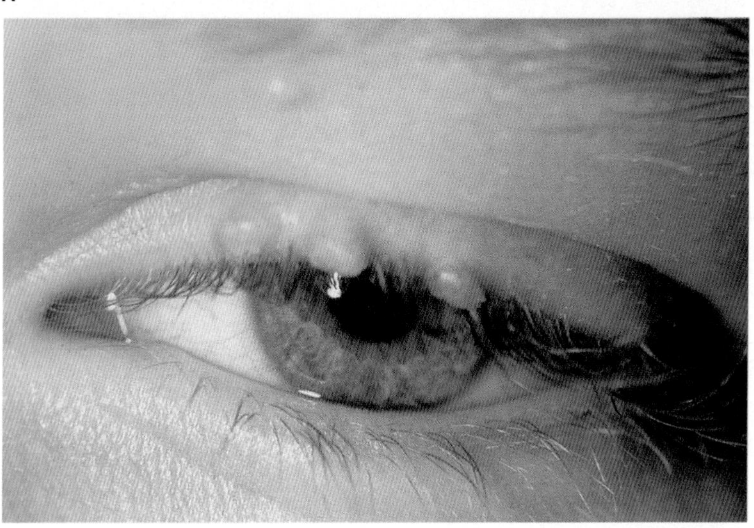

B

Figure 1-5 Molluscum contagiosum **A.** *There are 3 lesions on the upper eyelid. If the lesions are on the eyelid margin, the eye itself may be injected with a follicular conjunctivitis. This patient also had similar lesions on her leg.* **B.** *Multiple lesions of the eyelid margin. There was a mild follicular reaction in the inferior fornix. (Courtesy of Jurij Bilyk, MD.)*

XANTHELASMA

Xanthelasma are yellowish plaques that occur medially on the upper or lower lids and are classic in appearance. They tend to enlarge with time and may or may not be associated with hyperlipidemia. *Synonyms:* xanthoma

Epidemiology and Etiology

Age Over 50 years of age. If younger, must consider a familial lipoprotein disorder.

Gender Either.

Etiology May or may not be associated with hyperlipoproteinemia.

History

The lesions are noted for months to years with slow enlargement.

Examination

Soft, yellow-orange plaques located medially on the upper and/or lower eyelids. (Fig. 1-6A and B).

Special Considerations

If LDL is elevated in the lipid profile, it is a sign of a familial lipoprotein disorder.

Differential Diagnosis

- If the xanthelasmas are present bilaterally no other lesions look like this. Early, a xanthelasma can look like an inclusion cyst or syringoma.

Laboratory Tests

Laboratory evaluation of lipid profile.

Pathophysiology

Macrophages containing droplets of lipids form xanthoma cells. These xanthoma cells then accumulate forming the xanthelasma.

Treatment

Excision most commonly. Electrodesiccation, laser, and application of trichloroacetic acid are other treatments.

Prognosis

Good but with time additional deposition may occur and the lesions reappear.

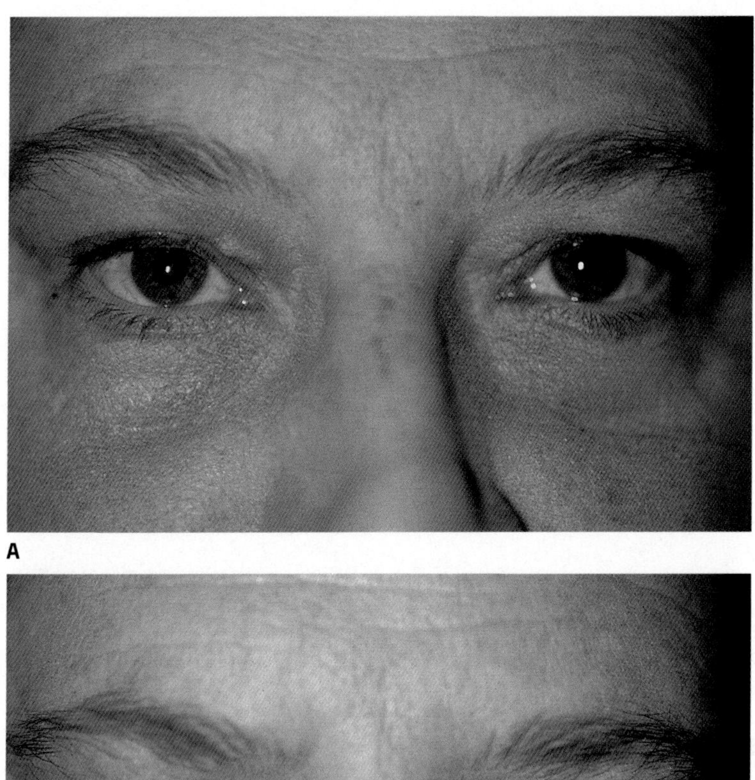

A

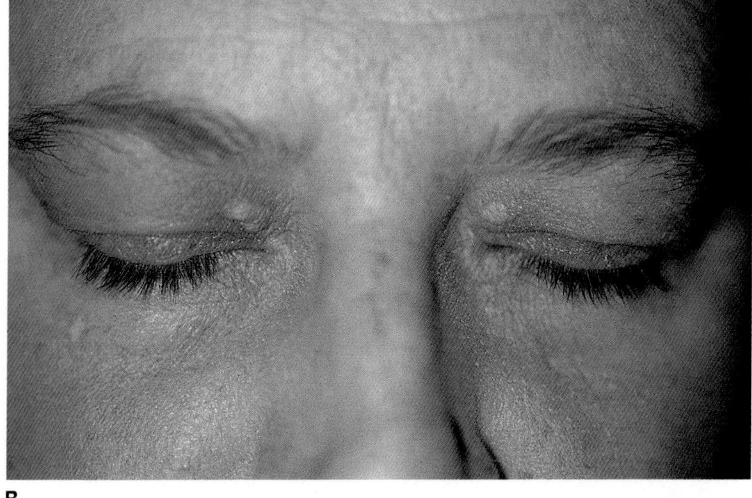

B

Figure 1-6 Xanthelasma **A** *and* **B.** *These lesions are in the classic area of the upper eyelids. They are still relatively small but with time, the lipid deposition will continue and they will enlarge. Less commonly, they can occur in a similar position on the lower eyelids.*

SYRINGOMA

Syringoma present as multiple lesions on the lower lids of women. The onset is usually insidious. Patients typically present with cosmetic concerns because of the numerous "bumps" on the lower eyelids. The challenge can be excision of the large number of lesions present without causing scarring or an ectropion.

Epidemiology and Etiology

Age Begins in puberty.

Gender Occur in women and may be familial.

Etiology An adenoma of the intraepidermal eccrine ducts.

History

Lesions noted on the lower eyelids with insidious onset. May be present elsewhere on the face, axillae, umbilicus, upper chest, and vulva.

Examination

Lesions are 1 to 2 mm, skin colored or yellowish, and usually multiple (Fig. 1-7). They occur commonly on the lower eyelids but may occur elsewhere on the face, axillae, umbilicus, upper chest, and vulva.

Differential Diagnosis

- Very few other lesions look similar or present with numerous lesions on the lower eyelids. A single lesion can look like an inclusion cyst, basal cell carcinoma, or trichoepithelioma.

Pathophysiology

Benign adenoma of the intraepithelial eccrine ducts. Pathology shows many small ducts in the dermis with comma-like tails with the appearance of tadpoles.

Treatment

Patients often request removal on a cosmetic basis. Removal is by electrosurgery or direct excision.

Prognosis

A large number on the face can be difficult to remove. Additional lesions may grow after excision.

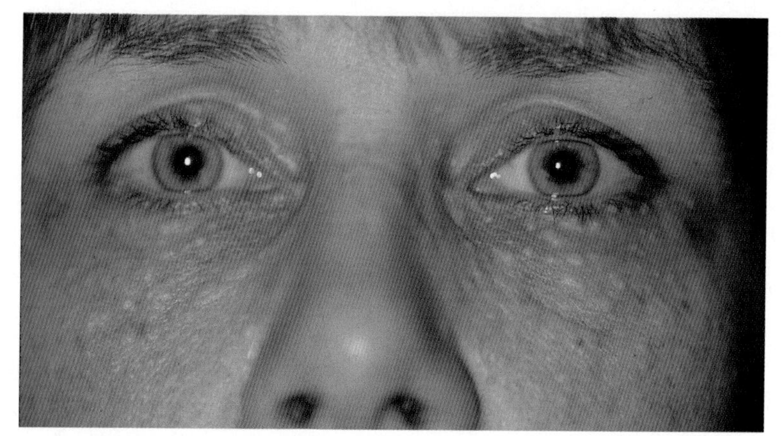

Figure 1-7 Syringoma *Multiple lesions in the classic area of the lower eyelids. There can be just a few lesions or even more than in this patient.*

APOCRINE HYDROCYSTOMA

Apocrine hydrocystoma is a very common lesion arising along the eyelid margin. It is a clear, cystic lesion that transilluminates although the overlying skin may give it a bluish color.

Epidemiology and Etiology

Age Adults.

Gender Equal.

Etiology Cyst formation from the glands of Moll along the eyelid margin.

History

Cyst noted and may slowly enlarge.

Examination

Cystic lesion near or on the eyelid margin (Fig. 1-8A and B). These lesions are translucent or bluish and transilluminate. There may be multiple lesions.

Differential Diagnosis

- Cystic basal cell carcinoma
- Eccrine hydrocystoma (retention cyst of eccrine glands)

Pathophysiology

This lesion is an adenoma of the secretory cells of Moll and not a retention cyst.

Treatment

Marsupialization of the cyst may be adequate for superficial lesions but deeper lesions require complete cyst wall excision.

Prognosis

Excellent. Rare recurrence after excision.

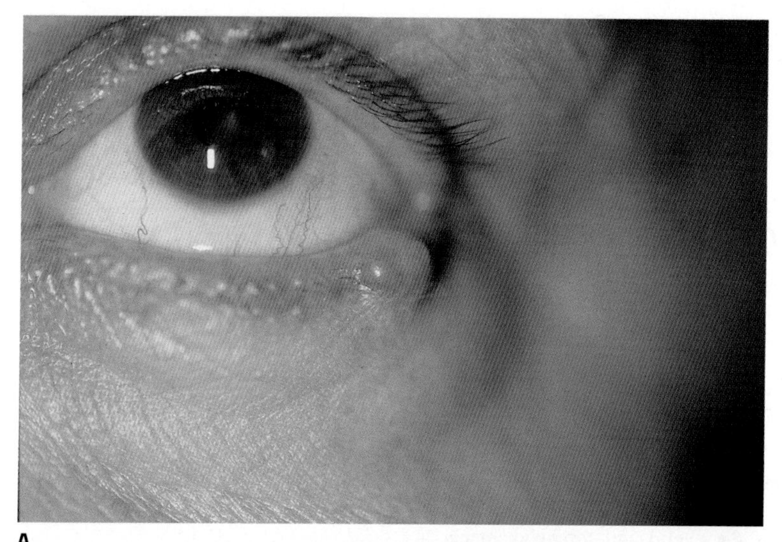

A

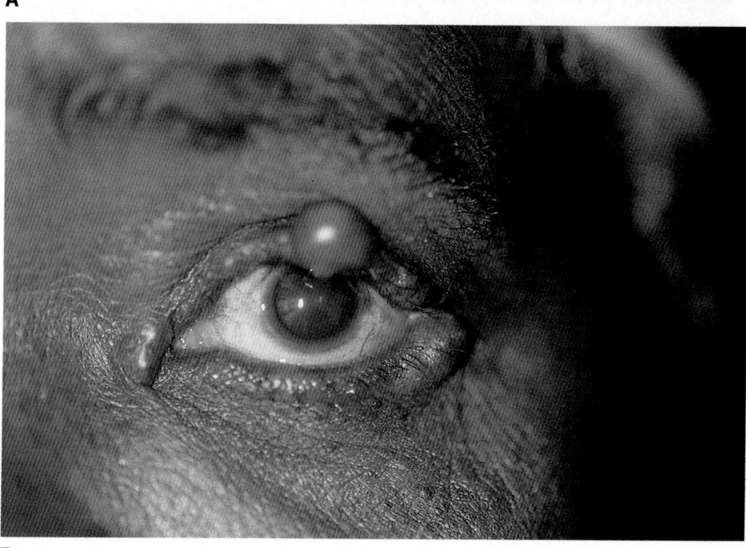

B

Figure 1-8 Apocrine hydrocystoma **A.** *This lesion on the upper eyelid transilluminates with the slit beam. On excision there will be a gush of clear fluid.* **B.** *Multiple lesions. Lesions are often smaller than these and are difficult to photograph.*

TRICHOEPITHELIOMA

Trichoepithelioma is a benign flesh-colored papule that arises from an immature hair follicle. It can occur on the eyelid margin but more commonly elsewhere on the face, scalp, neck, and upper trunk.

Epidemiology and Etiology

Age First appears at puberty.

Gender More common in males.

Etiology Benign appendage tumor with hair differentiation.

History

Lesions of the eyelid and forehead appear at puberty and can slowly increase in size and number.

Examination

Small pink or skin-colored papules that can increase in size and become quite large (Fig. 1-9).

Special Considerations

May be confused with a basal cell carcinoma, especially if it appears as a solitary tumor.

Differential Diagnosis

- Epidermal inclusion cyst
- Basal cell carcinoma
- Syringoma

Treatment

Excision with pathologic evaluation.

Prognosis

Excellent.

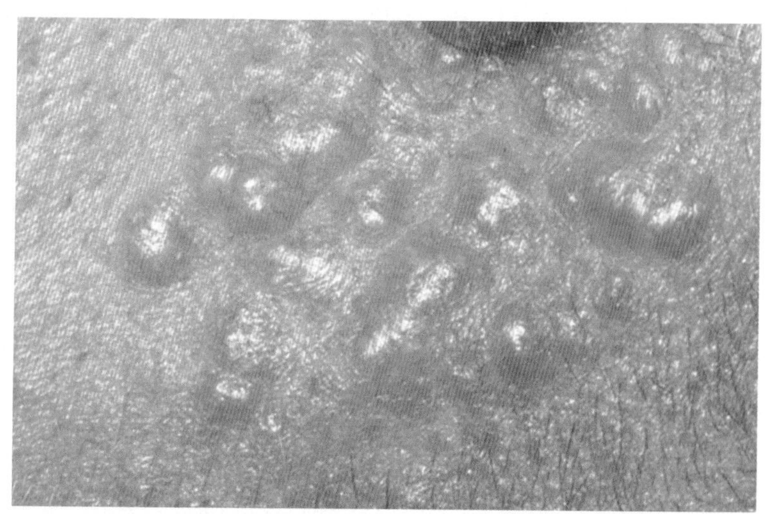

Figure 1-9 Trichoepithelioma *These pink or skin-colored lesions can occur on the skin or eyelid margin. They can enlarge and be confused with a basal cell carcinoma. (From Fitzpatrick TB et al.* Color Atlas & Synopsis of Clinical Dermatology, *4th ed. New York, McGraw-Hill, 2001.)*

NEVI (NEVOCELLULAR NEVI)

Nevocellular nevi are small (less than 1 cm), circumscribed, acquired pigmented lesions that are made up of melanocytic nevus cells located in the epidermis, dermis, and rarely deeper.

Epidemiology and Etiology

Age Appear in early childhood and reach a maximum size in young adulthood. These lesions gradually involute and disappear by age 60 years. The exception is the dermal nevus, which does not involute.

Gender Equal.

Etiology Groups of melanocytic nevus cells located in the epidermis, dermis, or, rarely, in the subcutaneous tissue.

History

Pigmented lesion that is stable or involuting. The lesions are asymptomatic.

Examination

Nevi can be grouped as follows (Fig. 1-10A and B).

Junctional nevi: round or oval, flat or very slightly raised lesion, less than 1 cm in diameter. Tan or brown in color with smooth regular borders.

Compound nevi: round, elevated, dome-shaped lesion with smooth or papillomatous surface. Dark brown in color but becomes mottled as this lesion evolves into a dermal nevus; often has hairs growing out of the lesion.

Dermal nevi: round, dome-shaped, elevated nodule, skin colored, tan, or brown with telangiectasias. These do not disappear with age and may become more pedunculated.

Special Considerations

Any enlarging lesions, those changing color, or becoming irritated in any way after age 20 years need to be biopsied to rule out malignant change.

Differential Diagnosis

- Seborrheic keratosis
- Malignant melanoma
- Dermatofibroma
- Basal cell carcinoma

Laboratory Tests

Histologic examination if biopsied.

Treatment

Observation, unless the lesion changes color, its borders become irregular, or the lesion begins to itch, hurt, or bleed. Any of these are indications for excisional biopsy with histologic evaluation.

Prognosis

Rare chance of malignant transformation.

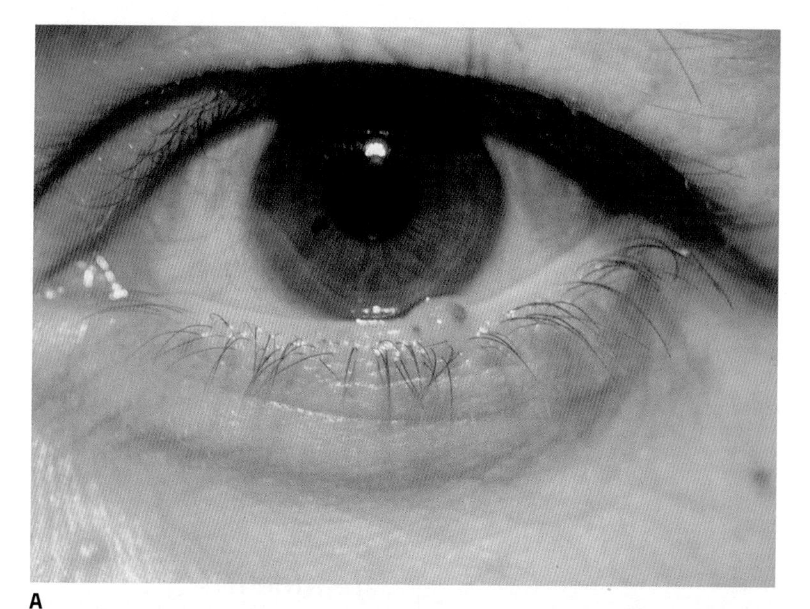

A

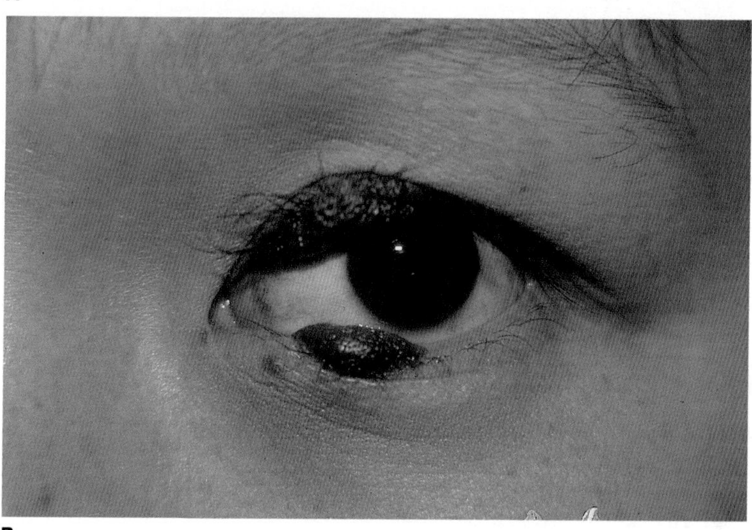

B

Figure 1-10 Nevi **A.** *This small nevus of the lower eyelid is amelanotic except for a few pigmented spots. Nevi on the eyelid margin will often mold against the eyeball, as in this picture, but cause no discomfort or corneal changes.* **B.** *A split nevus where nevi cells were split congenitally as the eyelid fissure formed. This nevus is very dark and shows the variation that can occur in the color of these lesions.*

KERATOACANTHOMA

Keratoacanthoma presents as an isolated lesion on the face with a very unique appearance. The lesion is dome shaped with a central keratin filled crater. It grows rapidly over weeks and may undergo spontaneous regression over months.

Epidemiology and Etiology

Age Most often over 50 years of age, rare younger than 20.

Gender More common in males than females by a ratio of 2 to 1.

Etiology Unknown; ultraviolet radiation and chemical carcinogens may have a causative role.

History

Rapid onset of growth over a few weeks. The lesion is often asymptomatic except for cosmetic changes. There may be occasional tenderness.

Examination

Single, dome-shaped nodule with a central keratotic plug. The lesion is firm and is slightly red to light brown in color (Fig. 1-11A and B).

Special Considerations

Differentiation from a squamous cell carcinoma may not be possible both clinically and even sometimes pathologically. If the differentiation cannot be made, the lesion must be treated as a squamous cell carcinoma.

Differential Diagnosis

- Squamous cell carcinoma
- Hyperkeratotic actinic keratosis

Laboratory Tests

Histopathology of the excised lesion.

Treatment

Excision with pathologic evaluation. These lesions will sometimes spontaneously regress over a few months to a year. The need to rule out a squamous cell carcinoma and the cosmetic appearance almost always leads to excision prior to spontaneous regression, especially around the eyelids.

Prognosis

Good. Depending on the size of the lesion, reconstruction of the defect may leave some eyelid changes.

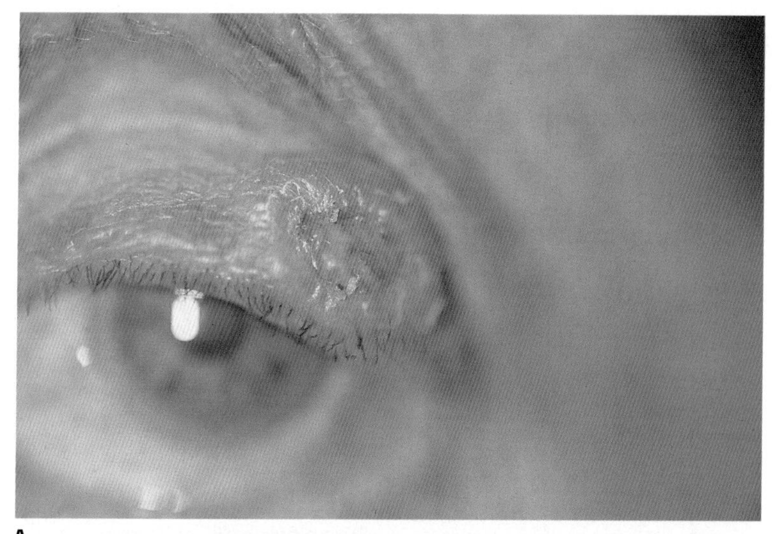
A

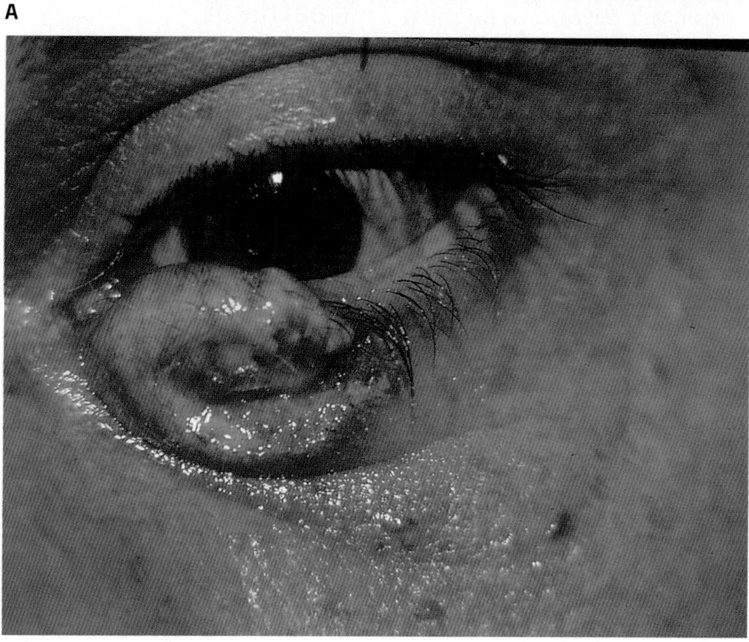
B

Figure 1-11 Keratoacanthoma **A.** *Lesion of the left upper eyelid that grew over 2 to 3 weeks. It was excised without recurrence.* **B.** *Large lesion of the left lower eyelid in a 40-year-old patient. The appearance could be that of a squamous cell carcinoma, however, the history of growth over 4 weeks and the patient's age point to a keratoacanthoma. This lesion was excised without recurrence.*

HEMANGIOMA OF THE EYELID (CHERRY ANGIOMA)

Hemangiomas of the eyelid are raised, red, benign lesions that appear on the eyelids in adulthood and can increase in size but usually remain less than 3 to 5 mm.

Epidemiology and Etiology

Age Adulthood.

Gender Equal.

Etiology Unknown.

History

Usually appear spontaneously and can increase in size over a short time. Patients may have other similar lesions elsewhere on their body.

Examination

Raised, bright red, blood-filled lesions that can occur anywhere on the body (Fig. 1-12A). They may be single or multiple.

Differential Diagnosis

- Pyogenic granuloma (Fig. 1-12B).
- Melanoma

Laboratory Tests

Pathologic evaluation after excision.

Treatment

Excision usually for cosmetic reasons, less commonly to have the lesion evaluated pathologically.

Prognosis

Excellent.

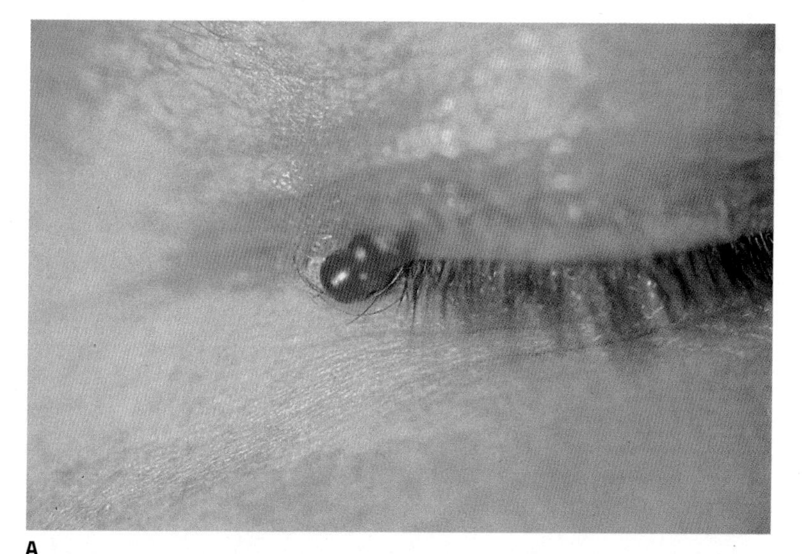

A

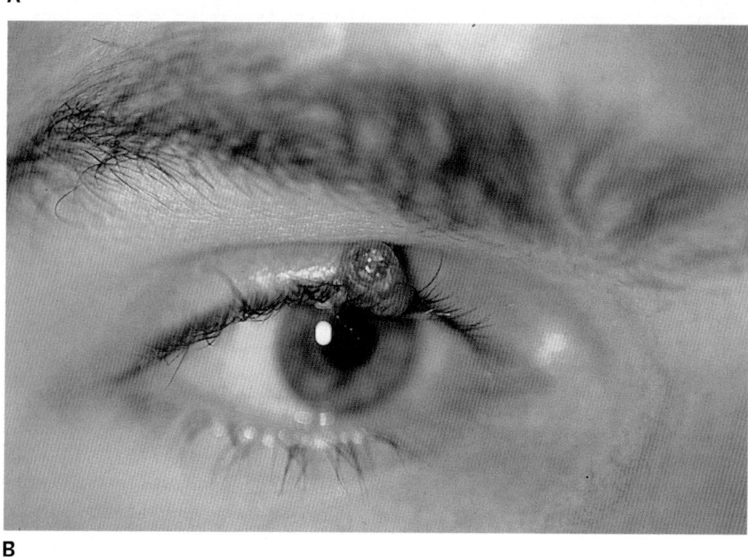

B

Figure 1-12 Eyelid hemangioma **A.** *Very red, blood-filled lesion that may be just slightly raised or very elevated as in this picture. On excision, there is usually a small gush of blood but these lesions usually do not bleed excessively. Rarely, these can bleed actively so the surgeon must be prepared.* **Pyogenic granuloma** **B.** *A pyogenic granuloma can look similar to a hemangioma but it usually is solid, not blood filled, and often somewhat papillomatous.*

Chapter 2

EYELID INFLAMMATION

CHALAZION

A type of focal inflammation of the eyelid; it is a common lesion of the eyelid. The most common cause is blockage of a meibomian gland of the eyelid. Chalazia can present with an inflamed, tender, red eyelid or as a discrete nontender lump in the eyelid.

Epidemiology and Etiology

Age Any.

Gender Equal.

Etiology Focal inflammation of the eyelid resulting from the obstruction of the meibomian glands.

History

Often present with acute onset of focal eyelid inflammation. The inflammation will resolve but may turn into a chronic cyst-like lesion. The onset may be more insidious with appearance of the cyst-like lesion with minimal inflammation.

Examination

In the acute process, the eyelid may be diffusely inflamed with pain focally over the involved area (Fig. 2-1A). There may be pointing over the blocked meibomian gland. As the inflammation resolves, the resulting lesion is a firm mass in the tarsal plate with or without residual inflammation (Fig. 2-1B).

Special Considerations

Chronic, nonresolving chalazion needs to be biopsied to rule out a carcinoma.

Differential Diagnosis

- Sebaceous adenocarcinoma
- Squamous cell carcinoma
- Basal cell carcinoma

Pathophysiology

Blockage of the eyelid glands results in release of the gland contents into the tarsus and eyelid resulting in an inflammatory process. The inflammatory process is then walled off with time, resulting in the cyst-like lesion. The exact role of bacteria in this process is unclear.

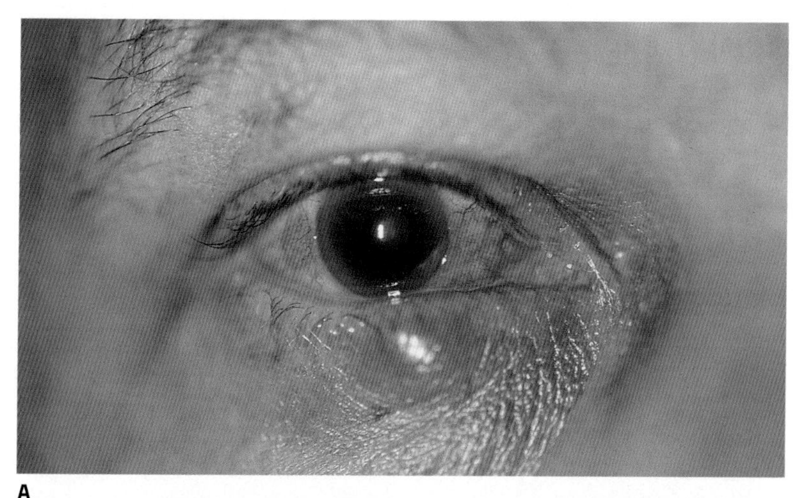

A

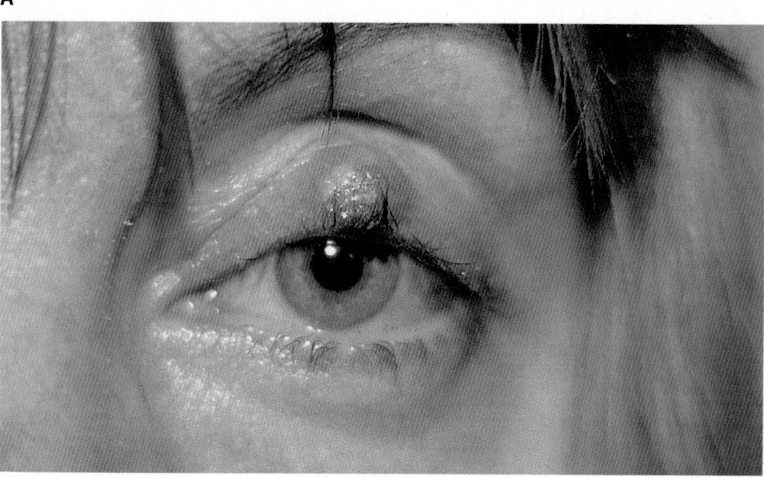

B

Figure 2-1 Chalazion **A.** *A firm, formed lump of the left lower eyelid. There is still some inflammation of the chalazion. The eye is red from blepharoconjunctivitis, which often is part of a chalazion. Most of the time, the eye is white and quiet.* **B.** *A chronic chalazion of the left upper eyelid with some crusting over the chalazion from external drainage.*

Treatment

When in the inflammatory phase, initial treatment is warm compresses and steroid antibiotic drops or ointment. As the lesion becomes cystic, treatment is then excision via a conjunctiva incision. Injection of steroid into the lesion may also be effective. Steroid injections need to be used cautiously in patients with darkly pigmented skin as they can cause depigmentation.

Prognosis

Good. These lesions can be multiple and are rarely resistant to treatment.

HORDEOLUM

An acute infection of the glands of Zeis (external hordeolum) or meibomian glands (internal hordeolum). It presents as a red, inflamed, tender eyelid. In practice, the terms chalazion, hordeolum, and stye are often used interchangeably (and incorrectly).
Synonym: stye

Epidemiology and Etiology

Age Any.

Gender Equal.

Etiology Acute bacterial infection of the glands of Zeis or the meibomian glands.

History

Sudden onset of focal inflammation of the eyelid centered around a gland of the eyelid.

Examination

Red, swollen, tender eyelid often with a focal area of infection around a gland of the eyelid (Fig. 2-2A and B).

Differential Diagnosis

- Preseptal cellulitis
- Eyelid abscess

Pathophysiology

Eyelid gland becomes infected probably associated with blockage of the gland.

Treatment

Warm compresses and topical steroid/antibiotic drops or ointment. Rarely, this can evolve into an abscess, which needs drainage, or a cellulitis that requires systemic antibiotics.

Prognosis

Excellent.

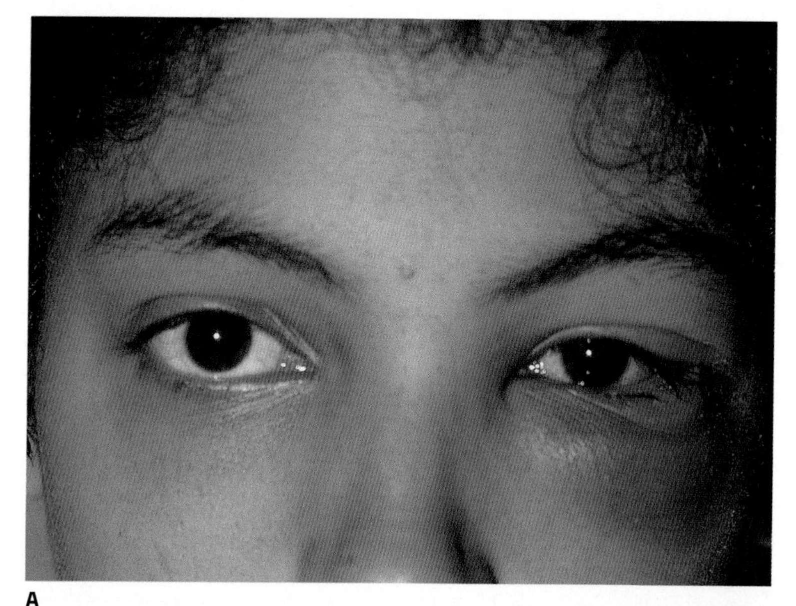

A

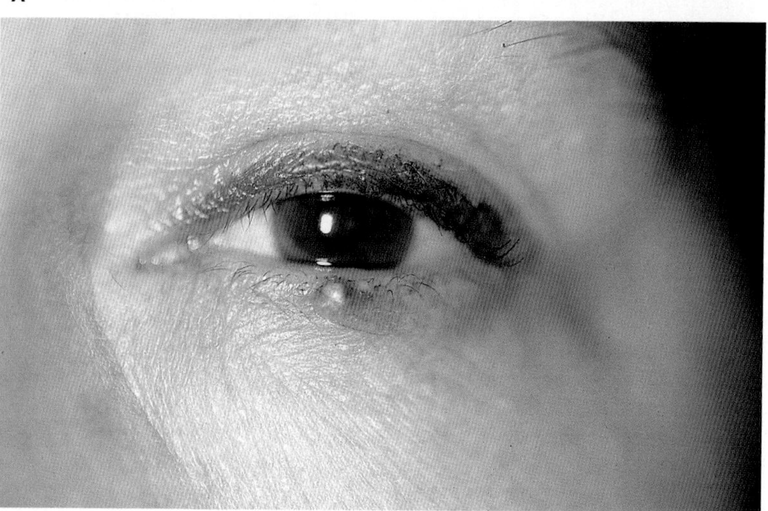

B

Figure 2-2 Hordeolum **A.** *Acute inflammation of the left lower eyelid caused by blockage and infection/inflammation of a meibomian gland. This lesion may resolve as the acute inflammation resolves or evolve into a chalazion.* **B.** *Blockage with infection/inflammation of the glands of Zeis is involved in this eyelid lesion. Note this lesion is on the external eyelid in the area of the eyelash follicles. Hordeola usually resolve without sequelae but can sometimes become chronic and take many weeks to resolve.*

FLOPPY EYELID SYNDROME

Floppy eyelid syndrome is seen in obese patients, many of whom have sleep apnea. The eyelids become very loose and floppy either as a primary process or secondary to chronic rubbing of the eyelids at night. This syndrome must be considered as a cause for a chronic, papillary conjunctivitis.

Epidemiology and Etiology

Age Adults.

Gender Males more commonly affected.

Etiology Unknown. The eyelid laxity and loss of structure may be related to chronic mechanical eyelid rubbing or due to some innate abnormality of the patient's eyelids.

History

Patient presents with chronic papillary conjunctivitis that is usually bilateral and may give the history of his eyelids spontaneously everting at night. The patient may complain of chronic nonspecific irritation. The symptoms are often worse on the side the patient sleeps on.

Examination

Eyelids are flaccid and easily everted (Fig. 2-3A–C). There is chronic papillary conjunctivitis with a keratitis often with diffuse superficial punctate keratitis (SPK). Typically, the palpebral conjunctiva has a velvety appearance. There is a high incidence of obesity in these patients.

Special Considerations

There is a significant incidence of sleep apnea in patients with floppy eyelid syndrome. All patients need to have sleep studies.

Differential Diagnosis

- Other forms of conjunctivitis in a patient with eyelid laxity.

Pathophysiology

There is loss of elastin fibers in the tarsus but the cause remains speculative.

Treatment

Patching or a shield over the eye can be attempted but is usually not helpful long term. Horizontal eyelid tightening is usually required.

Prognosis

The laxity will recur with time. Horizontal tightening will relieve symptoms for a period of time.

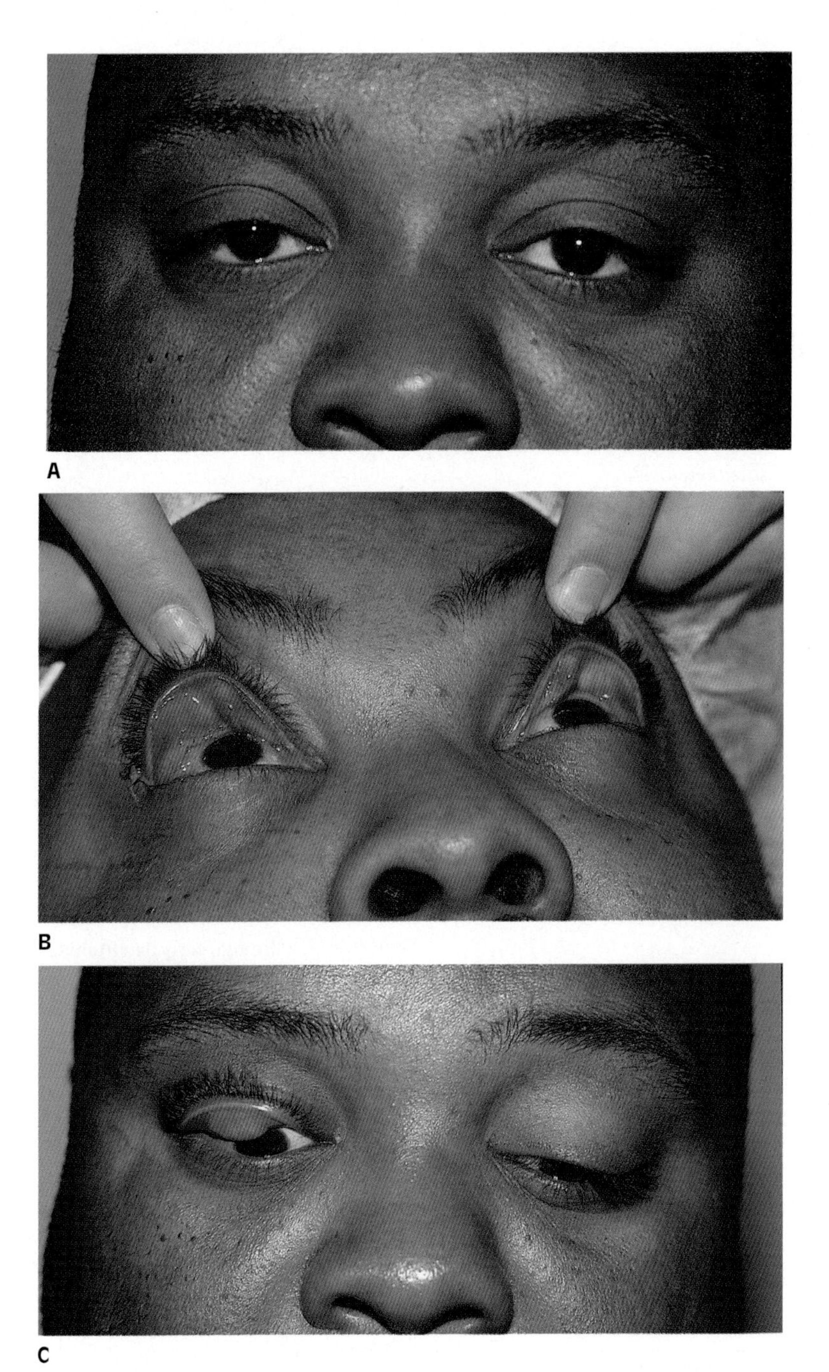

Figure 2-3 Floppy eyelid syndrome **A.** *Patient with mild ptosis but complains of chronic irritation of the eyes. His eyes are white but he has moderate corneal SPK.* **B.** *Upper eyelids are easily everted and the undersides of the eyelids are red with a diffuse papillary reaction. The eyelids are very loose and, once everted, will often remain everted even with blinking (***C***).*

Chapter 3

EYELID NEOPLASMS

ACTINIC KERATOSIS

These lesions may be single or multiple on chronically sun-exposed skin. They appear as dry, rough, scaly lesions that are stable but can rarely disappear spontaneously.
Synonym: solar keratosis

Epidemiology and Etiology

Age Over age 40; rare under 30 years.

Gender Higher incidence in males.

Etiology Sun exposure over time in a fair-skinned white population results in actinic keratosis.

History

Extensive sun exposure in youth. Lesions present for months.

Examination

Rough, slightly elevated, skin-colored or light brown lesions with hyperkeratotic scale (Fig. 3-1).

Special Considerations

It is estimated that one squamous cell carcinoma will develop per 1000 actinic keratoses.

Differential Diagnosis

- Squamous cell carcinoma
- Discoid lupus

Laboratory Tests

Pathologic evaluation if biopsied.

Pathophysiology

Repeated solar exposure results in damage to the keratinocytes by the cumulative effects of ultraviolet radiation.

Treatment

Prevention through early and lifelong use of sunscreen. Excise nodular lesions and submit for pathologic evaluation. Most flat lesions respond to liquid nitrogen or topical application of 5% 5-fluorouracil cream over a few days to weeks.

Prognosis

Some actinic keratoses may disappear spontaneously but most remain for years unless treated. Incidence of squamous cell carcinoma developing in these lesions is unknown but has been estimated to be one squamous cell carcinoma in every 1000 actinic keratoses.

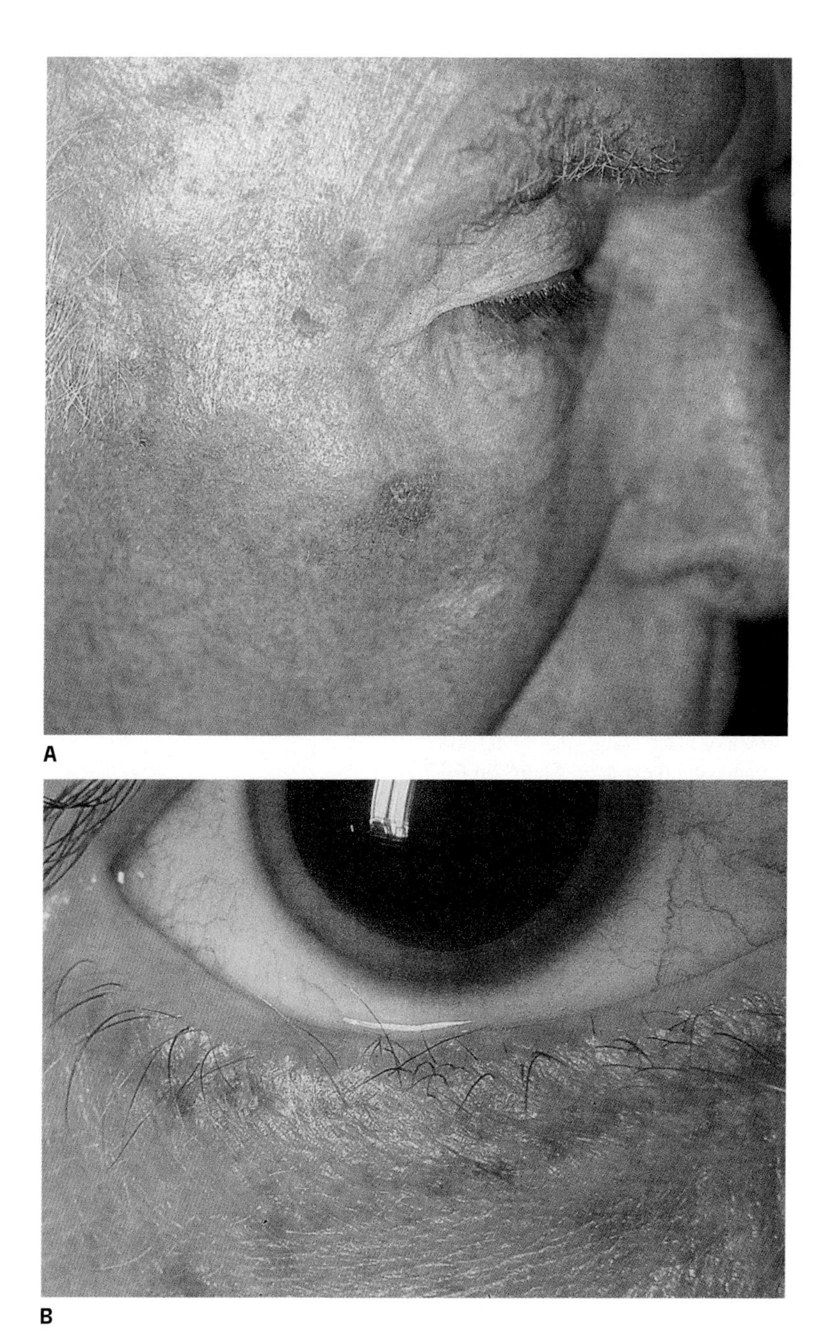

Figure 3-1 Actinic keratosis **A.** *Multiple actinic keratoses on the cheek and brow with signs of chronic sun damage.* **B.** *Lesion involving the lower eyelid. (Courtesy of Jurij Bilyk, MD.)*

LENTIGO MALIGNA

Lentigo maligna is a flat intraepidermal neoplasm and the precursor lesion of lentigo maligna melanoma. The lesion has striking variations of brown and black (Fig. 3-2), often described as a "stain."

Epidemiology and Etiology

Age Median age is 65 years.

Gender Equal incidence in males and females.

Etiology Sun exposure is a definite factor.

History

History is usually not helpful as exact onset of lesion is unclear.

Examination

Flat, dark brown or black color, sharply defined edges. Often appears like a dark "stain" on the skin.

Special Considerations

This is a premalignant lesion and should be excised because of the chance of development into a lentigo maligna melanoma.

Differential Diagnosis

- Seborrheic keratosis
- Actinic keratosis
- Malignant melanoma

Laboratory Tests

Histopathologic evaluation.

Treatment

Excision with margins sent for pathologic evaluation.

Prognosis

Excellent if excised before developing into a melanoma.

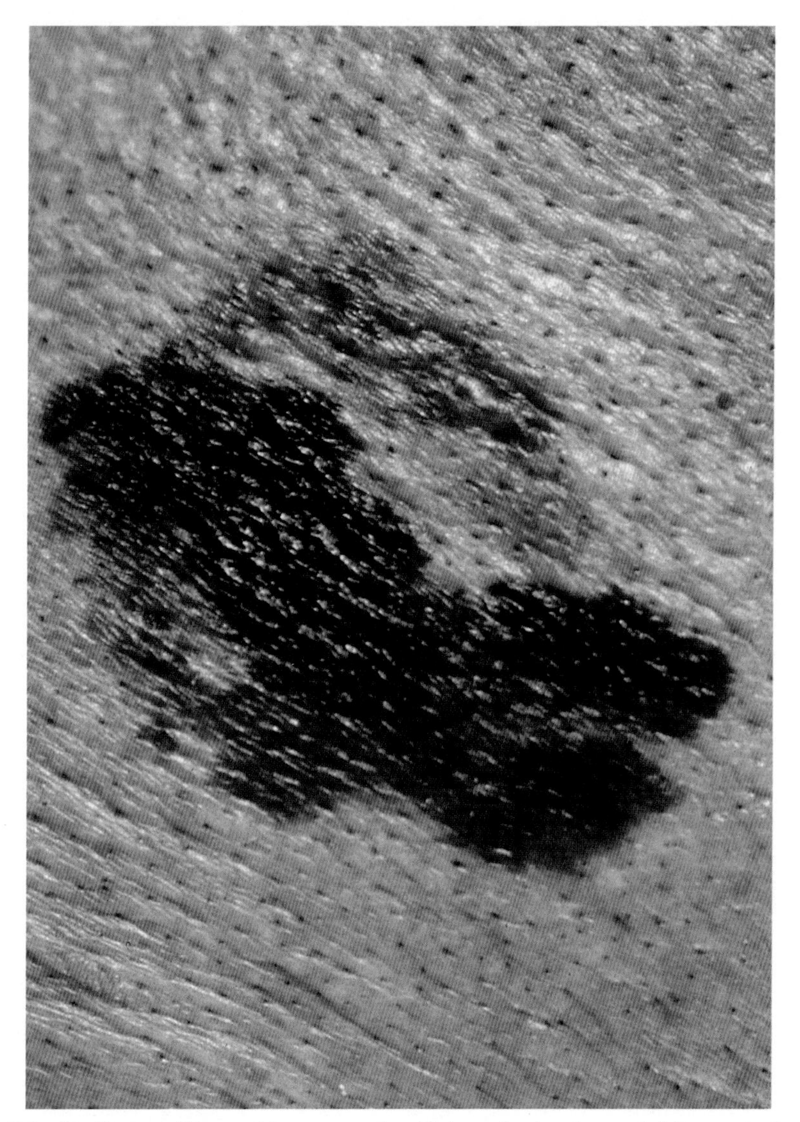

Figure 3-2 Lentigo maligna *A large macule with irregular borders and different shades of brown. (From Fitzpatrick TB et al.* Color Atlas & Synopsis of Clinical Dermatology, *4th ed. New York, McGraw-Hill, 2001.)*

BASAL CELL CARCINOMA

Basal cell carcinoma is the most common type of skin cancer. It is locally invasive and aggressive but has very limited capacity to metastasize. If neglected, it can invade the orbit, especially if located in the medial canthal area. Most commonly, it occurs on the lower eyelid and is treated by complete excision.

Epidemiology and Etiology

Age Over 40 years of age. Rare cases do occur in the 20s and 30s.

Gender Males more than females.

Etiology Sun exposure and fair skin with poor ability to tan are risk factors. Treatment with x-ray (for acne) increases the risk.

Incidence 500 to 1000 per 100,000 people.

History

Slowly enlarging lesions in sun-exposed areas. The lesions may be associated with bleeding.

Examination

Round or oval, firm lesions with depressed center. The lesions are pink or red with fine threadlike telangiectasia. The center may be ulcerated. Basal cell carcinoma may also appear scarlike or be cystic (Fig. 3-3A to D).

Special Considerations

Aggressive treatment of basal cell carcinoma of the medial canthal area is indicated because of the risk of orbital extension from the medial canthal area. Basal cell carcinomas almost never metastasize. Sclerosing basal cell carcinomas have poorly defined margins and may recur. Basal cell nevus syndrome is an autosomal dominate syndrome in which patients develop multiple basal cells at a very young age (Fig. 3-3E and F).

Differential Diagnosis

- Squamous cell carcinoma
- Trichoepithelioma

Laboratory Tests

Lesions are sent for pathologic evaluation.

Treatment

Complete surgical excision with pathologic evaluation. Frozen sections are often needed to assure complete excision. Reconstruction of the defect is then completed at the same time. Treatment with radiation should not be used for lesions around the eye unless the patient is not a surgical candidate.

Prognosis

Good when promptly and completely excised. Neglected cases can invade the orbit and brain and have the potential, in rare cases, to be fatal.

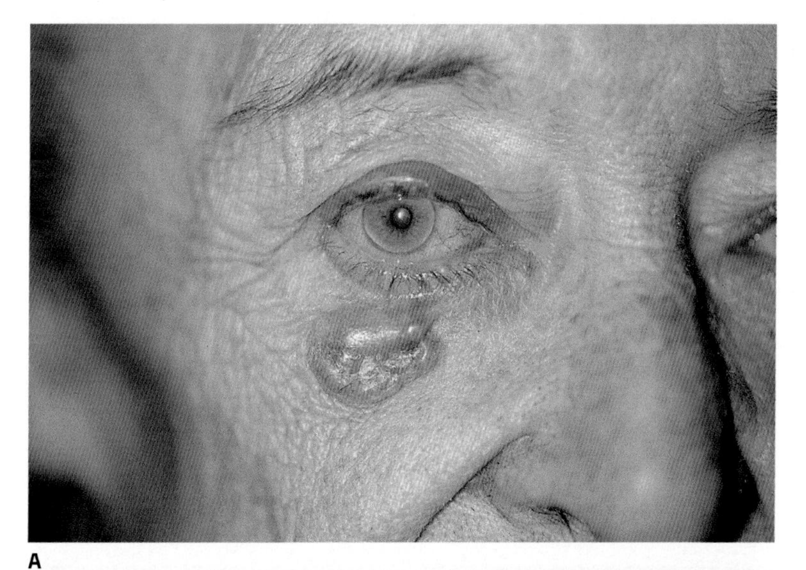

A

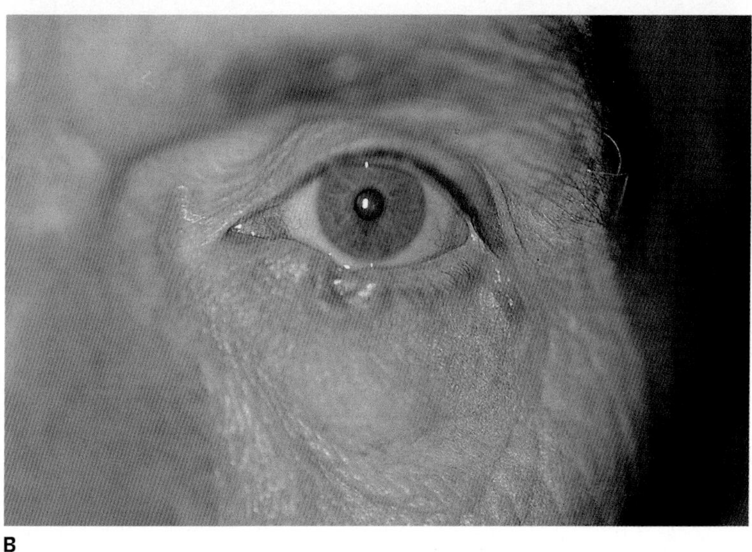

B

Figure 3-3 Basal cell carcinoma **A.** *This picture is the classic appearance of a basal cell carcinoma. This lesion does not involve the eyelid margin but large lesions such as this one are a challenge for reconstruction because of the chance of lower eyelid ectropion.* **B.** *Notching of the eyelid margin is a sign of an eyelid neoplasm. This basal cell carcinoma has caused a notch and demonstrates the smooth pearly borders of a basal cell carcinoma. (Continued.)*

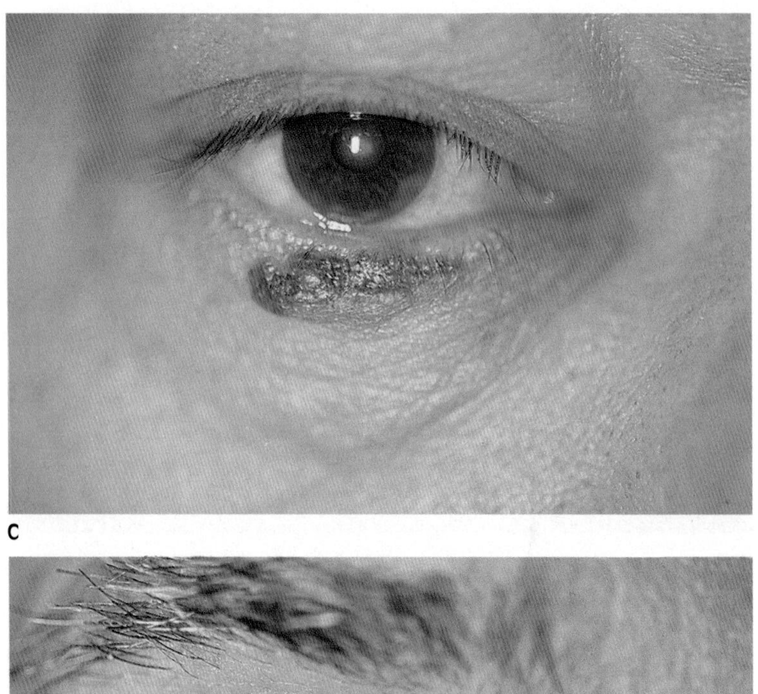

C

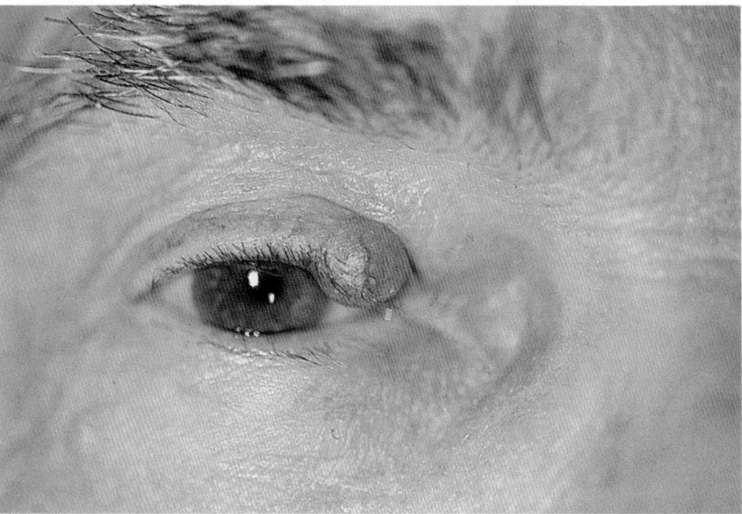

D

Figure 3-3 Basal cell carcinoma (cont.) **C.** *Basal cell carcinoma may present as pigmented lesions, especially in patients with darker pigmented skin. Note the pearly edges on the inferior part of the lesion.* **D.** *A cystic lesion can be a basal cell carcinoma. This lesion is larger than most hydrocystomas and has a slightly violaceous hue. This cystic basal cell carcinoma was filled with a thick clear gel-like material, which is classic. (Continued.)*

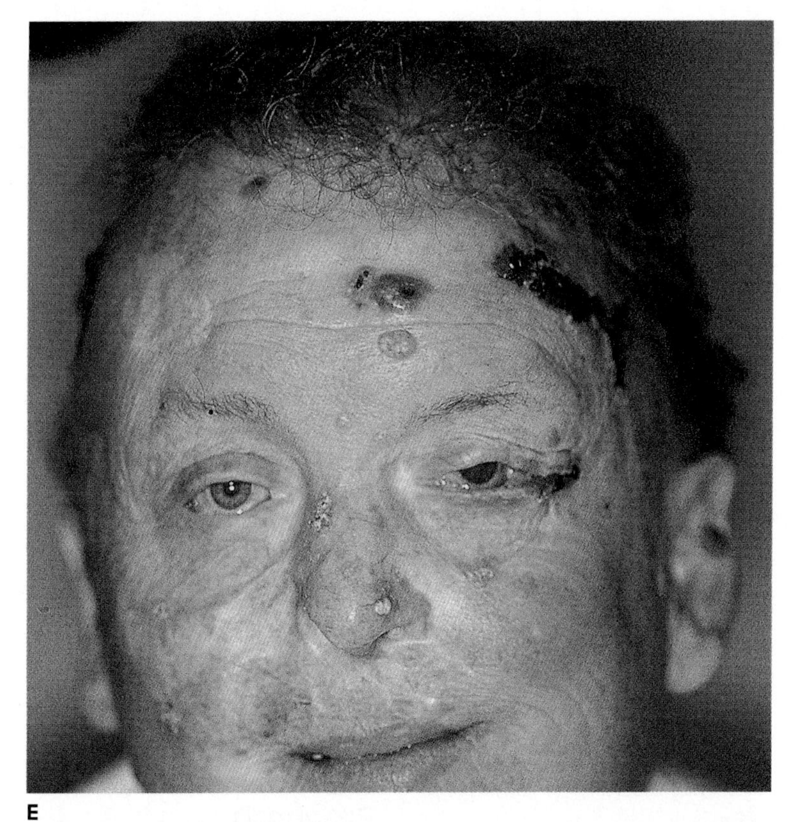

E

F

Figure 3-3 Basal cell nevus syndrome (cont.) **E.** *Basal cell nevus syndrome with many basal cell carcinomas all over the face occurring at a young age.* **F.** *Pits of the palms of the hands that are often seen in basal cell nevus syndrome.*

SQUAMOUS CELL CARCINOMA

Squamous cell carcinoma is a malignant tumor of epithelial keratinocytes. It is often the result of exogenous carcinogens (ultraviolet exposure, exposure to ionizing radiation, arsenic). These lesions are much less common than basal cell carcinoma on the eyelids and are usually successfully treated with excision.

Epidemiology and Etiology

Age Over age 55 years.

Gender Males more commonly involved than females.

Etiology Sun exposure and fair skin with poor ability to tan are risk factors. Treatment with x-ray (for acne) increases the risk.

Incidence 12 per 100,000 white males; 7 per 100,000 white females; 1 per 100,000 blacks.

History

Persistent keratotic lesion or plaque that does not resolve after 1 month must be considered a potential carcinoma, especially in sun-exposed areas.

Examination

Two types of lesions.

- Differentiated lesions are keratinized, firm, and hard.
- Undifferentiated lesions are fleshy, granulomatous, and soft.

These can present from very small to large. They may be crusted with bleeding or smooth (Fig. 3-4).

Differential Diagnosis

- Actinic keratosis
- Basal cell carcinoma
- Keratoacanthoma

Laboratory Tests

Pathologic evaluation.

Treatment

Complete surgical excision with controlled margins. Specimens are sent for pathologic evaluation.

Prognosis

Excellent unless the lesion is neglected. Squamous cell carcinoma does rarely spread via lymphatics, blood vessels, or along nerves.

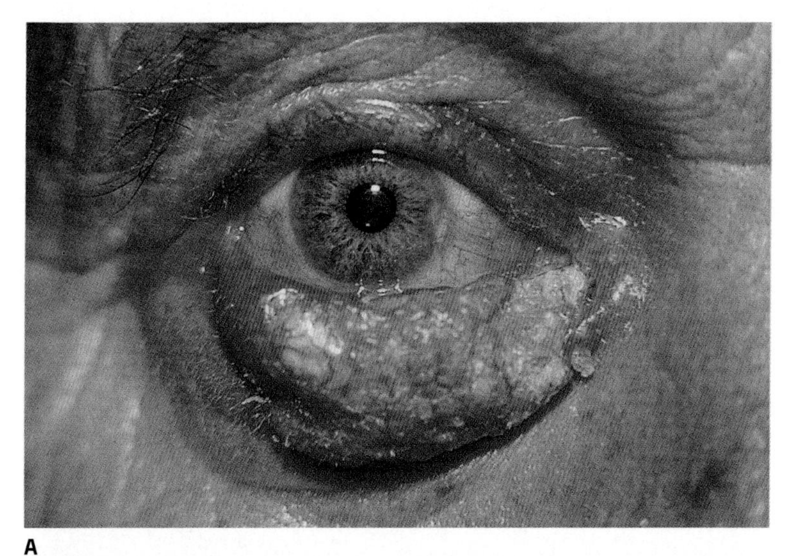

A

B

Figure 3-4 Squamous cell carcinoma **A.** *This is a very large squamous cell carcinoma that was neglected. It now infiltrates the entire lower eyelid. Note the crusting on the lesion, which is usually present with squamous cell carcinoma and is less common with basal cell carcinoma.* **B.** *Smaller lesion of the lower eyelid that shows crusting and an irregular, erosive central area.*

SEBACEOUS ADENOCARCINOMA

Sebaceous adenocarcinoma is a highly malignant and potentially fatal tumor that arises from the sebaceous glands of the eyelid. Early, this tumor can be difficult to recognize and once it grows, it is difficult to contain as it can have skip areas. Early recognition and aggressive excision are the keys to successful treatment.

Epidemiology and Etiology

Age Usually greater than 50 years of age.

Gender More common in females than males.

Etiology Arises from the meibomian glands, glands of Zeis, or from the sebaceous glands of the caruncle, eyebrow, or facial skin.

History

Often starts as a chronic blepharitis or nonresolving chalazion. Patients may have a chronic red, irritated eye for months to years.

Examination

Multiple potential presentations.

- Nodular lesion simulating a chalazion.
- Unilateral chronic blepharitis.
- Cellular membrane growing over the conjunctiva.
- Destructive, often ulcerated, lesion on the eyelid margin (Fig. 3-5).

Occurrence in the upper eyelid is twice as common as the lower eyelid.

Special Considerations

This lesion is the great masquerader and delay in diagnosis as a carcinoma and subsequent growth of the lesion add to the poor prognosis for this tumor.

Differential Diagnosis

- Basal cell carcinoma
- Squamous cell carcinoma
- Chronic blepharitis
- Chronic chalazion

Pathology

It is important to have special lipid stains performed on lesions that are suspected to be sebaceous adenocarcinoma. Without these stains, the lesion may be misdiagnosed.

Treatment

Diagnosing the lesion is often the biggest challenge. Biopsy of any suspicious lesion is the key. Once diagnosed, complete excision with wide, controlled margins is the treatment of choice. There can be skip areas so careful follow-up for recurrence is needed.

Prognosis

This is a potentially lethal tumor that must be treated aggressively.

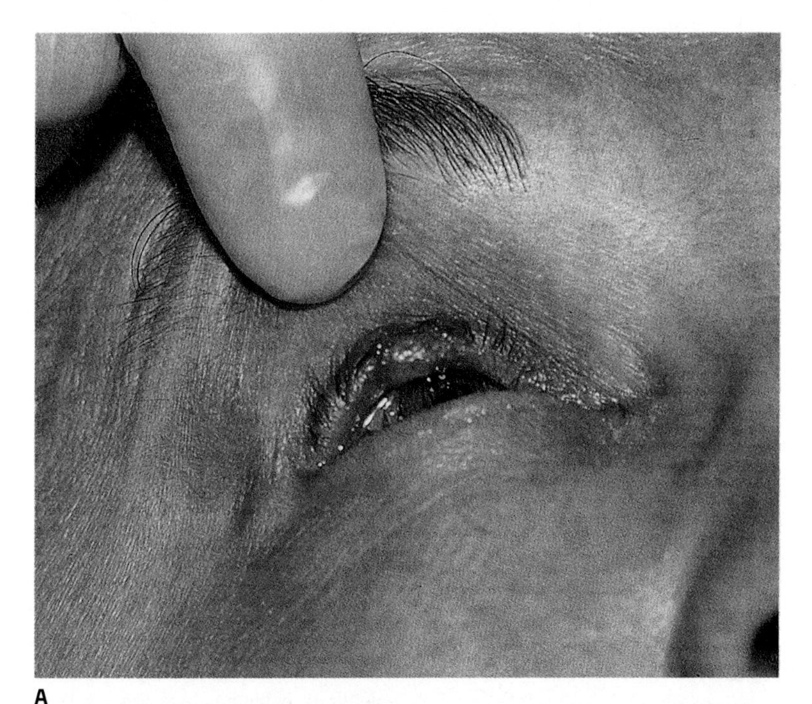

A

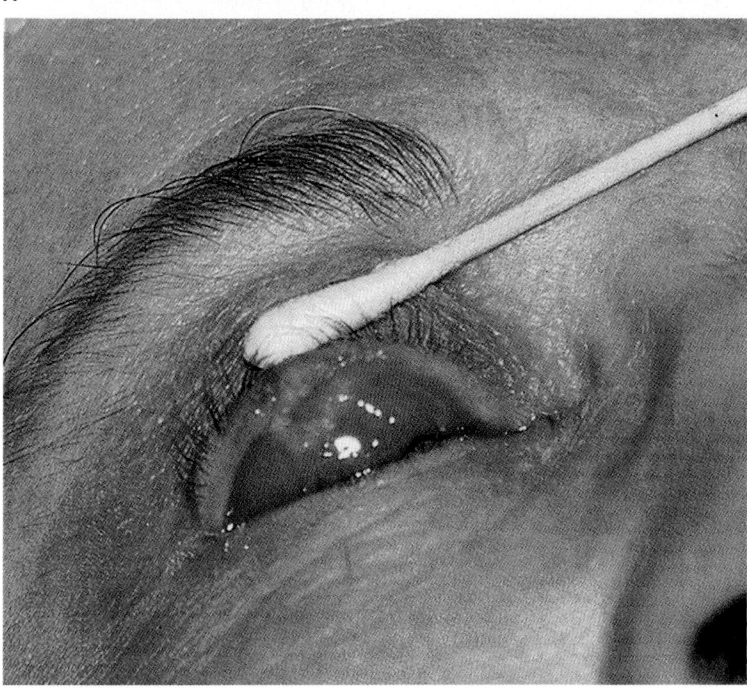

B

Figure 3-5 Sebaceous adenocarcinoma **A.** *The eyelid margin is red and inflamed with notching.* **B.** *When the eyelid is everted, there is an infiltrative lesion of the tarsal conjunctiva.*

MALIGNANT MELANOMA

Malignant melanoma is a rare but very dangerous malignant lesion of the eyelids. Sun exposure as a child is an etiologic factor. Despite aggressive surgical excision, this can still be a fatal tumor.

Epidemiology and Etiology

Age Third decade and beyond.

Gender Equal between males and females.

Etiology Sun exposure and genetic predisposition.

History

Pigmented lesion with recent growth or change in appearance.

Examination

Pigmented lesion with irregular pigment deposition, irregular margins, or just increase in size (Fig. 3-6). There may be ulceration and bleeding.

Differential Diagnosis

- Nevus
- Pigmented basal cell carcinoma

Laboratory Tests

Specimens are sent for pathologic evaluation.

Treatment

Complete excision with aggressive, controlled surgical margins. The deeper the lesion, the wider the margins required.

Prognosis

Dependent on the depth of the tumor. Eight-year survival rate is 33 to 93 percent depending on depth of melanoma invasion.

Depth (mm)	8-Year Survival (percent)
< 0.76	93.2
0.76–1.69	85.6
1.70–3.60	59.8
> 3.60	33.3

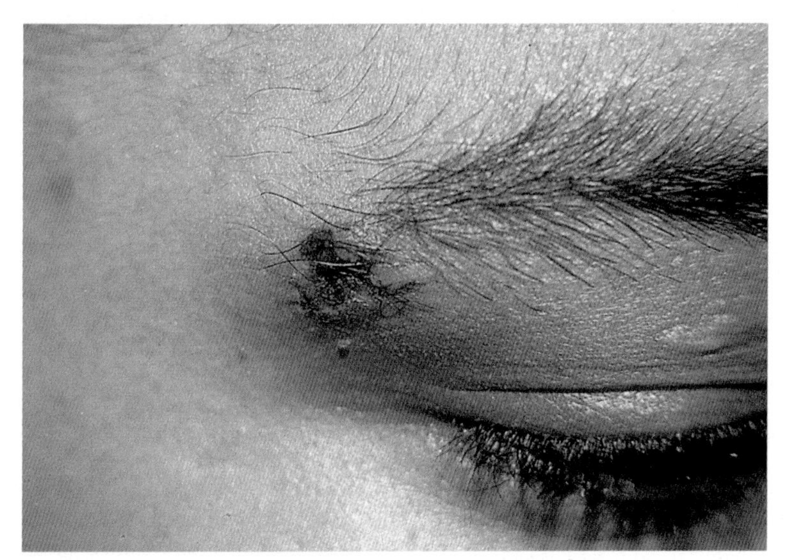

Figure 3-6 Malignant melanoma *Lesion of the right eyebrow that has grown over a few months. The lesion has irregular areas of lighter and darker pigmentation.*

KAPOSI'S SARCOMA

Kaposi's sarcoma is a vascular neoplasia that can involve multiple systems. It is a rare lesion of the eyelids but when present, is usually associated with a compromised immune system, most commonly HIV disease.

Epidemiology and Etiology

Age Any

Gender More common in males.

Etiology Vascular neoplasia often associated with immune compromise in the United States.

History

Rapid growth of lesion may occur. Patients most commonly are HIV positive although other forms of immune compromise may predispose patients to these lesions.

Examination

Elevated dermal lesions that are red or purple (Fig. 3-7).

Differential Diagnosis

- Pyogenic granuloma
- Chalazion
- Hemangioma
- Melanocytic nevus

Laboratory Tests

Pathologic evaluation if biopsied. Evaluation of immune system if indicated.

Treatment

Excision with pathologic evaluation. Cryotherapy or intralesional chemotherapeutic agents may be used for local control of the lesions. Radiation treatment for some large lesions.

Prognosis

Patients who develop lesions associated with HIV often have a short survival and die from advancement of the HIV disease. Patients with primary Kaposi's sarcoma may survive for years.

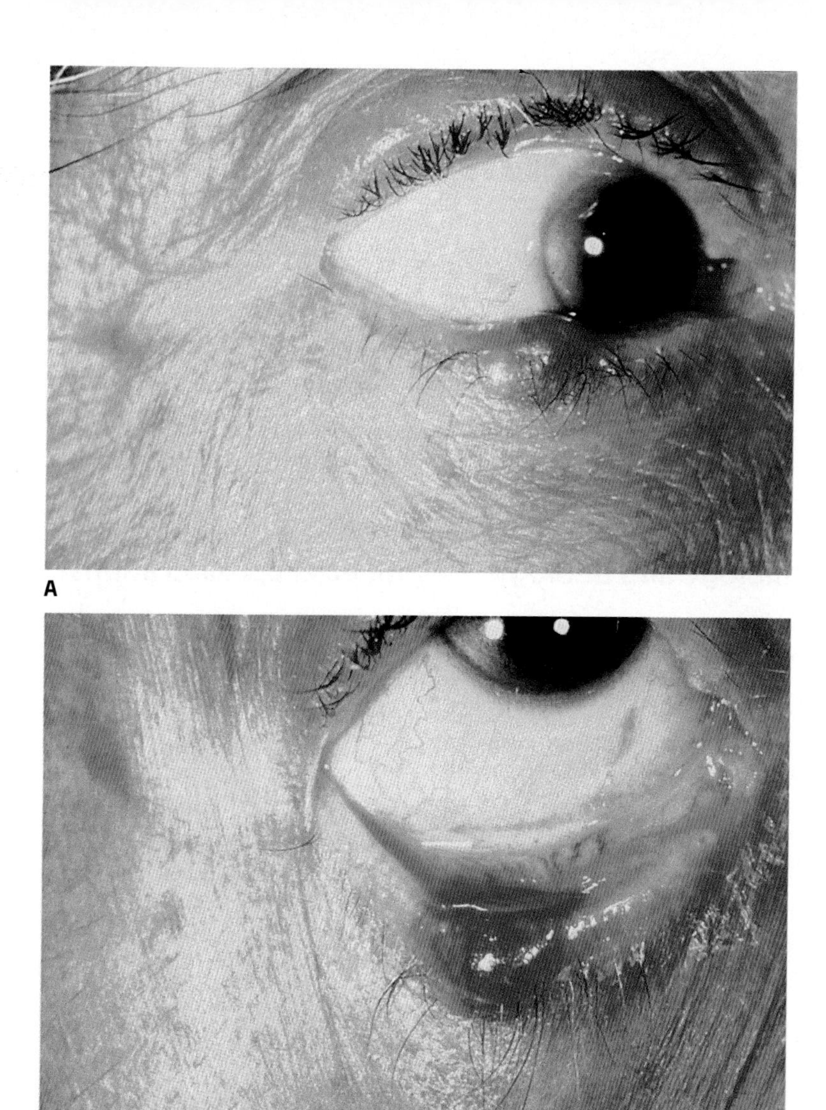

Figure 3-7 Kaposi's sarcoma **A** *and* **B.** *Lesion of the lower lid in a patient with AIDS.*

Chapter 4
EYELID TRAUMA

MARGINAL EYELID LACERATION

Marginal eyelid lacerations are most commonly associated with trauma to the entire orbital area and often, there are other associated injuries. The extent of laceration can vary greatly. Prompt, meticulous closure is the treatment of choice.

Epidemiology and Etiology

Age Any age. Second through fourth decades most common.

Gender Males more commonly affected.

Etiology Blunt trauma (e.g., fist), direct cut (e.g., glass, knife), or dogbite, most commonly.

History

Trauma history is variable from minor to major injuries. It is important to determine the cause of the trauma to know whether to suspect foreign bodies. The amount of force causing the injury will help determine the likelihood of more significant injuries of the orbit and globe.

Examination

Must evaluate globe and orbit for injuries. Evaluate the extent of the injury to the eyelid and be sure that the lacrimal system is not injured (Fig. 4-1). CT scanning may be required if other injuries or foreign bodies are suspected.

Special Considerations

Dogbites require copious irrigation of the wound and special care because of the great risk of infection. Tetanus immunization must be up to date.

Treatment

Meticulous closure of the wound within 24 to 48 hours. Surgery can be done in the office or emergency room setting unless the lacerations are complex or in children, where an operating room setting with general anesthesia is required.

Prognosis

Good. The more complex the wound, the greater the chance of scarring, which may then require secondary repair at a later date.

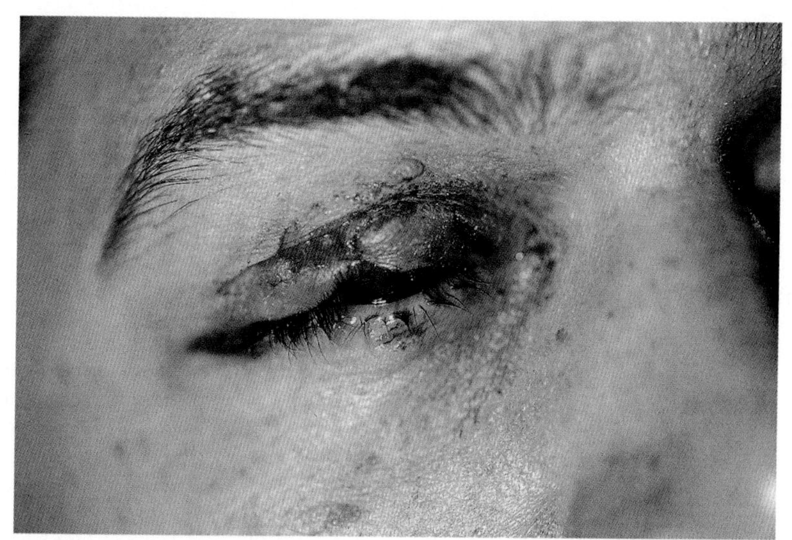

Figure 4-1 Marginal eyelid laceration *Central eyelid laceration from an umbrella catching under the eyelid. Isolated marginal lacerations without canalicular involvement are more likely due to some object directly tearing the eyelid. Canalicular lacerations are more often because of tearing and stretching as the medial lid is the weakest area and the first to tear.*

CANALICULAR EYELID LACERATION

The medial eyelid is the weakest area of the eyelid, so any horizontal traction on the eyelid is most likely to result in damage to the medial eyelid and the canaliculus. Eyelid trauma requires careful inspection of the medial canthal area to note the lacerated canaliculus. Repair with silicone intubation is the treatment of choice.

Epidemiology and Etiology

Age Any age. Second through fourth decades most common.

Gender Males more commonly affected.

Etiology Usually a tearing injury as the medial eyelid is the weakest area of the eyelid.

History

Trauma history is variable including blunt force, dogbites, and, rarely, sharp objects.

Examination

Evaluate eye and orbit for injuries. Any cut medial to the lacrimal puncta must be evaluated for a canalicular laceration. Probing of the canalicular system may be necessary if a laceration is suspected (Fig. 4-2).

Special Considerations

The farther the laceration is medially from the lacrimal puncta, the more difficult it is to find the distal cut end.

Treatment

Surgical repair with anastamosis of the canalicular ends and intubation of the lacrimal system. Locating the distal end of the canaliculus may be difficult and often requires loupes or an operating microscope. Depending on the severity of the injury and the patient's cooperation, surgical repair is usually performed in the operating room setting with local or general anesthesia. The tubing is left in the lacrimal system for 6 weeks to 6 months depending on severity and the individual practitioner.

Prognosis

Good. Even the injuries that result in a scarred canaliculus usually do well as most patients do well with one functioning canaliculus.

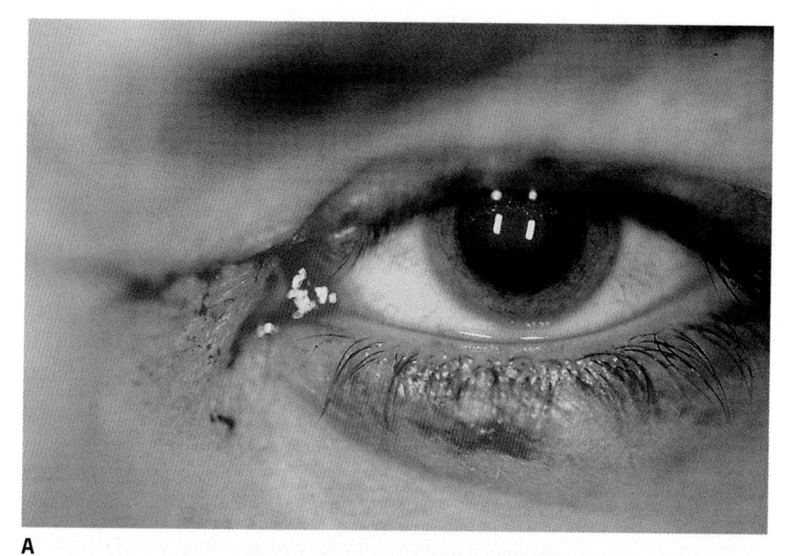

A

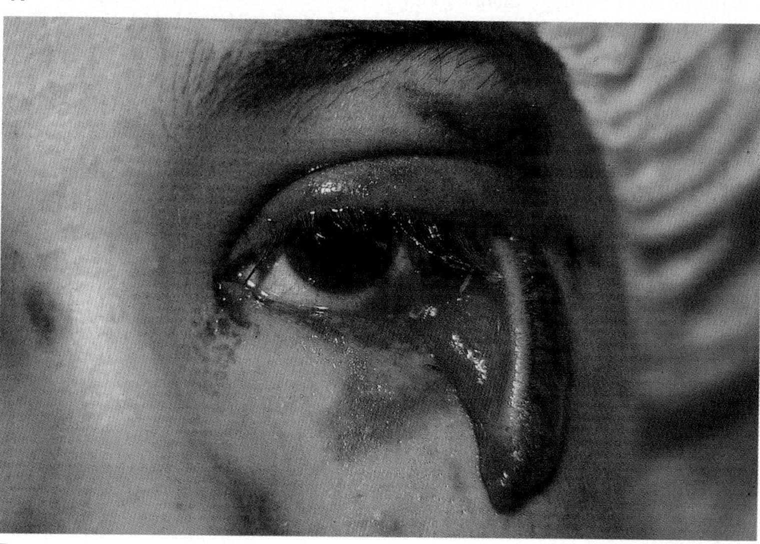

B

Figure 4-2 Canalicular laceration **A.** *Any cut or tear medial to the punctum, no matter how superficial it appears, needs to be explored for involvement of the canaliculus. This laceration involved both the upper and lower canaliculi.* **B.** *The punctum and cut canaliculus can be seen at the medial edge of the cut eyelid. This eyelid was nearly completely avulsed.*

DOG BITES

Dog bites are highly variable in their extent but generally do not involve injury to the globe itself. Prompt repair with copious irrigation often gives fairly good results depending on the extent of the original injury.

Epidemiology and Etiology

Age Most commonly children, adults less common.

Gender Equal.

Etiology In children, the dog may be trying to bite the child on the nose to show domination, which is what happens between dogs, and usually does not represent an attack. The eyelid laceration is the result of the dog's canine tooth catching the eyelid and tearing the medial lid rather than a true bite to the eyelid.

History

Often, the child knows the dog and there is a single bite and not a vicious attack.

Examination

Evaluation of the eye and orbit for other injuries. There is most commonly a single bite with multiple areas of injury. There may be puncture wounds or larger tears and gashes (Fig. 4-3).

Special Considerations

The bite must be reported to the health department for follow up to be sure the dog is properly vaccinated for rabies. Tetanus immunization must be up to date.

Treatment

The eyelid laceration must be treated as outlined previously. The risk of infection in animal and human bites is high because of the bacteria in the mouth. Copious irrigation of the wounds is the only treatment of proven benefit to decrease the risk of infection. The use of broad-spectrum, systemic antibiotics has not been proven to lessen the chance of infection but should be considered.

Prognosis

Good. The more severe the injury the greater the risk of postoperative deformity.

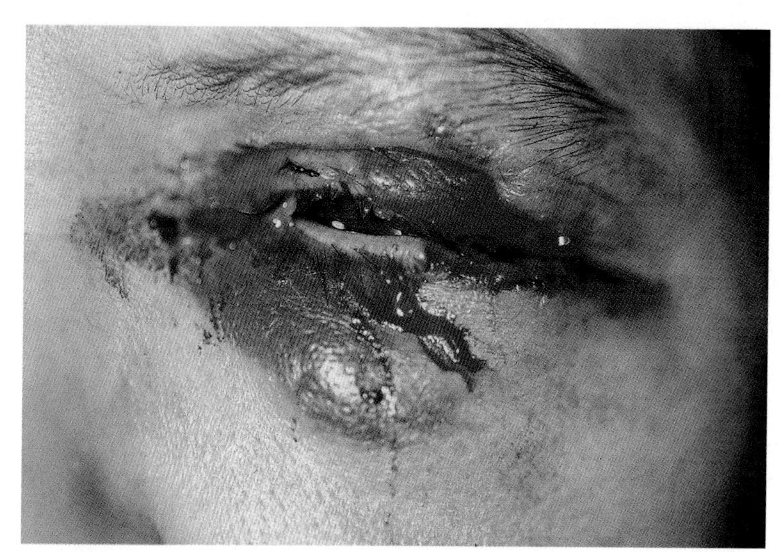

Figure 4-3 Dog bite with eyelid lacerations *Dog bites are usually a single bite but the amount of damage can be highly variable from mild to severe. The eyelid damage is usually related to tearing as the dog pulls away and the teeth get caught on the eyelid. Both the medial and lateral canthi are torn and multiple puncture wounds are seen.*

EYELID BURNS

Eyelid burns are usually associated with significant burns to the rest of the face and body unless they are electrical or chemical. All burns take days to weeks for the full tissue death and necrosis to manifest itself. Reconstruction can be very difficult because of poor vascularization.

Epidemiology and Etiology

Age Any.

Gender Males more commonly affected.

Etiology Burns that involve the eyelids are usually associated with burns over a large percentage of the body.

History

Generally associated with other facial burns unless the etiology is electrical or chemical.

Examination

Burns of the eyelid vary in depth and severity. The concern is to protect the cornea with lubrication. With time, the eyelids will scar resulting in poor closure and more corneal exposure (Fig. 4-4).

Treatment

Antibiotic ointment and copious corneal lubrication. Systemic antibiotics are usually part of the systemic care. As the burns heal, cicatricial changes become more prominent and the use of skin grafts is required.

Prognosis

Dependent on the severity of the burns. Severe burns may require multiple surgeries and skin grafts to protect the cornea.

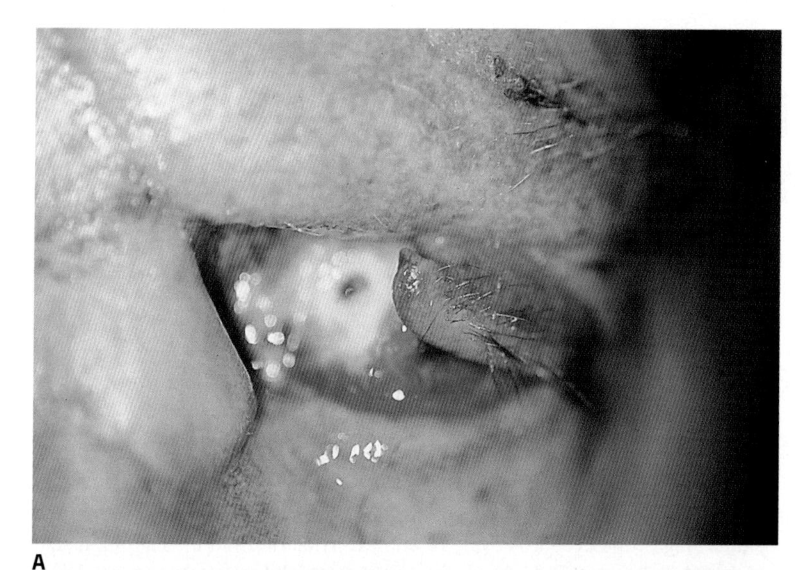

A

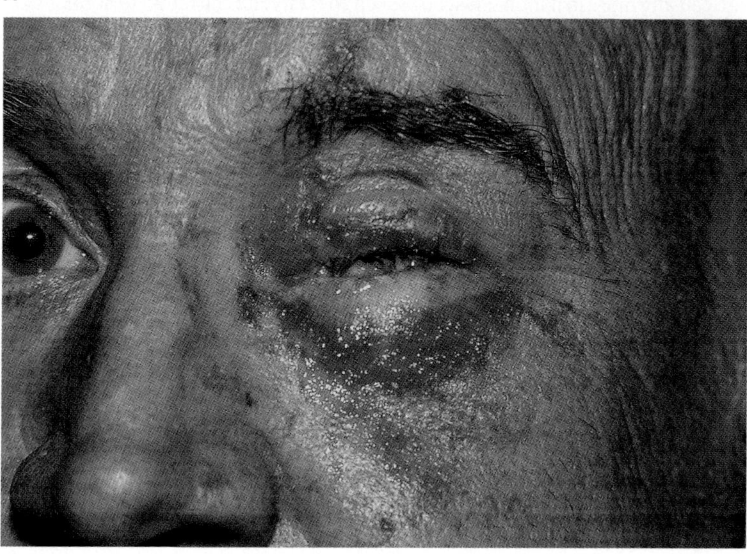

B

Figure 4-4 Eyelid burn *Electrical burn with necrosis of the upper eyelid and underlying scleral necrosis. Electrical burns can take weeks for the total amount of tissue necrosis to be come apparent.* **B.** *Molten lead was splashed onto the eyelid and into the eye. With thermal burns, the extent of damage is evident more quickly. Note the relative lack of vascularization along the lower eyelid margin from the burn. There was partial necrosis and loss of part of the eyelid margin over time.*

Chapter 5

EYELID MALPOSITIONS

ENTROPION

ACUTE SPASTIC ENTROPION

Acute spastic entropion is the result of eyelid swelling along with orbicularis spasm that results in a temporary inturning of the eyelid. A cycle of corneal irritation from the entropion, causing more eyelid spasm, causing more irritation, must be broken so the eyelid can return to normal. Some of these patients will have underlying involutional changes (laxity) that may result in a recurrent entropion.

Epidemiology and Etiology

Age More common in older patient population.

Gender Equal occurrence in males and females.

Etiology Ocular irritation or inflammation causes continued forced blinking and closure of the eye. This will lead to inturning of the lower eyelid in eyelids that have involutional changes predisposing them to entropion (see Section "Involutional Entropion").

History

Recent surgery on the eye or recent onset of ocular irritation.

Examination

Lower eyelid entropion (Fig. 5-1) with associated involutional factors such as horizontal laxity and orbicularis override. In addition, there is a separate identifiable irritant to the eye. This irritant may be keratitis, foreign body, suture, or just inflammation postoperatively.

Differential Diagnosis

- Involutional entropion
- Cicatricial entropion

Pathophysiology

Involutional changes of the eyelid allow the forced closure of the eyelid orbicularis muscle to override the tarsus and drive the eyelid margin inward toward the eye.

Treatment

Treatment of the underlying ocular irritation or inflammation will resolve some cases. This involves treating the ocular irritation and stabilizing the eyelid to halt the additional irritation the eyelid is causing. Stabilizing the eyelid may involve taping the eyelid out or Quickert sutures. Some cases will then resolve, others will become an involutional entropion and need more extensive surgery.

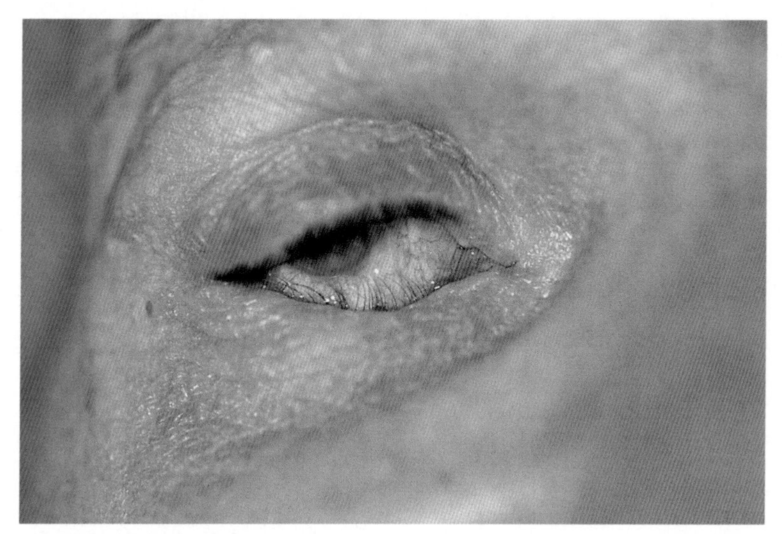

Figure 5-1 Acute spastic entropion *Patient with a corneal abrasion. Continued irritation and blinking leads to an entropion.*

Prognosis

Excellent. Recurrence in patients with significant involutional factors of the eyelid may develop an involutional entropion at a later time.

INVOLUTIONAL ENTROPION

Eyelid laxity both horizontally and vertically predisposes to the instability of the lower eyelid. The additional factor required is the ability of the patient's orbicularis muscle to override the tarsus and drive the eyelid inward. Patients present with red, irritated eyes from the eyelid margin and tarsus in contact with the eye itself.

Epidemiology and Etiology

Age More common in older patient population.

Gender Equal occurrence in males and females.

Etiology Horizontal laxity and orbicularis override result in inversion of the eyelid.

History

Acute onset of eye irritation. This irritation is sometimes intermittent in nature and becomes more constant.

Examination

Inverted lower eyelid with inferior corneal superficial punctate keratitis (SPK) or corneal abrasion (Fig. 5-2). Entropion is usually associated with horizontal eyelid laxity. Orbicularis muscle override is usually noted as fullness over the tarsal plate when the lid is entropic. The entropion can be intermittent and not always present on examination. Placing topical anesthetic drops in the eye, having the patient close the eyes forcefully, and look downward will usually bring out the entropion.

Differential Diagnosis

- Cicatricial entropion
- Acute spastic entropion

Pathophysiology

Aging of eyelid tissues results in laxity and stretching of supporting structures.

Treatment

Surgical correction is based on correcting the factors contributing to the entropion; usually horizontal shortening of the eyelid and tightening the eyelid retractors in any of multiple ways.

Prognosis

Excellent. There is a 5 to 10 percent chance of recurrence over 5 to 10 years.

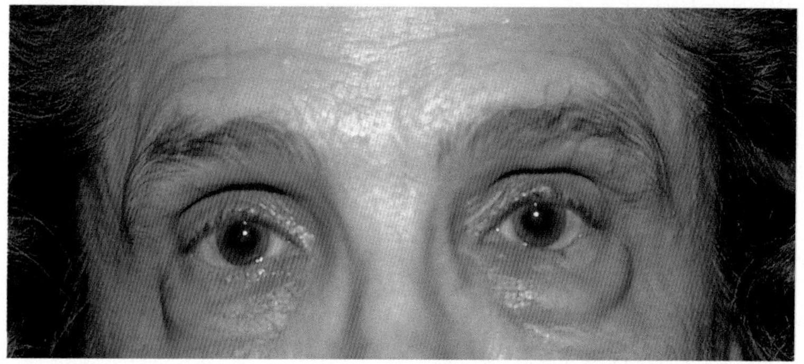

Figure 5-2 Involutional entropion *Bilateral entropions with involutional changes. The rolled in orbicularis muscle can be seen driving the eyelid margin inward on the left.*

CICATRICIAL ENTROPION

Cicatricial entropion is caused by conjunctival scarring pulling the eyelid inward. Generally, treatment is surgical but defining and treating the cause of the conjunctival scarring must be done first or most cases will recur. Occurs in the upper or lower eyelid.

Epidemiology and Etiology

Age Any age.

Gender Equal occurrence in males and females.

Etiology Scar tissue on the conjunctival surfaces results in shortening of the posterior lamella, physically pulling in the eyelid. Factors include:

- Surgery
- Conjunctival scarring diseases (e.g., ocular cicatricial pemphigoid, Stevens–Johnson syndrome, trachoma)
- Trauma
- Conjunctival burns (e.g., chemical)
- Antiglaucoma drops

History

Chronic low-grade inflammation over months to years results in the entropion that then causes more irritation. The other scenario is a history of trauma or surgery resulting in an entropion and associated irritation.

Examination

Careful evaluation of the conjunctiva for signs of scarring causing inversion of the eyelid. This may include evaluation of the other eyelids to determine if the entropion is isolated or involving all four eyelids, which may help determine the etiology (Fig. 5-3A and B).

Special Considerations

Must determine etiology of conjunctival scarring before treating. Any progressive disease must be quieted before surgery can be done on the eyelids.

Differential Diagnosis

- Acute spastic entropion
- Involutional entropion

Laboratory Tests

Conjunctival biopsy with immunofluorescence testing if ocular cicatricial pemphigoid is suspected.

Treatment

Determine the etiology of the conjunctival scarring. Quiet any active disease. Surgical correction of the entropion with a marginal rotation or buccal mucosal graft is then the treatment of choice.

Prognosis

Variable depending on the etiology. Entropion secondary to trauma and surgery usually do very well. Progressive disease processes, such as ocular cicatricial pemphigoid, can make it much more difficult to prevent recurrence of the entropion.

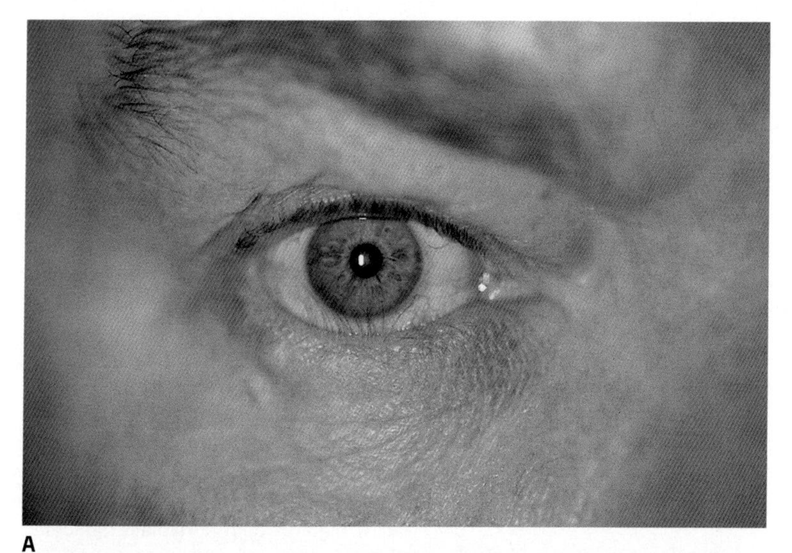

A

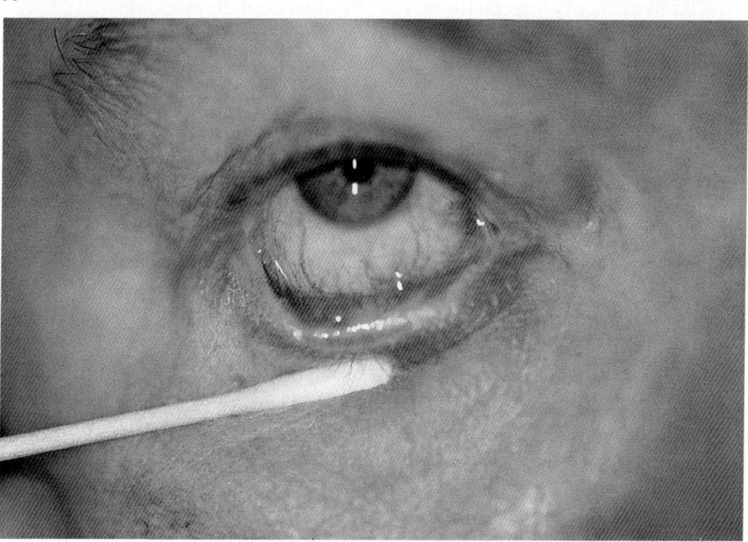

B

Figure 5-3 **A** *and* **B. Cicatricial entropion** *Externally, it is difficult to differentiate this cicatricial entropion from an involutional entropion until the eyelid is everted* **(B)** *and the cicatricial changes are noted pulling the eyelid inward.*

ECTROPION

INVOLUTIONAL ECTROPION

Involutional ectropion has the same involutional factors as in an involutional entropion (e.g., horizontal laxity and vertical instability). These patients do not have hypertrophic, spastic orbicularis muscle to override and so the unstable eyelid sags outward instead of being driven in. Symptoms are less acute and not as severe as in involutional entropion. Many patients will have mild involutional ectropions and may be asymptomatic.

Epidemiology and Etiology

Age Incidence increases as age increases.

Gender Equal occurrence in males and females.

Etiology Eyelid tissue laxity, especially horizontal laxity.

History

Insidious onset of ocular irritation and/or tearing. Patient may note redness and inflammation of the eyelid margin.

Examination

Eyelid sagging inferiorly and away from the globe surface (Fig. 5-4). Must look for the amount of horizontal laxity, corneal exposure, and stenosis of the lacrimal puncta.

Special Considerations

Tarsal ectropion is complete eversion of the eyelid and indicates detachment of the lower eyelid retractors. This condition must be recognized as it requires both horizontal tightening and reattachment of the retractors.

Differential Diagnosis

- Cicatricial ectropion
- Paralytic ectropion

Treatment

Mild ectropion with only mild exposure symptoms can sometimes be treated with ocular lubrication. Definitive treatment involves horizontal eyelid shortening and possible punctoplasty.

Prognosis

Excellent. Recurrence after surgery is estimated at 5 to 10 percent but is higher the longer the follow up is done and the more severe the ectropion was at the time of the repair.

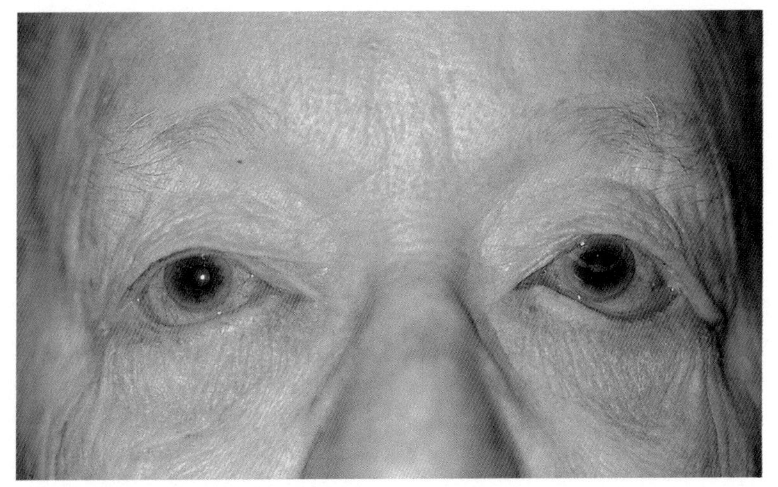

Figure 5-4 Involutional ectropion *Bilateral ectropions with very lax eyelids. Note the red palpebral conjunctiva from chronic exposure.*

PARALYTIC ECTROPION

Paralytic ectropion is the result of temporary or permanent seventh cranial nerve palsy. The lower eyelid sags away from the globe resulting in loss of protection of the eye and inability of the lacrimal system to collect tears. Patients with less severe palsy and other eye protective mechanisms intact present with tearing. Patients with more severe palsies and poor eye protection mechanisms present with corneal breakdown.

Epidemiology and Etiology

Age Any age.

Gender Equal occurrence in males and females.

Etiology Facial palsy etiologies include:

- Bell's palsy
- Surgery: intracranial or facial
- Stroke
- Tumor

History

Previous onset of facial palsy. Depending on the severity of the facial palsy, the ectropion may have onset at the same time or the eyelid may slowly sag with time. The severity of the condition depends on the severity of the paralysis, corneal sensation, and ocular lubrication.

Examination

The lower eyelid is found to be sagging away from the globe (Fig. 5-5). Evaluate severity of facial palsy, degree of ectropion, amount of corneal exposure, amount of lagophthalmos, and presence of Bell's phenomenon.

Special Considerations

Must check for corneal sensation as loss of corneal sensation will make all exposure symptoms much worse. Any unexplained facial palsy must be worked up.

Differential Diagnosis

- Bell's palsy versus nonresolving facial palsy.

Treatment

Treatment depends on the anticipated duration of the paralysis. If spontaneous improvement is anticipated then treatment with lubrication and a temporary tarsorrhaphy if severe corneal problems are present is indicated. If corneal exposure is still a problem with lubrication use and the paralysis is long term then horizontal eyelid tightening is used to treat the paralytic ectropion. Placing a gold weight in the upper eyelid may also be required. Rarely, a permanent tarsorrhaphy may be needed.

Prognosis

Variable. The ectropion tends to recur over time if the paralysis is permanent.

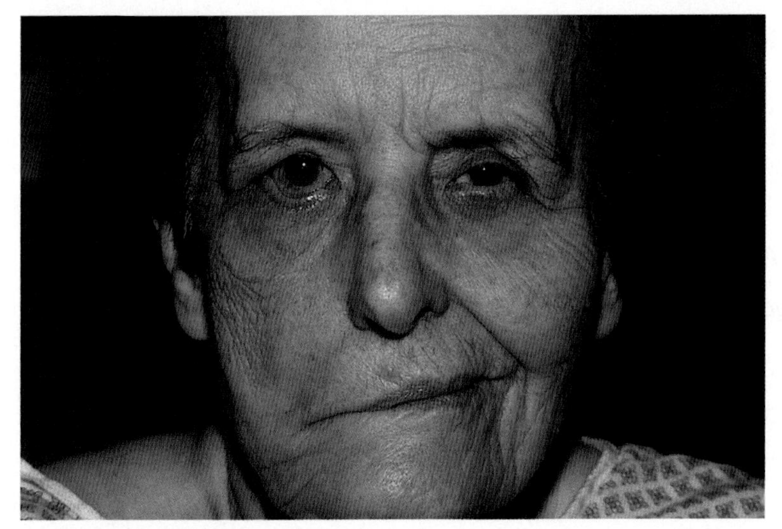

Figure 5-5 Paralytic entropion *Right lower eyelid ectropion as the result of a facial palsy.*

CICATRICIAL ECTROPION

Cicatricial ectropion is caused by mechanical shortening of the anterior lamellae of the eyelid pulling the eyelid down and outward. This results in tearing and corneal exposure. More common in the lower eyelid but can occur in the upper eyelid.

Epidemiology and Etiology

Age Any age.

Gender More common in males because of higher incidence of traumatic events.

Etiology Scarring of the anterior lamellae of the eyelid pulls the eyelid outward. The etiologies include:

- Trauma
- Surgery
- Dermatitis
- Skin carcinoma

History

May include a specific history such as trauma or surgery. If a chronic dermatologic condition is the cause of the scarring, this may be a known or a previously unrecognized condition.

Examination

External scarring or skin changes are noted on the upper or more commonly the lower eyelid. This scarring results in shortening of the eyelid skin and outturning of the eyelid margin (Fig. 5-6A).

Special Considerations

Must always consider a skin carcinoma as the possible cause of scarring of the skin. If the cause is unclear, a biopsy is needed.

Differential Diagnosis

- Important to differentiate involutional ectropion from those with cicatricial changes.

Treatment

Treatment of any underlying dermatologic condition is important. In traumatic or post-surgical cases, the scarring should be left for 6 months or longer unless exposure or other problems necessitate earlier treatment. Treatment involves lysis of any deep scar tissue with horizontal tightening. If the skin shortening is severe, full thickness skin grafts will be required. Skin grafts have the potential for scarring and a cosmetically noticeable area at the graft site (Fig. 5-6B).

Prognosis

Trauma or surgically induced cases do well with repair. Chronic conditions of the skin tend to result in recurrences.

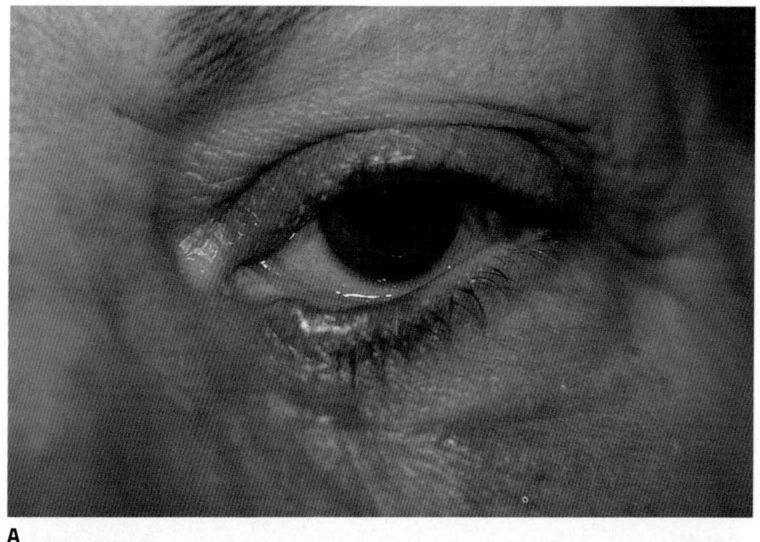

A

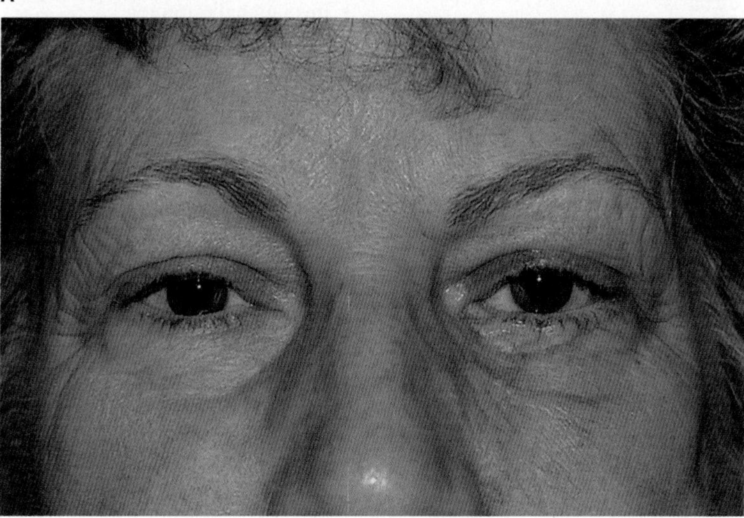

B

Figure 5-6 Cicatricial ectropion **A.** *Trauma to the left lower eyelid results in scarring of the skin with vertical shortening as well as scarring internally within the eyelid.* **B.** *After repair using a skin graft.*

MECHANICAL ECTROPION

Mechanical ectropion is a rare cause of ectropion in which a mass of some type pushes the eyelid outward. There are usually associated involutional changes, which allow the eyelid to be pushed outward.

Epidemiology and Etiology

Age Older patients.

Gender Equal occurrence in males and females.

Etiology Gravity pulls the eyelid away from the eye or pushes the eyelid away from the eye secondary to a mass. Causes of the mass effect include:

- Dermatochalasis
- Edema
- Chalazion
- Eyelid tumor (hemangioma, inclusion cyst, etc.)

History

Patient may be asymptomatic, have symptoms of corneal irritation, or have redness and irritation of the eyelid.

Examination

Must determine the degree of involutional changes of the eyelid as well as the etiology of the mass distorting the eyelid. The amount of corneal exposure and any corneal scarring should also be noted (Fig. 5-7).

Differential Diagnosis

- Involutional ectropion
- Cicatricial ectropion
- Paralytic ectropion

Treatment

Excision of the mass and correction of the involutional factors of the eyelid.

Prognosis

Good if the mass can be eliminated.

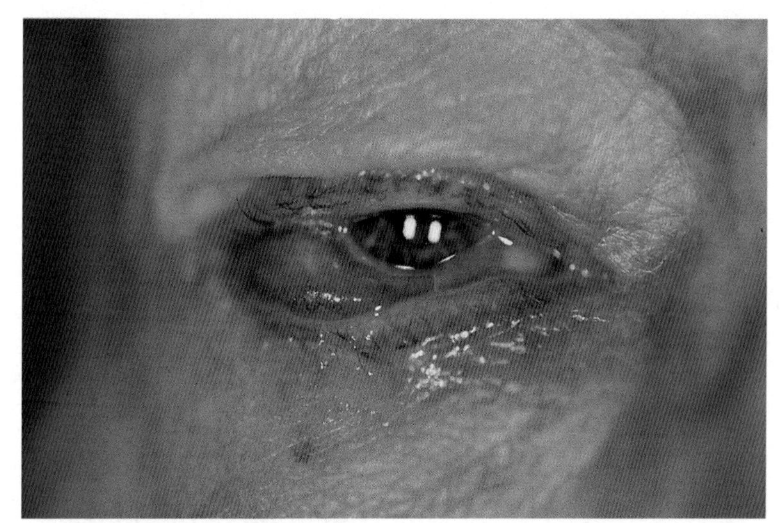

Figure 5-7 Mechanical ectropion *Chemosis from an inflammatory process mechanically pushes the lower eyelid outward. There are usually some involutional changes present to allow the eyelid to be pushed out. Resolution of the chemosis allowed the eyelid to return to a normal position.*

SYMBLEPHARON

Symblepharon is scarring between the bulbar and palpebral conjunctiva. This may be associated with active inflammation or there may be no inflammatory signs.

Epidemiology and Etiology

Age Any age.

Gender More frequent in women.

Etiology The following can result in scarring of two conjunctival surfaces.

- Chronic blepharitis
- Previous trauma
- Conjunctival scarring diseases (e.g., ocular cicatricial pemphigoid, Stevens–Johnson syndrome)
- Atopic disease
- Eyelid surgery
- Conjunctival burns
- Chronic glaucoma drops, especially miotics

History

There may be no history, just asymptomatic symblepharon noted on examination. Patients with history of eye or eyelid trauma or inflammation may also have symblepharon.

Examination

Scarring of the conjunctival surfaces may be very subtle with slight inferior fornix shortening or it may be very obvious with large conjunctival bands between the eye and eyelid (Fig. 5-8A and B). Must be sure to examine under the upper lid for conjunctival scarring as early signs are sometimes more obvious there.

Special Considerations

It is important to determine the cause of the symblepharon. If asymptomatic, the symplepharon may require no treatment except looking for the cause of the scarring. Ruling out a progressive conjunctival scarring disease, such as ocular cicatricial pemphigoid, is important.

Differential Diagnosis

- The differential diagnosis involves determining the cause of the symblepharon, not whether the process is a symblepharon.

Laboratory Tests

Conjunctival scarring of unknown etiology requires a conjunctival biopsy with immunofluorescence testing to rule out ocular cicatricial pemphigoid. In rare cases, squamous cell carcinoma may cause symblepharon, thus pathologic evaluation should be considered in select cases.

Treatment

None for mild symblepharon. Monitoring for progression is important. Significant symblepharon may cause trichiasis and cicatricial entropion that then may require treatment.

Prognosis

Variable depending on the cause of the symblepharon.

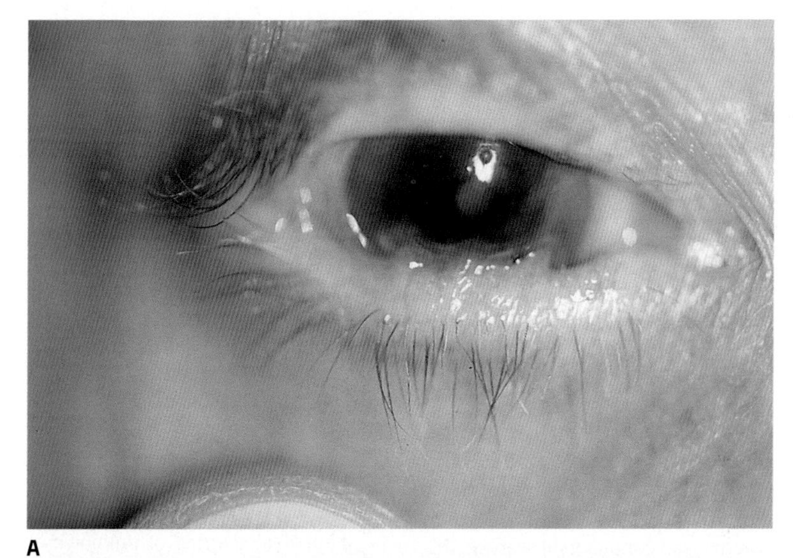
A

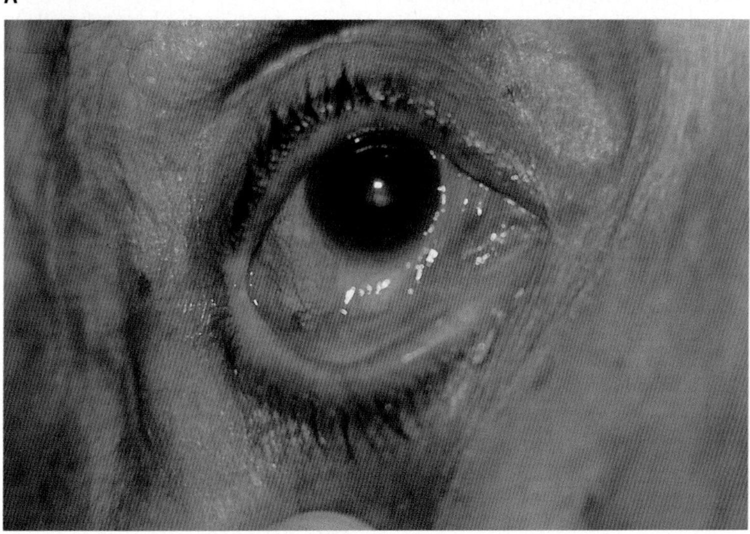
B

Figure 5-8 Symblepharon **A.** *Scarring is seen between the eyelid and the inferior cornea. Early symblepharon* (**B**) *may only be noted as shortening of the fornix.*

TRICHIASIS

Trichiasis is an acquired misdirection of eyelashes. Trichiasis may be focal as is seen after eyelid trauma in the area of the laceration. The process may be diffuse with eyelid scarring and lashes along the entire lid.

Epidemiology and Etiology

Age Any age. Nontraumatic causes are rare in childhood. More common with increasing age.

Gender More common in females.

Etiology Lash follicles are distorted and become misdirected with scarring of the eyelid. Chronic eyelid inflammation may result in growth of misdirected lashes. Chronic blepharitis, eyelid trauma, and conjunctival scarring diseases can all cause trichiasis.

History

Patients will often have a history of chronic eye irritation and inflammation. They may also have a long history of eyelash problems. There may be a history of eyelid trauma or surgery.

Examination

Eyelashes are seen rubbing on the eyelid surface (Fig. 5-9). The amount of corneal changes depends on the number of lashes and duration. There may be just SPK or there may be corneal scarring.

Special Considerations

Important to differentiate trichiasis from abnormal eyelid positions, such as entropions, which secondarily result in eyelashes rubbing on the cornea.

Differential Diagnosis

- Spastic entropion
- Involutional entropion
- Cicatricial entropion
- Congenital distichiasis

Laboratory Tests

Conjunctival scarring of unknown etiology requires a conjunctival biopsy with immunofluorescence testing to rule out ocular cicatricial pemphigoid.

Treatment

Lashes can be epilated for temporary relief but they always grow back. Electrolysis or cryotherapy will ablate lashes on a more "permanent" basis. At best 50 percent of the lashes will not regrow so multiple treatments are required. In cases of severe scarring, eyelid surgery will be needed to correct the problem. This may include marginal rotation, excision of the abnormal lashes, and a buccal mucosal graft.

Prognosis

Dependent on the cause of the trichiasis. Chronic progressive inflammatory diseases, such as ocular cicatricial pemphigoid, will often have recurrent lashes that can be very difficult to completely eradicate. Trichiasis related to trauma or other nonprogressive scarring usually responds well to treatment.

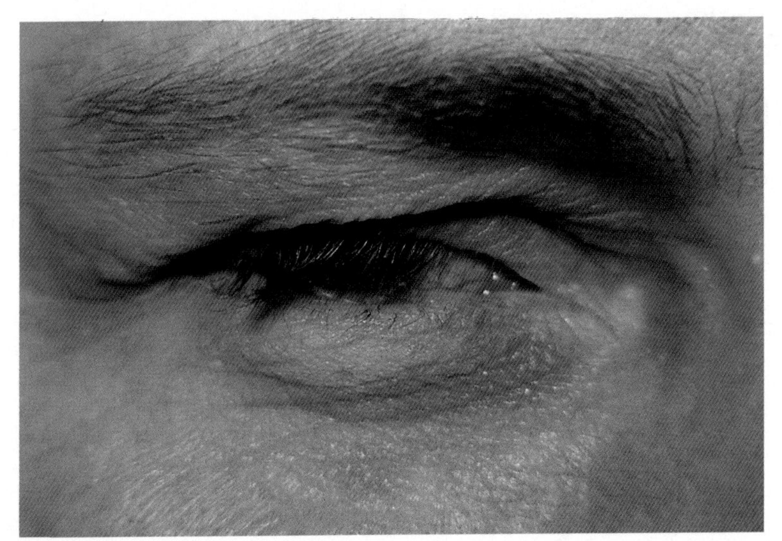

Figure 5-9 Trichiasis *Eyelashes are growing posteriorly, contacting the cornea from the upper eyelid. In true trichiasis, the eyelid margin is normal. Often, with conjunctival scarring disease, there will be some accompanied inturning of the eyelid margin.*

PTOSIS

CONGENITAL MYOGENIC PTOSIS

Congenital myogenic ptosis is the most common congenital ptosis and results from a dysgenesis of the levator muscle. It may be unilateral or bilateral and can vary in severity from very mild ptosis to very severe.

Epidemiology and Etiology

Age Birth.

Gender Equally affects males and females.

Etiology The levator muscle development is abnormal resulting in fibrosis and fatty infiltration of the levator muscle.

History

Ptosis noted at birth or soon after. Child may have chin up head position, especially if bilateral. Parents may note the child's eyes are open while asleep.

Examination

Ptosis is noted to be either unilateral or bilateral. There is little or no levator function resulting in a fibrotic, stiff eyelid with a fairly fixed position as the eye moves from up to down gaze. The lid crease is often poorly formed. Depending on the severity of the ptosis, there may be amblyopia with unilateral ptosis (Fig. 5-10).

Special Considerations

There will be abnormal superior rectus function in 16 percent of patients; this makes exposure problems after repair and strabismus a concern.

Differential Diagnosis

- If the ptosis is congenital with poor levator function there is little else in the differential. Birth trauma can result in a ptosis but there is usually good levator function and the levator muscle is not fibrotic. Marcus Gunn jaw wink needs to be considered in all cases of congenital ptosis (see section, Marcus Gunn Jaw Wink).
- There are other forms of myogenic ptosis that are acquired, not congenital, such as in muscular dystrophy, chronic progressive external ophthalmoplegia (CPEO), myasthenia gravis, or oculopharyngeal dystrophy.

Laboratory Tests

Skeletal muscle biopsy and electrophysiologic testing may be needed. An ECG should be done if CPEO is suspected.

Treatment

Frontalis suspension surgery using suture or fascia lata. The age to do surgery depends on the severity of the ptosis and any underlying amblyopia. Amblyopia may need treatment with patching once the eyelid is lifted. There is controversy in treating unilateral congenital ptosis regarding whether to do a frontalis suspension only on the ptotic eye or if the normal eye should have excision of the levator and a frontalis suspension as well to provide symmetry.

Prognosis

Surgery is very successful in lifting the lid above the pupillary axis. The eyelid will sometimes fall with time and repeat surgery may be needed later.

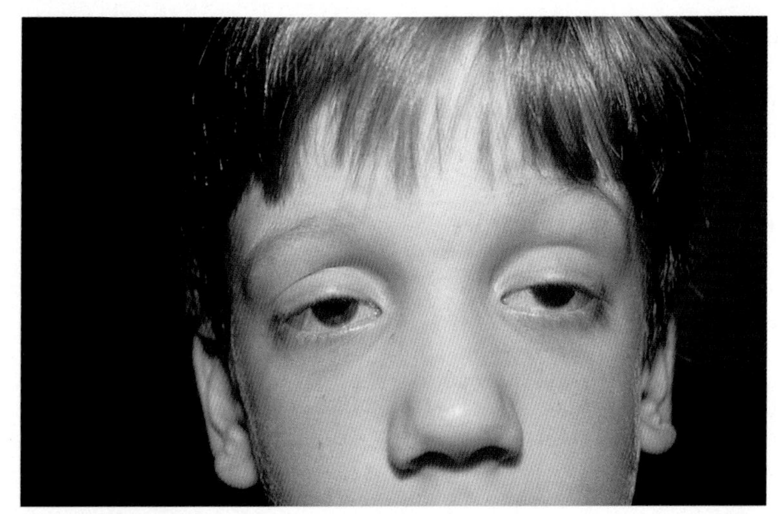

Figure 5-10 Congenital myogenic ptosis *Moderate congenital ptosis in a child. Note the extreme use of the eyebrows to lift the eyelids. There is a prominent eyelid crease in this child but it is usually poorly defined in congenital ptosis. Levator function was 3 mm.*

ACQUIRED MYOGENIC PTOSIS

Acquired myogenic ptosis is an unusual cause of ptosis related to development of a muscular disease that can be localized or may be systemic.

Epidemiology and Etiology

Age Acquired but can present in children or adults.

Etiology Systemic muscular diseases that can cause acquired myogenic ptosis include muscular dystrophy, chronic progressive external ophthalmoplegia (CPEO), myasthenia gravis, and oculopharyngeal dystrophy.

History

Progressive ptosis that is often associated with other muscular dysfunction.

Examination

Ptosis is noted with decreased levator function. There may be abnormal eye movements and abnormal facial tone. Myasthenia gravis may have double vision as part of the presentation. Chronic progressive external ophthalmoplegia has decreased eye movements but there is no diplopia. Careful evaluation of the ability to close the eyes is needed as poor closure will increase the risk of postoperative corneal exposure (Fig. 5-11A and B).

Special Considerations

Chronic progressive external ophthalmoplegia is a gradual, bilateral ptosis that begins in childhood or young adulthood and is progressive with involvement of extraocular muscles. It is hereditary in 50 percent of the cases. It is progressive until the eyes are fixed in a slightly downward direction with a severe ptosis. Heart block, retinitis pigmentosa, abnormal retinal pigmentation, and various neurologic signs have been associated with this syndrome.

Differential Diagnosis

- Congenital ptosis
- Neurogenic ptosis

Laboratory Tests

Skeletal muscle biopsy and electrophysiologic testing may be needed. An ECG should be done if CPEO is suspected.

Treatment

Surgery is needed for correction. Evaluation and treatment of any systemic abnormalities must be addressed first. Depending on the severity of the ptosis and the amount of levator function, either levator resection or frontalis suspension is indicated. Frontalis suspension with a silicone rod will work well in many of these patients.

Prognosis

Most patients can achieve an eyelid level that is functional. Most will not be able to achieve an eyelid level or function that is considered normal.

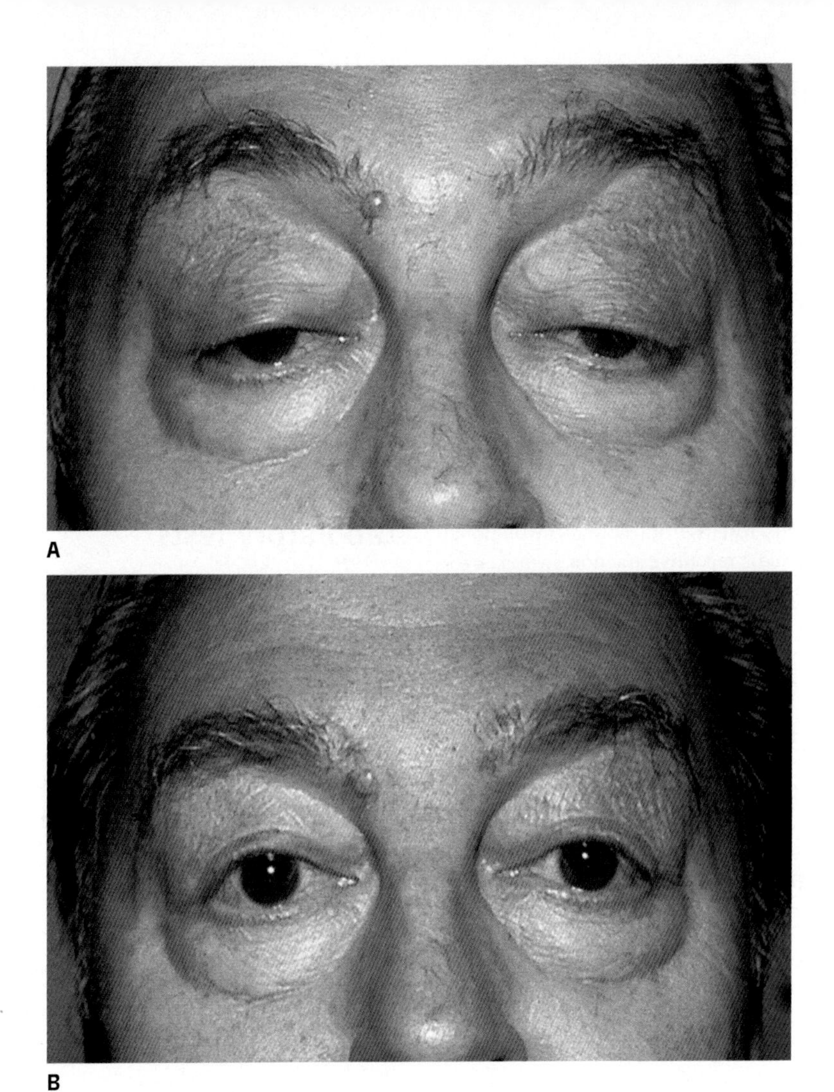

Figure 5-11 Acquired myogenic ptosis **A.** *Patient with muscular dystrophy and severe ptosis. There is very little levator function and the patient is barely able to keep his eyelids above the pupil with extreme eyebrow elevation.* **B.** *The same patient after frontalis suspension surgery. He can now effectively lift his eyelids by elevating his eyebrows.*

APONEUROTIC PTOSIS

Aponeurotic ptosis is the most common type of ptosis and is the result of disinsertion of the levator aponeurosis. This type of ptosis may be caused by normal aging changes, swelling, or repetitive stretching. The onset of ptosis is gradual.

Epidemiology and Etiology

Age Rarely congenital. Most common in older patients.

Gender Equal.

Etiology Aponeurotic ptosis is due to an abnormality of the levator aponeurosis or its insertion. This results from normal involutional changes and/or repetitive traction such as eyelid rubbing, eyelid swelling, and eye surgery.

History

Gradual, progressive droopiness of the eyelids is the most common history. Recent eye surgery or eyelid swelling can exacerbate the ptosis.

Examination

Mild to severe ptosis with normal levator function and often a high eyelid crease or less commonly a poor eyelid crease. The ptosis may be worse in downgaze (Fig. 5-12).

Special Considerations

Myasthenia gravis must be considered in all cases.

Differential Diagnosis

- Congenital ptosis (differentiate by poor levator function)
- Myasthenia gravis
- Traumatic ptosis

Laboratory Tests

None.

Treatment

External levator resection and müllerectomy are both good surgical approaches for successful repair. Dry eyes, poor eye closure, and poor Bell's phenomenon must all be recognized preoperatively. These conditions make postoperative corneal exposure more likely.

Prognosis

Excellent prognosis for successful surgical correction.

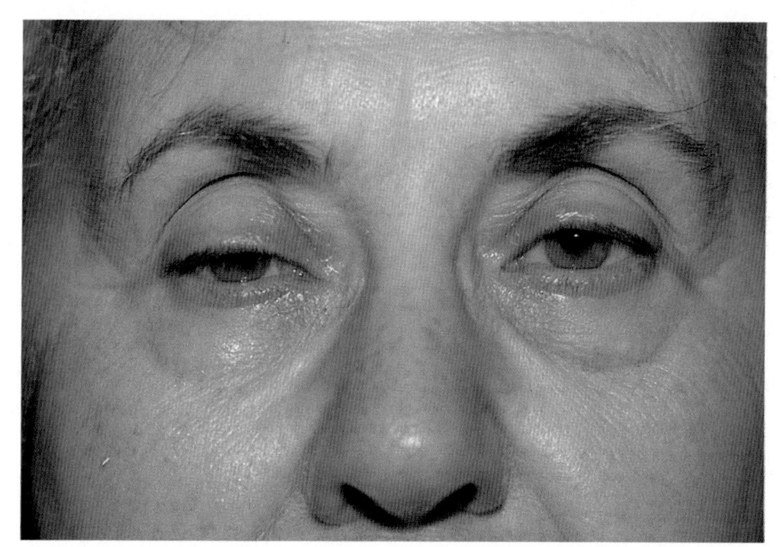

Figure 5-12 Aponeurotic ptosis *Bilateral ptosis from dehiscence of the levator aponeurosis. Note the high, very defined upper eyelid crease. Levator function was 18 mm.*

NEUROGENIC PTOSIS

THIRD NERVE PALSY

Third cranial nerve palsy is usually manifest as sudden or progressive onset of ptosis with an underlying strabismus. Determining the etiology is the first priority as some causes of a third cranial nerve palsy are life-threatening. Treatment is difficult.

Epidemiology and Etiology

Age Any age. Rare in children.

Gender No female and male difference noted.

Etiology

- Ischemic microvascular disease
- Compressive: aneurysm, tumor
- Trauma
- Ophthalmoplegic migraine: children

History

Acute onset of ptosis with double vision when the eyelid is lifted. May or may not be associated with pain.

Examination

Complete ptosis with the eye positioned down and out (Fig. 5-13A and B). There is an inability to elevate, depress, or adduct the eye. The pupil may or may not be dilated. Abberant regeneration of the third nerve should be ruled out.

Special Considerations

If the pupil is dilated the patient needs emergent neuroimaging to rule out a posterior communicating artery aneurysm. Nonresolving third nerve palsies, incomplete third nerve palsies, and any third nerve palsy with aberrant regeneration requires neuroimaging. Patients under 50 years of age need neuroimaging unless they have significant vascular disease. Vasculopathic causes of third nerve palsies should resolve within 3 months.

Differential Diagnosis

- Myasthenia gravis
- Chronic progressive external ophthalmoplegia

Laboratory Tests

MRI with MRA, or an angiogram if the third nerve palsy involves the pupil.

Pathophysiology

Interruption of the third nerve may be caused by compression of the nerve or ischemia. Ischemia will not cause pupillary dilation and will resolve within 3 months.

Treatment

The majority of pupil-sparing third nerve palsies will resolve in 3 months. These patients should be given adequate time for spontaneous resolution before surgical correction is performed. The underlying strabismus must be treated before attempting to lift the eyelid. Ptosis surgery requires frontalis suspension but there is risk of corneal exposure. Frontalis suspension with a silicone rod is a safe surgical approach.

Prognosis

Many third nerve palsies will resolve in 3 to 6 months. Those that do not resolve are difficult to get into normal eyelid position without causing an unacceptable amount of corneal exposure. Patients will often have residual diplopia from the motility problems when the eyelid is raised.

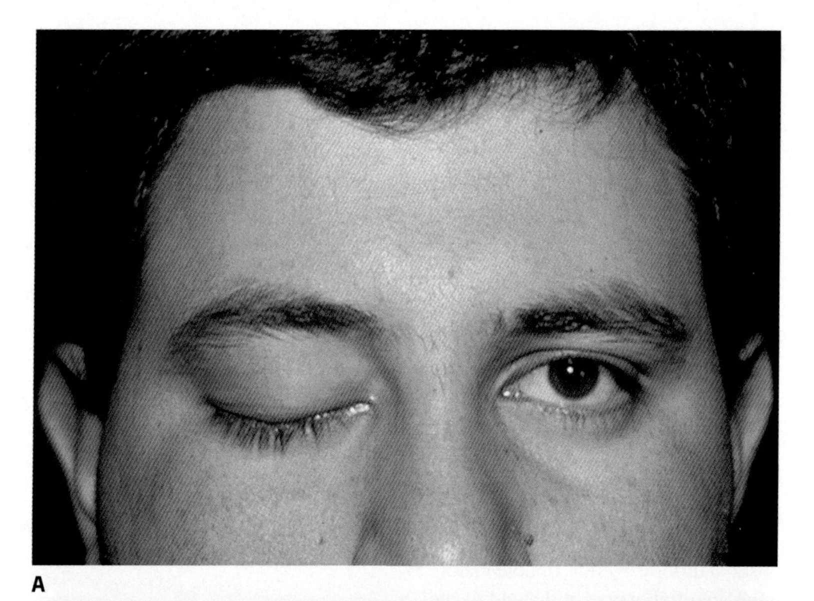

A

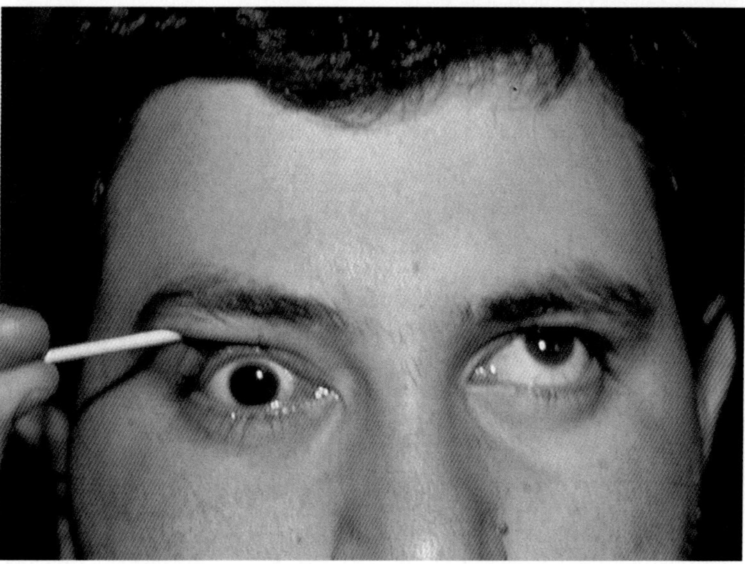

B

Figure 5-13 Third nerve palsy **A.** *Complete ptosis of the upper eyelid with no levator function.* **B.** *Elevation of the ptotic eyelid reveals ocular misalignment consistent with a third nerve palsy.*

MYASTHENIA GRAVIS

Myasthenia gravis is an autoimmune disorder in which autoantibodies attack the receptors of the neuromuscular junction. The result is usually a systemic muscular weakness that can be life-threatening due to respiratory compromise. Ptosis with or without diplopia can often be the initial presentation. Treatment of the systemic disease is maximized before any surgery is done on the eyelids.

Epidemiology and Etiology

Age Any age.

Gender More common in females.

Etiology Autoimmune disease; may be associated with thymoma or antecedent infection.

History

Insidious onset of droopy eyelids, double vision, or both, which are often worse at the end of the day. Patients may have facial weakness, proximal limb weakness, or difficulty swallowing and breathing. Symptoms are typically intermittent.

Examination

The disease is most often generalized and systemic but may present initially with ptosis and/or double vision. Ptosis is worsened with sustained upgaze and diplopia is worse with continual eye movements (fatigue). Weakness of the orbicularis muscles is usually found. There may also be facial and proximal limb weakness. Diagnosis may be made with the ice test or Tensilon testing. The ice test involves placing an ice pack on the eyelids for 2 min, if the ptosis is secondary to myasthenia gravis, it will improve. Tensilon testing involves IV administration of edrophonium chloride (Tensilon). Improvement of the ptosis or diplopia indicates the etiology is myasthenia gravis. The usefulness of Tensilon testing is limited because of the potential adverse effects including bradycardia and even respiratory arrest (Fig. 5-14).

Special Considerations

Patients with newly diagnosed myasthenia gravis need a CT or MRI of the chest to rule out thymoma. Patients with any signs or symptoms of respiratory compromise need immediate neurologic evaluation for possible hospital admission and treatment.

Differential Diagnosis

- Eaton–Lambert syndrome
- Chronic progressive external ophthalmoplegia
- Third nerve palsy

Laboratory Tests

Acetylcholine receptor antibody assay and single fiber EMG.

Pathophysiology

An autoimmune disorder in which autoantibodies attack the receptors of the neuromuscular junction.

Treatment

Treatment of the disease is systemic and may include pyridostigmine bromide (Mestinon), prednisone, and possible thymectomy. Treatment should be coordinated by a neuro-ophthalmologist or neurologist. Once maximum medical improvement has been achieved, surgical correction of the ptosis can be attempted. Frontalis suspension is usually required.

Prognosis

Variable depending on the severity of the disease.

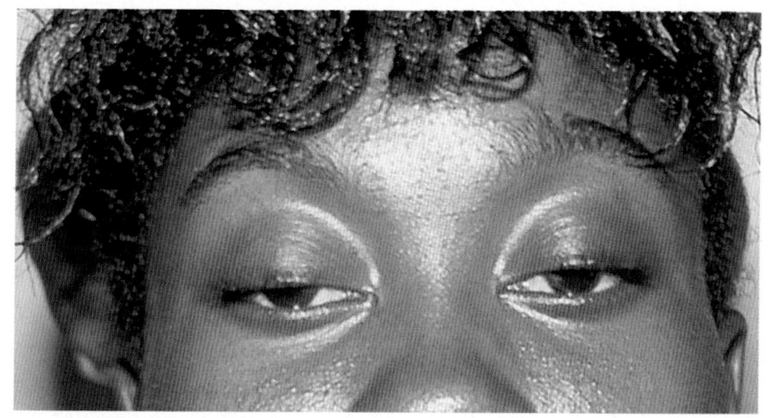

Figure 5-14 Myasthenia gravis *Bilateral ptosis with inability to keep the lids from covering the pupils. There is also decreased tone of the facial muscles.*

MARCUS GUNN JAW WINKING SYNDROME

This syndrome may be very mild or very dramatic with elevation of the eyelid with each jaw movement when chewing food. Treatment is required if the ptosis or the eyelid movement is significant.

Epidemiology and Etiology

Age Present at birth.

Etiology A congenital synkinetic syndrome caused by a congenital aberrant connection of the oculomotor nerve fibers that innervate the levator muscle and the trigeminal nerve fibers to the muscles of mastication.

History

A caretaker often first notices this condition when feeding the baby. The affected eyelid will move up and down with the jaw movement during feeding.

Examination

A unilateral ptosis with poor levator function. The unilaterally ptotic eyelid elevates with movement of the jaw. Movement of the mandible laterally, to the contralateral side most commonly, results in elevation of the eyelid (Fig. 5-15 A and B).

Special Considerations

The amount of ptosis and the amount of synkinetic movement will determine the treatment.

Differential Diagnosis

- Congenital ptosis

Laboratory Tests

None.

Treatment

If the amount of synkinetic movement is small then a frontalis suspension is done. If the synkinetic movement is large then the levator muscle must be disinserted and excised before the frontalis suspension can be done.

Prognosis

It may be difficult to get good symmetry in the eyelids unless both eyes are operated on.

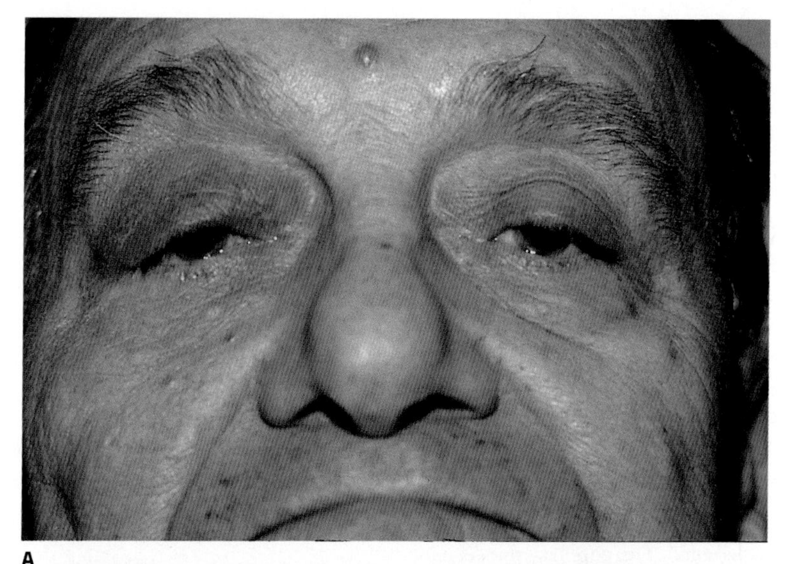
A

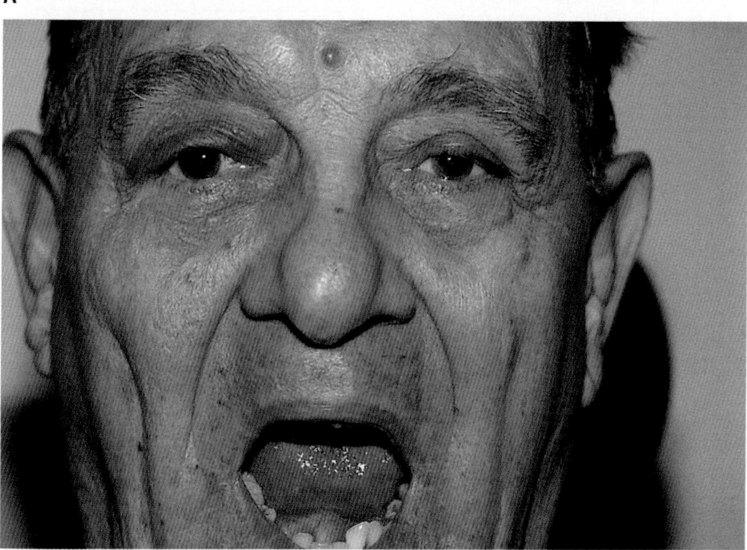
B

Figure 5-15 Marcus Gunn jaw winking syndrome **A.** *Patient with severe ptosis with full eyebrow elevation and chin up position to keep his eyelids above the pupil.* **B.** *With opening of his mouth, the eyelids go up and he is able to normalize his head position.*

HORNER'S SYNDROME

Horner's syndrome classically presents with mild ptosis (2 mm) and pupillary miosis. Once any serious etiology has been ruled out, these cases respond very well to surgical correction with a müllerectomy.

Epidemiology and Etiology

Age May be congenital or acquired.

Etiology Etiology of acquired cases includes trauma, surgical procedures in the neck area, apical lung malignancies, aneurysm, dissection of the carotid artery, and idiopathic.

History

Mild ptosis is noted. The pupillary miosis may or may not be noted until the examination.

Examination

Ptosis, pupillary miosis, and anhidrosis are the three findings. The ptosis is usually mild (1 to 2 mm). In congenital Horner's syndrome, there is also decreased pigmentation of the iris on the involved side (Fig. 5-16A and B).

Special Considerations

Cocaine testing is used to confirm the diagnosis. A 4 to 10 percent cocaine solution will dilate a normal pupil but will fail to dilate a pupil affected by Horner's syndrome. Other pharmacologic testing will differentiate first- and second-order neuron interruption from third-order neuron. Hydroxyamphetamine drops will not dilate the pupil of a third-order neuron Horner's syndrome. A third-order neuron Horner's syndrome is generally of benign etiology.

Differential Diagnosis

- Aponeurotic ptosis with pupillary anisocoria.

Laboratory Tests

Chest CT and MRI with gadolinium of the neck and brain in all patients with first- or second-order neuron involvement. Many neurologists will image all patients with Horner's syndrome.

Pathophysiology

Interruption of the sympathetic innervation of Müller's muscle results in the ptosis while the dilator muscle of the iris results in the miosis.

Treatment

Once determined to be of benign etiology, a müllerectomy is the procedure of choice.

Prognosis

The ptosis responds well to surgical correction.

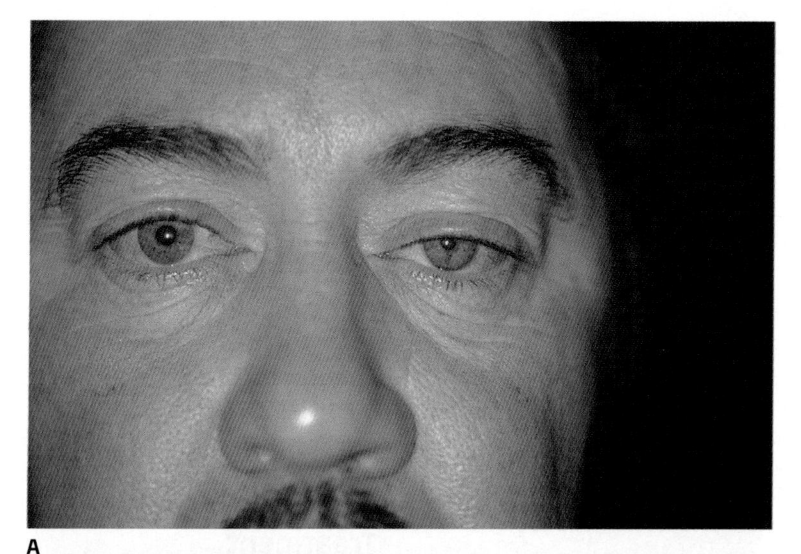

A

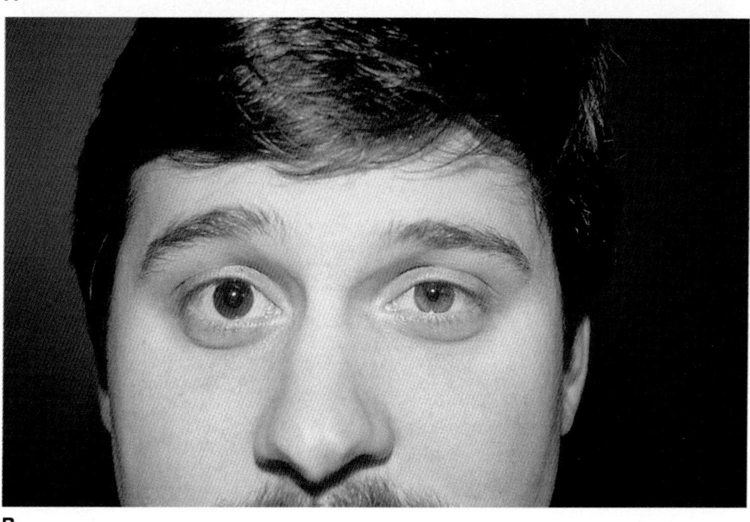

B

Figure 5-16 Horner's syndrome **A.** *Ptosis with miosis on the left side. The amount of ptosis is more than is often seen in Horner's syndrome and there may be some aponeurotic dehiscence as well.* **B.** *Congenital Horner's syndrome with ptosis, miosis, and iris hypopigmentation.*

MECHANICAL PTOSIS

Mechanical ptosis is drooping of the eyelid related to restriction of the eyelid from either scar tissue or the weight of a mass or swelling.

Epidemiology and Etiology

Age Any age.

Gender Equal.

Etiology The increased weight of any mass will weigh the eyelid down. This can include chalazion, skin carcinoma, giant papillary conjunctivitis, hemangiomas, neurofibromas, and so forth. Restriction of eyelid movement by scar tissue will also produce this form of ptosis.

History

Rapidity of onset varies according to the process. Chalazion will have rapid onset, whereas a large basal cell carcinoma may slowly worsen over years.

Examination

Ptosis with an eyelid mass or evidence of scar tissue (Fig. 5-17). The cause can be external or under the eyelid and difficult to see such as in severe giant papillary conjunctivitis. Eyelid scarring internally requires palpation and stretching and erosion of the eyelid to identify it.

Special Considerations

Imaging, such as CT, may be needed to determine the extent of the mass or to rule out a foreign body or a fracture after trauma.

Differential Diagnosis

- Traumatic ptosis
- Aponeurotic ptosis

Laboratory Tests

None.

Treatment

Addressing the cause is the primary treatment. Management can include medical treatment or surgical excision of a lesion or scar tissue. Some patients may require a second surgery to correct the ptosis if removing the mechanical cause is not curative.

Prognosis

Related to prognosis of the mass or swelling that is causing the ptosis. If it is due to a recurrent process the prognosis is poor.

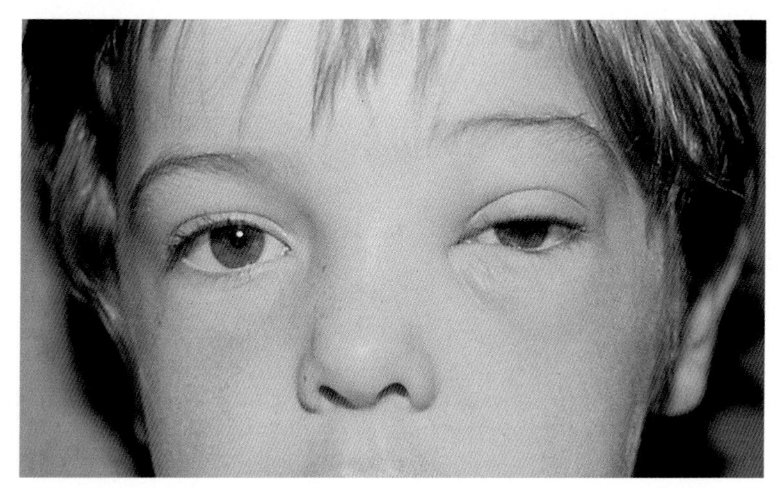

Figure 5-17 Mechanical ptosis *Neurofibroma of the left upper lid weighing down the eyelid and causing a ptosis.*

TRAUMATIC PTOSIS

Traumatic ptosis has multiple causes; however, exactly which causes are present in each case is difficult to determine. Allowing 6 months for spontaneous resolution before correction is the rule in all traumatic cases.

Epidemiology and Etiology

Age All ages.

Gender Males more common.

Etiology May include multiple causes including myogenic, neurogenic, and aponeurotic injuries.

History

Trauma to the eyelid with residual ptosis after the swelling resolves.

Examination

Documentation of the severity of ptosis will allow monitoring for improvement. Assessment of levator function also helps determine etiology. Any residual swelling, scarring, and lagophthalmos should also be documented (Fig. 5-18).

Special Considerations

Must wait 6 months for possible resolution of the ptosis before repairing. A number of cases will improve or resolve during this time. Any injury that suggests direct cutting of the levator should have exploration of the levator at the time of trauma repair if possible.

Treatment

Monitor for improvement over the 6 months following the trauma. If the lid is still ptotic after 6 months, surgical correction with external levator resection or frontalis suspension depending on levator function is indicated.

Prognosis

Good if there is good levator function. If there is poor levator function with scarring the prognosis is not as good.

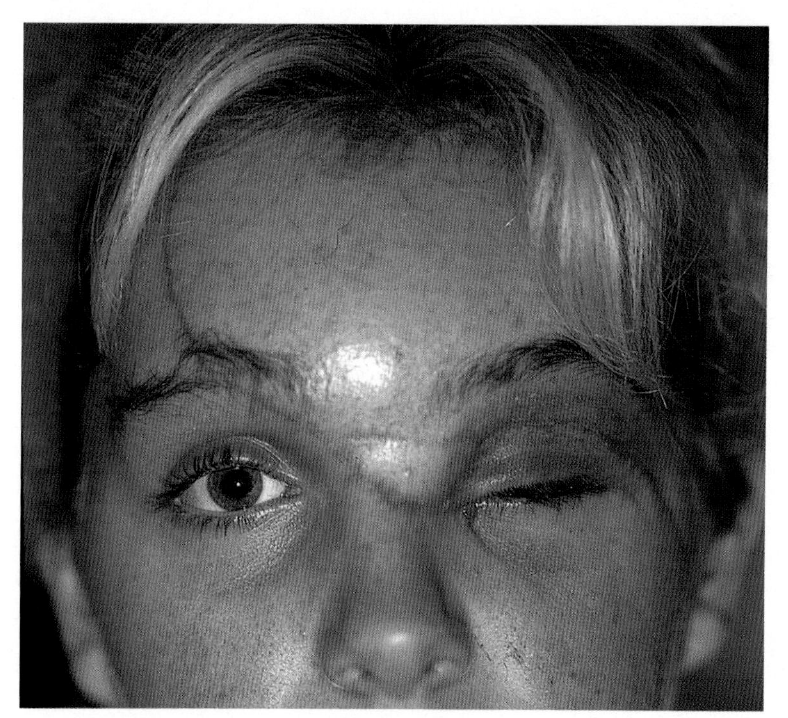

Figure 5-18 Traumatic ptosis *Eyelid and eyebrow lacerations resulting in a traumatic ptosis. This ptosis did not improve over 6 months and required surgical repair.*

PSEUDOPTOSIS

Pseudoptosis is the false illusion of ptosis caused by malposition of the eye, contralateral eyelid, or lack of orbital volume. It is very important to recognize a pseudoptosis to avoid doing unnecessary or the wrong surgery.

Epidemiology and Etiology

Age Any age.

Gender Equal.

Etiology The eyelid position is normal but other factors result in the appearance of ptosis. The most common is an abnormal position of the eye. Elevation of the eye or the eye sinking in will both give a false ptosis. Dermatochalasis (see section, "Dermatochalasis") is also a common cause of pseudoptosis.

History

Patient presents with the complaint of a droopy eyelid for a variable period of time.

Examination

In all patients with ptosis, evaluation must include noting the position of the eye. Enophthalmos, hypertropia, and a globe pushed superiorly all cause pseudoptosis. Evaluation of the eyelid skin relative to the true eyelid margin position is important (Fig. 5-19A). Eyelid retraction on the contralateral side must also be considered.

Special Considerations

CT scanning may be needed if a mass pushing the globe up is suspected.

Differential Diagnosis

- Enophthalmos (Fig. 5-19B)
- Hypertropia
- Globe malposition
- Lid retraction of the contralateral eyelid
- Dermatochalasis

Treatment

Depends on the cause of the pseudoptosis.

- Enophthalmos, microphthalmos, phthisis bulbi: build up the orbit
- Hypertropia: consider strabismus surgery
- Globe elevation: remove mass
- Contralateral eyelid retraction: correct eyelid retraction
- Dermatochalasis: blepharoplasty

Prognosis

Good.

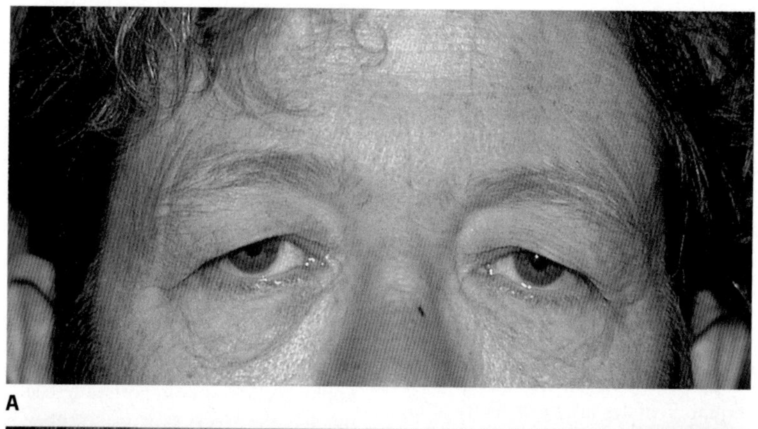

A

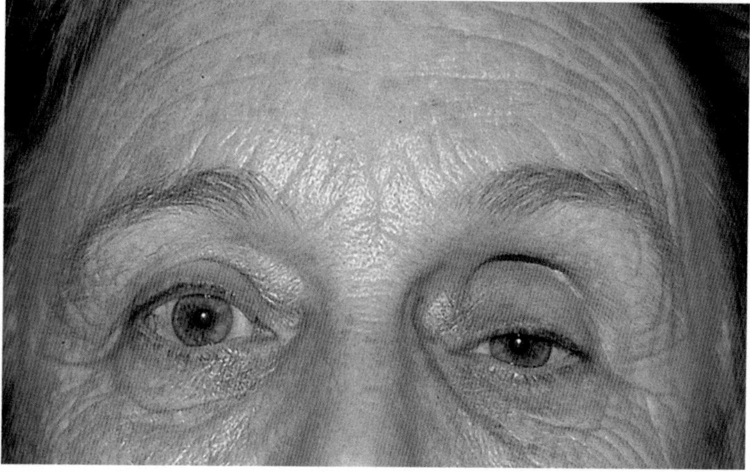

B

Figure 5-19 Pseudoptosis **A.** *Dermatochalasis is the most common cause of pseudoptosis. If the eyelid skin is elevated the eyelid is in a normal position under the skin.* **B.** *Another form of pseudoptosis is enophthalmos resulting in drooping of the eyelid. This patient may also have some component of levator aponeurosis disinsertion.*

BROW PTOSIS

Brow ptosis is drooping of the eyebrows. It is often a part of dermatochalasis but must be recognized and treated separately for the best results. Many patients will have some degree of brow ptosis and not have symptoms. Symptoms can include loss of superior visual field, brow ache and fatigue, and rhytids of the forehead and brow. Those with significant brow ptosis may require eyebrow surgery with or without eyelid surgery.

Epidemiology and Etiology

Age More common as patients age.

Gender Equal. Females are more likely to be symptomatic.

Epidemiology With aging, gravity, involutional changes, and loss of elasticity result in drooping of the eyebrows. Depending on multiple factors, this drooping will become symptomatic in those 50 years of age or older.

History

Patients will attempt to lift their eyebrows resulting in deep furrows of the forehead, brow ache, and even headaches.

Examination

Eyebrows sit below the superior orbital rim. This may give the appearance of excess upper eyelid skin. Patients will also develop furrows of the forehead from chronically elevating their eyebrows (Fig. 5-20).

Special Considerations

Brow droop will add to redundant skin of the upper eyelids. It is important to recognize how much of the excess skin on the upper eyelids will go away if the eyebrows are elevated. This excess from the brow droop should not be excised during blepharoplasty or the eyebrows will appear too close to the eyelids. Ideally, the brow should be lifted and then the blepharoplasty performed.

Treatment

Brow lift using one of the following techniques; each has its own indications and advantages.

- Endoscopic eyebrow lift
- Coronal eyebrow lift
- Midforehead eyebrow lift
- Direct eyebrow lift

Prognosis

Good.

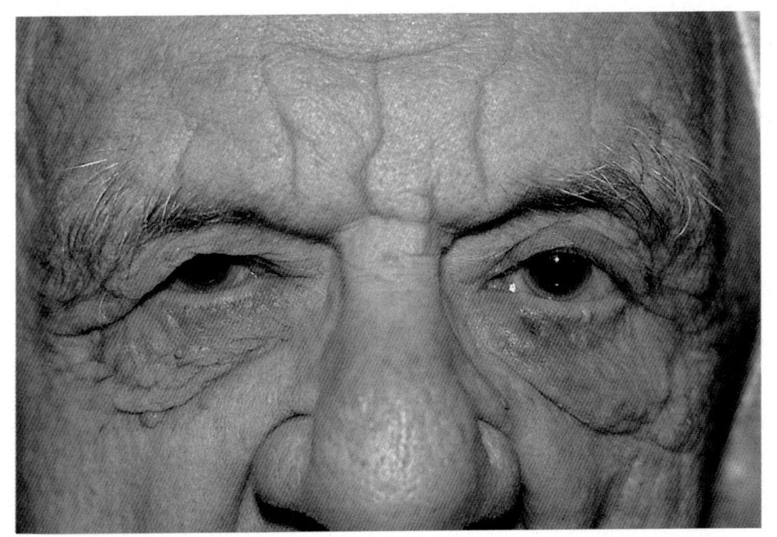

Figure 5-20 Brow ptosis *The eyebrows are well below the orbital rim in this patient, adding to the apparent amount of dermatochalasis.*

DERMATOCHALASIS

Dermatochalasis is a very common condition as people age. Loss of elasticity from ultraviolet exposure and aging results in excess skin of the upper and lower lids. If severe enough, the upper eyelid skin may cause functional blockage of the superior visual field. More commonly, the excess skin and the associated anterior prolapse of orbital fat is a cosmetic deformity.

Epidemiology and Etiology

Age Older patients.

Gender Equal male to female ratio.

Etiology Etiology is loss of eyelid skin elasticity from aging and ultraviolet light exposure. There may be a hereditary component to dermatochalasis, especially when it occurs at a younger age.

History

Symptoms are brow ache, heaviness around the eyes, and loss of superior visual field. These have a slow, insidious onset.

Examination

Excess skin of the upper eyelids to varying degrees. It becomes especially bothersome once the skin contacts the eyelashes. Dermatochalasis is often associated with anterior prolapse of orbital fat. Underlying the excess skin, the possibility of a true ptosis must be evaluated (Fig. 5-21).

Treatment

Blepharoplasty, which may be functional or cosmetic in nature.

Prognosis

Good.

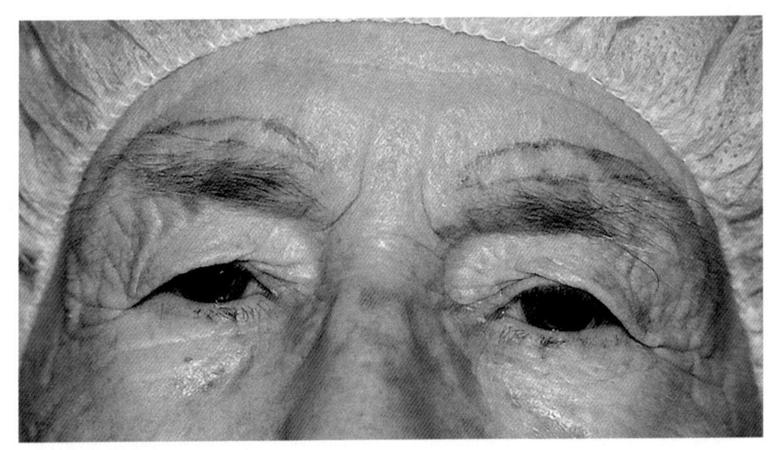

Figure 5-21 Dermatochalasis *There is a large amount of overhanging skin of both upper eyelids. The underlying eyelid position is normal. There is also some brow droop, which was addressed surgically at the same time as the blepharoplasty.*

BLEPHAROCHALASIS

Blepharochalasis is a rare, familial variant of angioneurotic edema that occurs in younger individuals. It is characterized by recurrent episodes of inflammatory edema of the eyelids that results in stretching of the tissues and, over time, the eyelids take on the appearance of dermatochalasis commonly seen in much older patients.

Epidemiology and Etiology

Age Onset in teens to 20s.

Gender More common in females.

Etiology Unknown. A variant of angioneurotic edema.

History

Recurrent episodes of eyelid swelling, usually unilateral.

Examination

Excess skin of the eyelids that is very thin and like paper (Fig. 5-22). There may also be true ptosis, lacrimal gland prolapse, and prominent vessels of the lids. Most commonly, these finding are unilateral. Patients may also be seen at the time of swelling with swollen, fluid-filled lids with very little inflammatory signs.

Differential Diagnosis

- Dermatochalasis
- Thyroid-related ophthalmopathy
- Orbital inflammatory disease

Pathophysiology

Unknown.

Treatment

Treatment is surgical excision of the skin and correction of ptosis. Surgical repair can be complicated by recurrent edema, which may result in recurrence of the problem.

Prognosis

Variable, depending on whether the edema continues to recur or burns out.

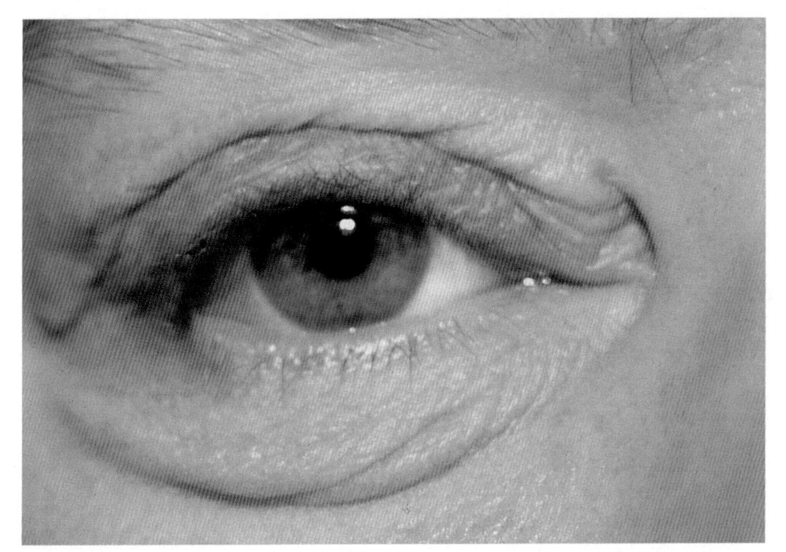

Figure 5-22 Blepharochalasis *This is a 25-year-old patient with recurrent swelling of the right eyelids resulting in the thin, stretched, redundant skin of the upper and lower eyelid.*

EYELID RETRACTION

Eyelid retraction is displacement of the eyelid toward the respective superior or inferior orbital rim resulting in scleral show. This condition can be mild and without symptoms or can result in corneal exposure. Thyroid ophthalmopathy is the most common cause and eyelid retraction is often the initial sign of this disease.

Epidemiology and Etiology

Age Adulthood. Rare in children. Age of onset dependent on etiology.

Gender Females more common.

Etiology Eyelid retraction is caused by thyroid ophthalmopathy most commonly, followed by over-aggressive eyelid surgery and vertical rectus muscle surgery (Fig. 5-23A and B). Upper eyelid retraction may be the result of contralateral ptosis. Lower lid retraction can be a normal anatomic variant. Parinaud syndrome is a central nervous system cause of upper eyelid retraction.

History

In thyroid ophthalmopathy, the patient notes slow onset of one or both eyes appearing too wide open or "starey eyed." Often, redness and irritation of the affected eye accompany these symptoms. Patients may have a history of systemic thyroid abnormalities. Those patients with a surgical cause will give the history of eyelid or eye muscle surgery.

Examination

Document the amount of eyelid retraction and whether there is retraction or ptosis on the other side. Upper eyelid lag on down gaze, proptosis, and dysmotility all go along with thyroid ophthalmopathy. Note signs of corneal exposure and previous eye or eyelid surgery.

Differential Diagnosis

- Malposition of the globe
- Hypotropia or hypertropia
- Contralateral ptosis

Laboratory Tests

Thyroid function tests unless patient has known, controlled thyroid abnormalities or there is a known surgical cause of the eyelid retraction.

Pathophysiology

Thyroid ophthalmopathy results in chronic inflammation of the lid retractors leading to scar tissue formation and retraction of the eyelids.

Treatment

In thyroid ophthalmopathy, the disease must be treated so it is inactive before any surgical correction. Treat corneal exposure with lubrication while waiting for the disease to become inactive. Most causes of eyelid retraction will require surgical treatment if they are significant. Recession of the retractors is the most common procedure used. This works for mild to moderate retraction. More severe retraction requires eyelid spacer material to be implanted. Excess excision of skin of the upper lids during blepharoplasty may require internal spacers or rarely skin grafts.

Prognosis

Generally, retraction can be treated successfully with surgery. Corneal exposure is often an ongoing problem that is improved with treatment but not completely cured.

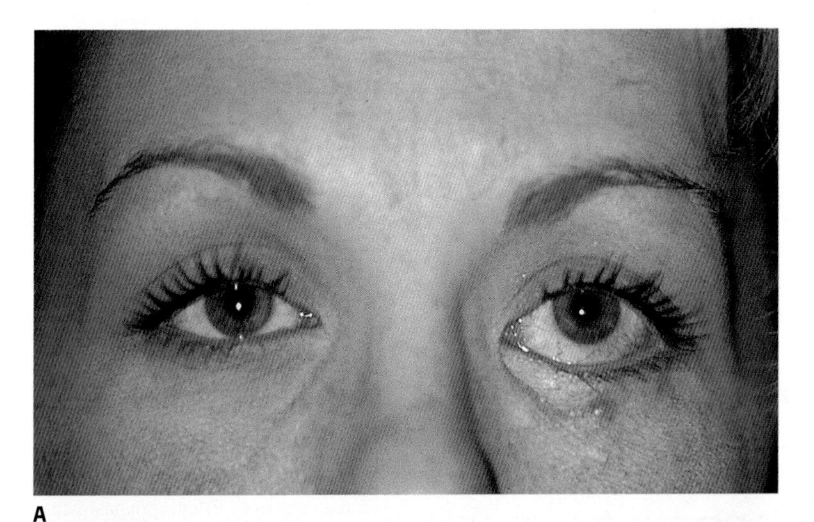

A

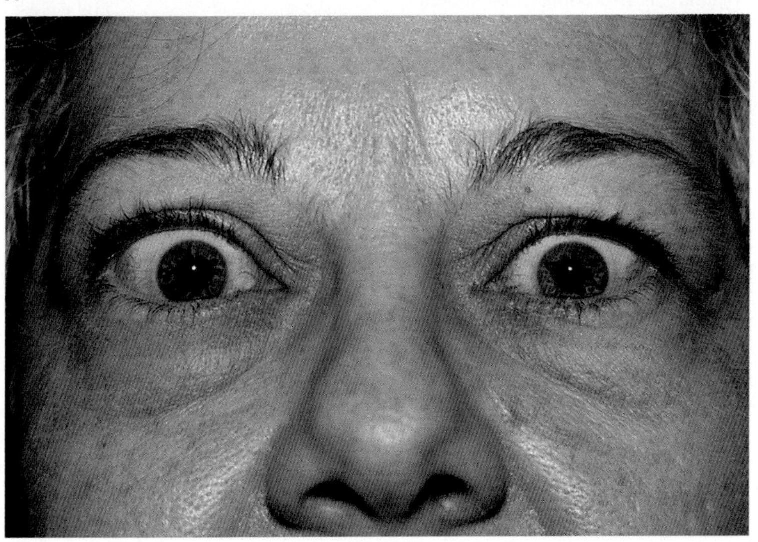

B

Figure 5-23 Eyelid retraction **A.** *Left, lower eyelid retraction from scarring of the eyelid to the orbital rim and a titanium plate after trauma.* **B.** *Thyroid-related ophthalmopathy with upper eyelid retraction.*

EYELID DYSKINESIS

BENIGN ESSENTIAL BLEPHAROSPASM

Benign essential blepharospasm is a bilateral condition characterized by involuntary spasms of the orbicularis oculi, procerus, and corrugator muscles. This condition may start as mild twitching of the eyelids and can progress so that these contractions leave the patients functionally blind during the contraction. Patients cannot predict when the spasms will occur and the forced closure of the eyelids can be life-threatening if they occur during driving, crossing streets, and so forth.

Epidemiology and Etiology

Age Onset is when patients are 40 years of age or older.

Gender Women more commonly affected than men.

Etiology Unknown, but probably of central nervous system origin, most likely in the basal ganglia. The process causes involuntary spasms of the orbicularis oculi, procerus, and corrugator muscles.

History

The spasms start as mild twitches and progressively worsen with time. Patients often do not present until the spasms are severe enough to interfere with activities of daily living.

Examination

Patient have intermittent episodes of forced eyelid closure that usually last for minutes (Fig. 5-24). Between spasms, the examination may be normal. Thus, the diagnosis is often based on history. The spasms are bilateral, although they can sometimes be more severe on one side than the other. Spasms can involve the lower face and neck with time. Spasms do not occur during sleep, unlike in hemifacial spasm.

Special Considerations

Must treat any condition that may cause ocular irritation and thus worsen the blepharospasm such as dry eyes. Blepharospasm can have fatal consequences if not controlled and the patient drives.

Differential Diagnosis

- Hemifacial spasm
- Severe dry eyes or other ocular irritation

Treatment

Botulinum toxin injection. These injections are effective for most patients and last 3 to 4 months before reinjection is required. With time, in some patients these injections may become less effective and partial surgical excision of orbicularis muscle and other protractors will be required. Botulinum toxin injection may still be needed but will be more effective after surgery. Muscle relaxants and sedatives are occasionally used in this disease but are of little benefit.

Prognosis

Good with botulinum toxin injection. Rare cases may not respond to treatment.

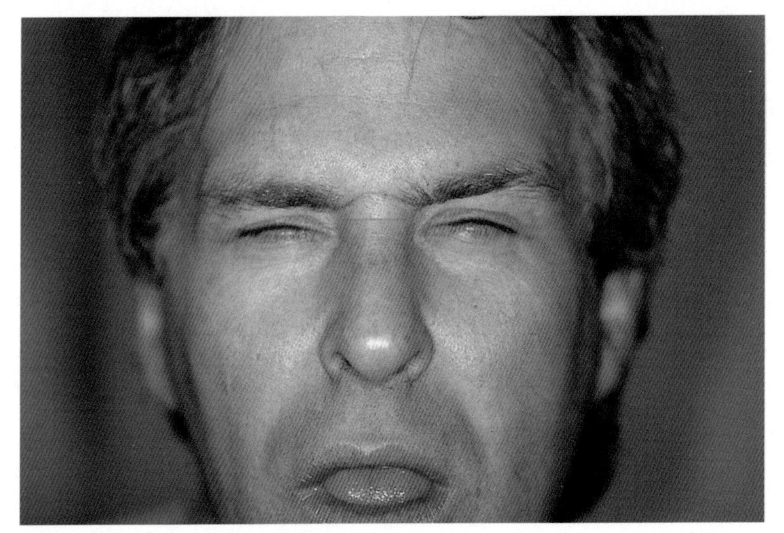

Figure 5-24 Benign essential blepharospasm *This patient would develop blepharospasm with any attempt to touch the eyes. The spasm can go on to involve other facial muscles.*

HEMIFACIAL SPASM

Epidemiology and Etiology

Age Adulthood.

Gender Equal male to female ratio.

Etiology Vascular compression of the facial nerve at the level of the brainstem.

History

Unilateral spasm of one side of the face.

Examination

The patient may have mild facial palsy on the affected side. The spasm may be seen on examination or noted by the patient's history (Fig. 5-25).

Special Considerations

Spasms are present during sleep, unlike benign essential blepharospasm where they are absent.

Differential Diagnosis

- Benign essential blepharospasm

Treatment

The patient needs MRI of the cerebellar–pontine angle to rule out a mass lesion. Botulinum toxin is then generally the treatment of choice. Neurosurgical decompression of the facial nerve is sometimes considered.

Prognosis

Botulinum A toxin controls the spasm but requires repeat injection every 3 to 6 months.

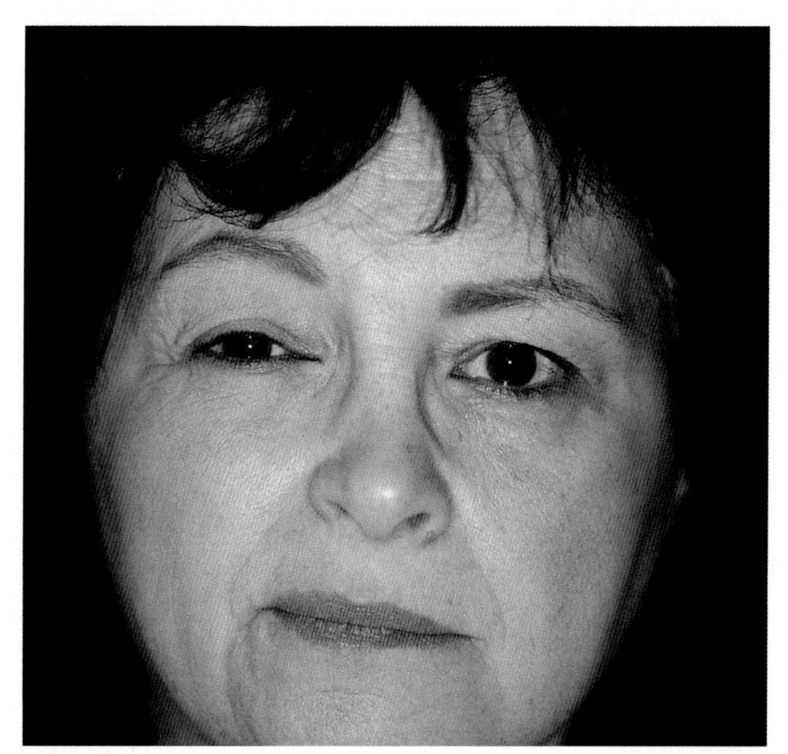

Figure 5-25 Hemifacial spasm *Hemifacial spasm of the left side of the face. The spasm is usually intermittent.*

Chapter 6

CONGENITAL EYELID ANOMALIES

BLEPHAROPHIMOSIS

Blepharophimosis is a congenital eyelid syndrome that has a characteristic eyelid appearance that includes telecanthus, epicanthus inversus, and severe myogenic ptosis.

Epidemiology and Etiology

Age Congenital.

Gender Equal.

Inheritance Autosomal dominant.

Etiology Unknown.

History

Often have family members with the same syndrome.

Examination

Characteristic eyelid findings include telecanthus, epicanthus inversus, and severe ptosis. Other findings, which may or may not be present, include lower eyelid ectropion, a poorly developed nasal bridge, hypoplasia of the superior orbital rims, hypertelorism, motility disorders, and various degrees of mental deficiency (Fig. 6-1A).

Differential Diagnosis

- No other syndrome gives these characteristic changes. Must differentiate from simple epicanthus (Fig. 6-1B) and telecanthus.

Treatment

Multiple stages of reconstruction are required. Initial surgery is aimed at the telecanthus and epicanthus inversus. This may require a simple Z-plasty, Y–V plasty, or transnasal wiring. The second stage is correction of the ptosis, which usually requires frontalis suspension. Finally, other eyelid abnormalities are addressed.

Prognosis

Significant improvement can be made with surgery. Depending on the severity, there will always be some eyelid changes that remain.

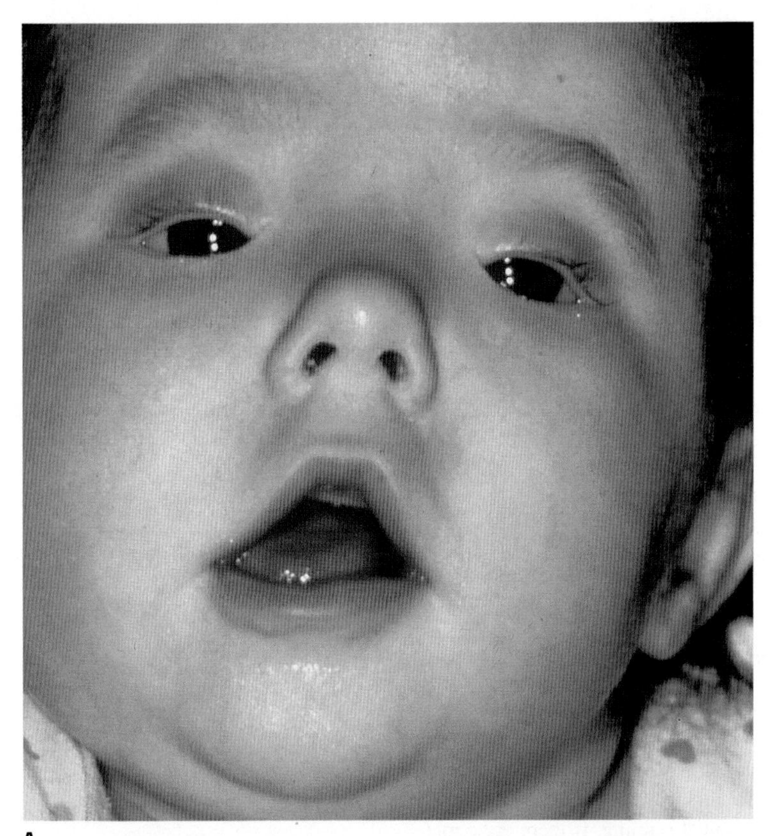

A

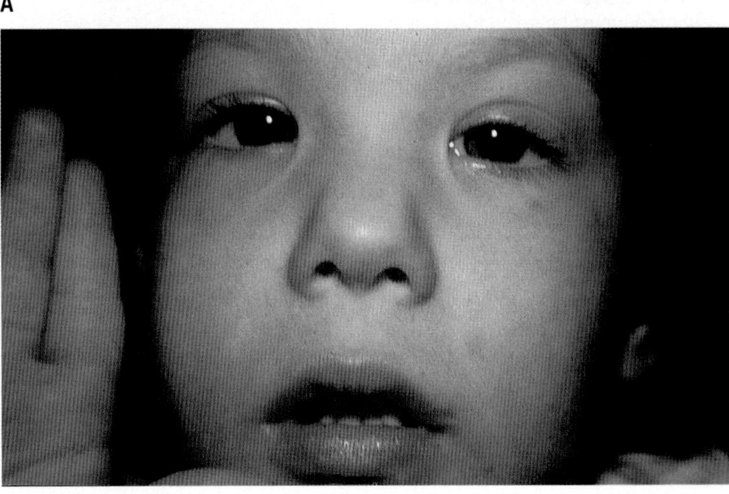

B

Figure 6-1 Blepharophimosis **A.** *This child has classic changes of blepharophimosis with ptosis, telecanthus, and epicanthus inversus.* **Epicanthal Folds** **B.** *These folds can often be seen as an isolated finding in young children. Unless severe, these epicanthal folds will lessen and even disappear as the child's face matures.*

EPIBLEPHARON

Epiblepharon is override of the pretarsal muscle and skin, which causes the cilia to assume a vertical position although the eyelid margin is in a normal position. This disorder is usually asymptomatic with no corneal staining and requires no treatment.

Epidemiology and Etiology

Age Congenital.

Gender Equal.

Etiology Immature facial bones are felt to allow for this excess skin and muscle.

History

There are usually no symptoms.

Examination

There is an excess of skin overriding the eyelid margin, which may even come in contact with the eye. If this skin can be pulled back, the eyelid margin under it is in a normal position. There is rarely any corneal staining. If there are corneal changes consideration must be given to surgical correction (Fig. 6-2).

Special Considerations

It is often very difficult to differentiate epiblepharon from congenital entropion, especially in an awake child who is squeezing their eyes shut. If there are significant corneal changes then it is likely the eyelid is entropic and surgery is required.

Differential Diagnosis

- Congenital entropion

Treatment

No treatment is needed in most cases. If there are corneal changes then excision of the excess skin and muscle is the treatment of choice.

Prognosis

Excellent. Most cases resolve as the facial bones mature. The rare case that requires surgery will respond well.

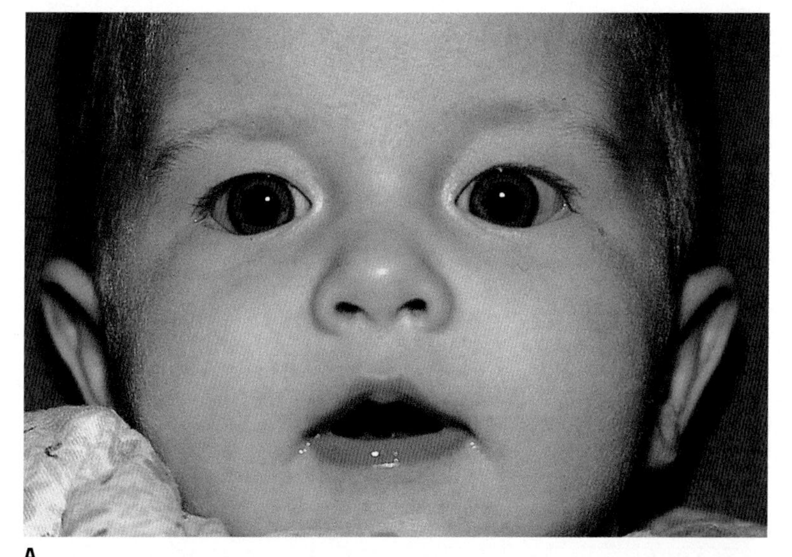

A

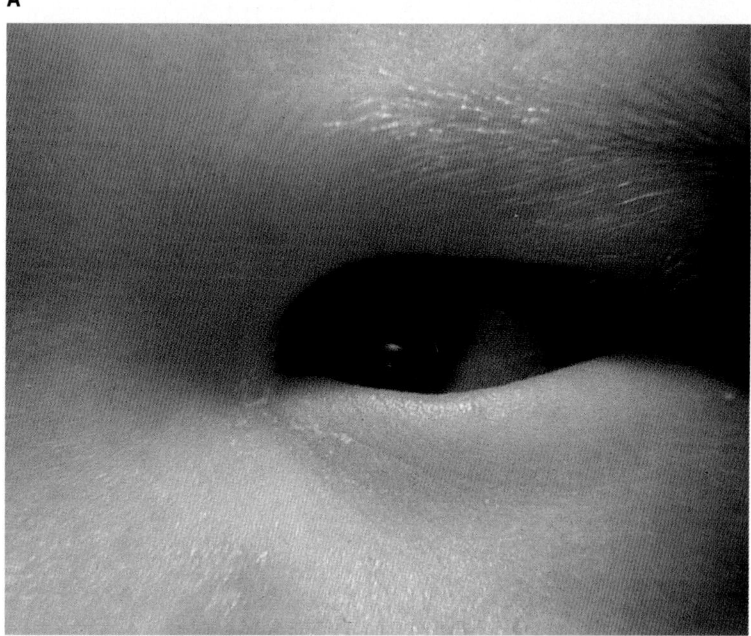

B

Figure 6-2 Epiblepharon **A** *and* **B.** *Excess skin of the lower eyelid rolls in and touches the cornea. The eyelid is in a normal position and the cornea is normal. This condition must be differentiated from congenital entropion (see Fig. 6-3).*

CONGENITAL ENTROPION

Congenital entropion is rare but can also be difficult to diagnose in an infant. An eye that is always irritated and that the child does not want to open is a clue to look for an epithelial defect or corneal scar.

Epidemiology and Etiology

Age At birth.

Gender Equal.

Etiology Usually related to an abnormality of the eyelid retractors or tarsus. Very rarely, there can be conjunctival scarring causing the entropion.

History

The child's eye is always irritated and the child does not want to open the eye.

Examination

It is difficult to examine the eyelid of an infant unless they are asleep. When the child is awake and an attempt is made to examine the eyelid, the child squeezes the eye shut and a normal eyelid may turn in. Evidence of corneal scarring or an epithelial defect on the inferior cornea is enough to suspect an entropion (Fig. 6-3).

Differential Diagnosis

- Epiblepharon

Treatment

Surgical correction is required. Excision of pretarsal skin and orbicularis with tightening of the retractors is the treatment of choice.

Prognosis

Good. Some chance of corneal scarring if not diagnosed early.

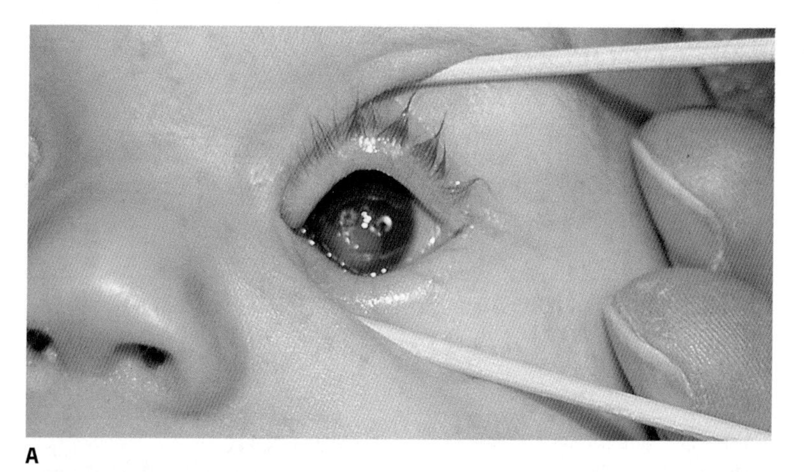

A

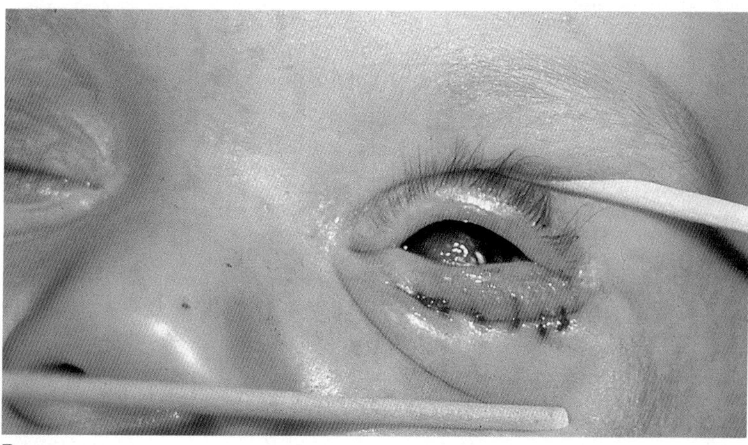

B

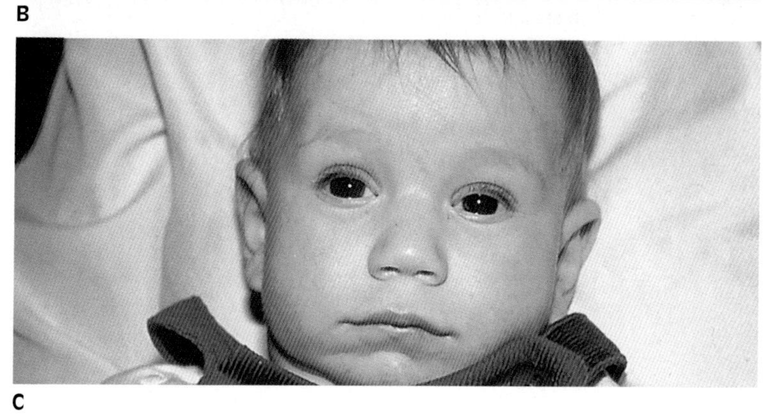

C

Figure 6-3 Congenital entropion **A.** *It is very difficult to examine a child's eyelid to try to determine if it is entropic, especially when the eye is already irritated. In this child, there is corneal scarring from a congenital entropion.* **B.** *Child immediately after placing rotating sutures in the lower eyelid.* **C.** *Postoperative picture 4 weeks after entropion surgery. The eyelid is in a normal position and the corneal opacity is resolving.*

CONGENITAL COLOBOMA

Congenital colobomas are full thickness defects in the eyelid. Even larger defects are usually well tolerated over the short term until the defect can be repaired. Upper eyelid colobomas are usually not associated with other systemic abnormalities, whereas lower eyelid colobomas are more commonly associated with facial cleft syndromes.

Epidemiology and Etiology

Age Apparent at birth.

Gender Equal.

Etiology Abnormal embryonic development results in these eyelid defects.

History

Eyelid defect is usually noted at birth or soon after. There are few symptoms.

Examination

The full thickness defect is most commonly medially on the upper eyelid. Colobomas in this location are not usually associated with any other abnormality. A coloboma of the lower eyelid is more likely to be part of a facial cleft syndrome and may have other facial defects and lacrimal abnormalities. Attention must be given to the cornea for signs of exposure although exposure is rare (Fig. 6-4).

Differential Diagnosis

- Birth trauma to the eyelid.

Treatment

Surgical repair of the coloboma is usually straightforward and can be done without any flaps that would occlude the eye and cause amblyopia.

Prognosis

Colobomas do very well with surgical repair. Other facial defects may not be as easy to repair.

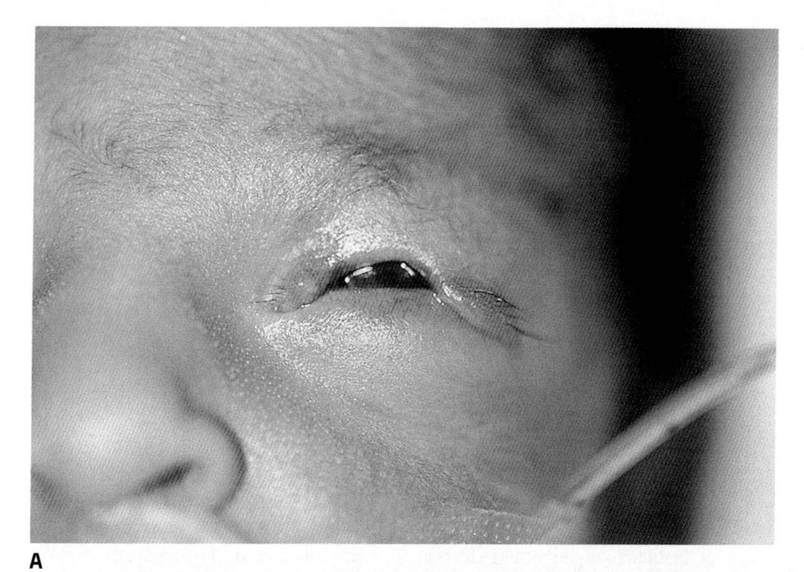

A

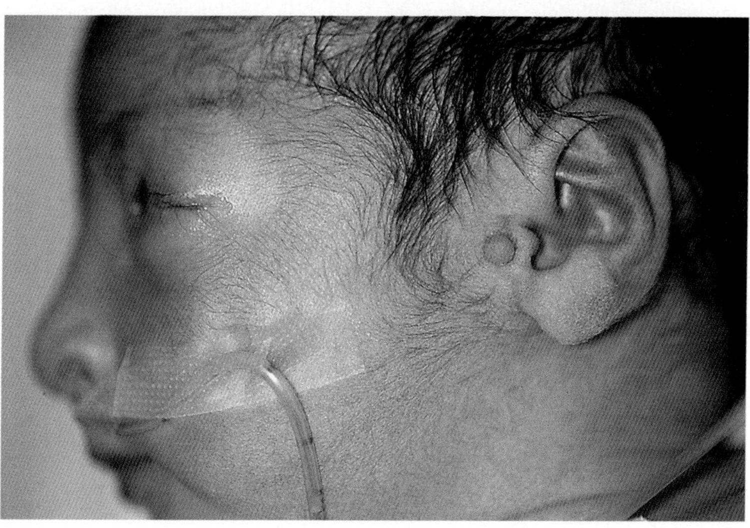

B

Figure 6-4 Congenital coloboma **A.** *Child born with a coloboma of the upper eyelid. This may be a totally isolated finding but coloboma and a preauricular skin tag* (**B**) *is consistent with Goldenhar's syndrome.*

CONGENITAL DISTICHIASIS

Distichiasis is a rare condition where an extra row of eyelashes replaces the meibomian gland openings on the eyelids.

Epidemiology and Etiology

Age Present at birth.

Gender Equal.

Etiology Embryonic pilosebaceous units improperly differentiate into hair follicles.

History

The extra row of lashes may be noted or eye irritation may prompt ophthalmic evaluation at which time the problem is discovered.

Examination

A second row of eyelashes is noted growing posterior to the normal eyelash position (Fig. 6-5). These lashes may be in contact with the cornea causing symptoms of eye irritation, corneal punctate staining, and scarring. A good corneal evaluation is important.

Differential Diagnosis

- Congenital entropion
- Conjunctival scarring causing trichiasis

Treatment

Treatment is based on the symptoms and individualized. If treatment is required, options are variable. Conservative treatment with lubrication and contact lenses is often not successful. Eyelash ablation with cryotherapy or electrolysis often result in recurrence of eyelashes but will be adequate in some patients. Surgical excision of the eyelashes and reconstruction sometimes using buccal mucosal grafts works in the most severe cases.

Prognosis

Usually good but multiple procedures may be required and there may be undesirable cosmetic defects after surgery.

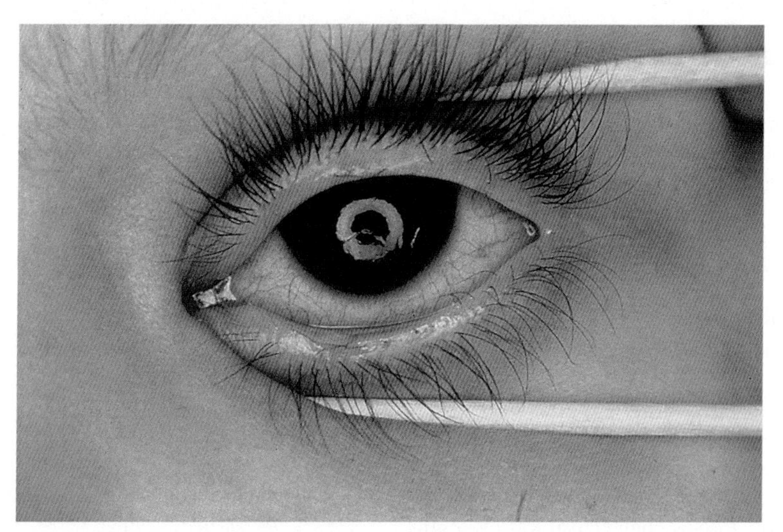

Figure 6-5 Congenital distichiasis *All four eyelids have these extra rows of eyelashes growing out of the position where the meibomian glands should be.*

ANKYLOBLEPHARON

Congenital ankyloblepharon is a failure of the eyelids to separate during embryonic development. Ankyloblepharon may also be acquired due to scarring which results in adherence of the eyelids to each other and to the globe.

Epidemiology and Etiology

Age Congenital. Acquired cases can occur at any age depending on the cause.

Gender Equal.

Etiology Congenital failure of the eyelids to separate during embryonic development. Acquired ankyloblepharon is most commonly the result of progressive conjunctival scarring resulting in fusion of the eyelids. Some causes include ocular cicatricial pemphigoid, Stevens–Johnson syndrome, chemical burns, and herpes zoster.

History

Congenital cases noted at birth. Acquired cases will usually have a history of progressive scarring related to the primary disease.

Examination

Congenital ankyloblepharon may have complete fusion of the eyelids or just a few bands holding the eyelids together. The eye and orbit may be normal or have associated abnormalities (Fig. 6-6A). Acquired ankyloblepharon shows fusion of the eyelids from scar tissue. The eye itself is not able to be seen (Fig. 6-6B).

Differential Diagnosis

- Cryptophthalmos
- Microphthalmos

Treatment

Congenital ankyloblepharon: lysis of the bands holding the eyelids together. Other reconstructive procedures may be needed depending on severity.

Acquired ankyloblepharon: determining the etiology of the scarring is done first. If this process needs treatment to quiet any inflammation, that must be done first. Attempts to reconstruct the eyelids and resurface the cornea can then be attempted. This requires coordination between oculoplastic and corneal surgeons.

Prognosis

Congenital ankyloblepharon: good.
Acquired ankyloblepharon: poor in most cases. The process causing the scarring will often hamper the healing after eyelid and corneal reconstructive surgery.

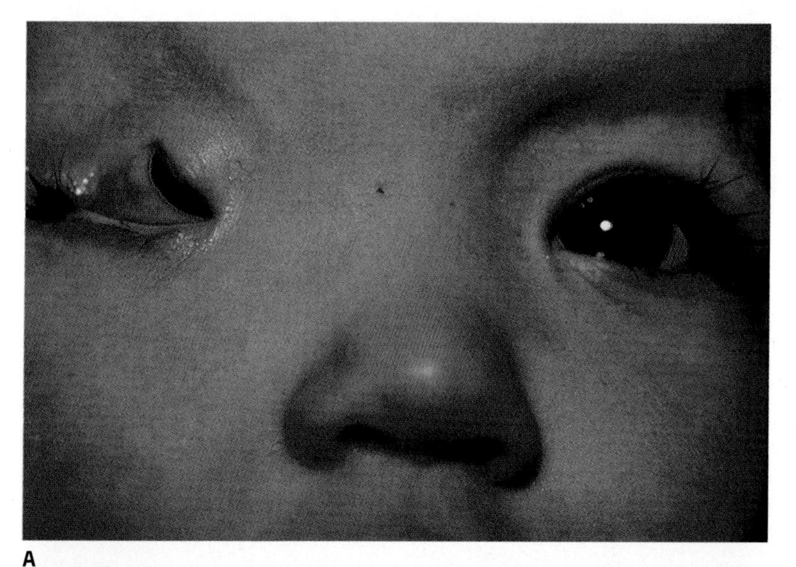

A

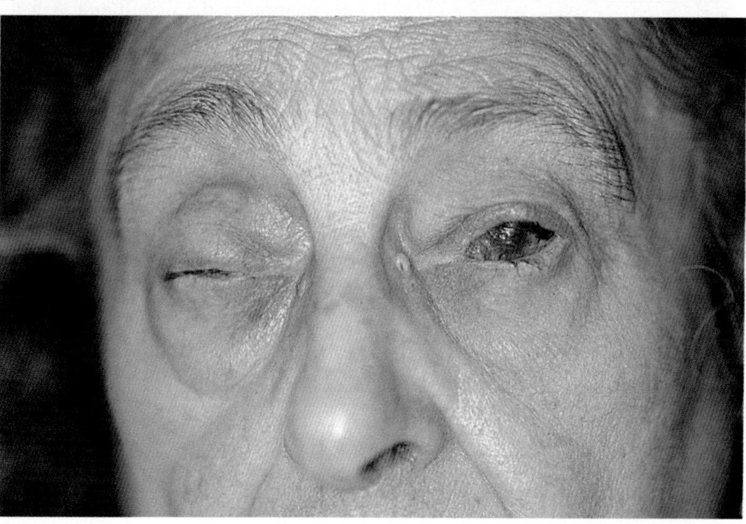

B

Figure 6-6 Congenital ankyloblepharon **A.** *Unilateral combined ankyloblepharon and cryptophthalmos. (Courtesy Richard W. Hertle, MD.)* **Ankyloblepharon** **B.** *Acquired ankyloblepharon as the result of scarring from ocular cicatricial pemphigoid. The eyelids are fused and there is likely scarring of the eyelids to the globe as well.*

Chapter 7

MISCELLANEOUS EYELID CONDITIONS

OCULAR CICATRICIAL PEMPHIGOID

Ocular cicatricial pemphigoid (OCP) is a conjunctival scarring disease that occurs in older adults. It can be mild or can be progressive and lead to corneal scarring and blindness. The disease continues to be a confusing, poorly understood condition that can be very difficult to treat in some patients.

Epidemiology and Etiology

Age Older adults.

Gender More common in females.

Etiology An autoimmune process where antibodies bind to the conjunctival basement membranes resulting in inflammation and scarring.

History

There may be a long history of ocular irritation and epilation of eyelashes over many years. The other extreme is rapidly progressive conjunctival and even corneal scarring with very red inflamed eyes. Some patients will have ulceration of other mucosal surfaces such as oral, esophageal, or genital lesions. Skin lesions may also be part of the presentation. A significant number of these patients has used or is currently using antiglaucoma drops.

Examination

Findings range from mild, subtle conjunctival scarring in the early stages to severe scarring where the eyelid is stuck to the cornea. Cicatricial entropion, trichiasis, and severe dryness all add to the poor ocular surface. The condition of the cornea is important in guiding treatment. Evaluation of the mouth and skin for other lesions is important (Fig. 7-1).

Special Considerations

Some patients on antiglaucoma medications will get conjunctival scarring that is not progressive if the medication is stopped. This finding was more common in patients using miotics, such as pilocarpine, but also seems to be associated with some of the more modern antiglaucoma drops. It is not clear whether these patients have OCP or if the scarring is entirely related to the drops.

Differential Diagnosis

- Stevens–Johnson syndrome
- Acid and alkali burns
- Previous eyelid surgery
- Trachoma
- Atopic disease

Laboratory Tests

Immunofluorescence testing of the conjunctiva will reveal immunoglobulins at the basement membrane in OCP. A positive biopsy is diagnostic but a negative biopsy does not rule out OCP, as there are a significant number of biopsy negative cases of OCP.

Pathophysiology

An autoimmune process in which immune complexes bind at the conjunctival basement membrane that results in inflammation and eventual scarring. This destroys the tear glands of the conjunctiva and causes inturned eyelids and lashes and corneal scarring.

Treatment

The inflammation must be quieted first. This may require only doxycycline in very mild cases or strong medications such as cyclophosphamide or azathioprine in refractory cases. Once the inflammation is quiet, eyelid problems, such as trichiasis or entropions, can be addressed surgically. All patients will require aggressive lubrication and/or punctal occlusion.

Prognosis

Variable. Some patients' disease will burn out or respond to treatment without significant ocular injury. In other patients, the disease can progress no matter what treatment is used.

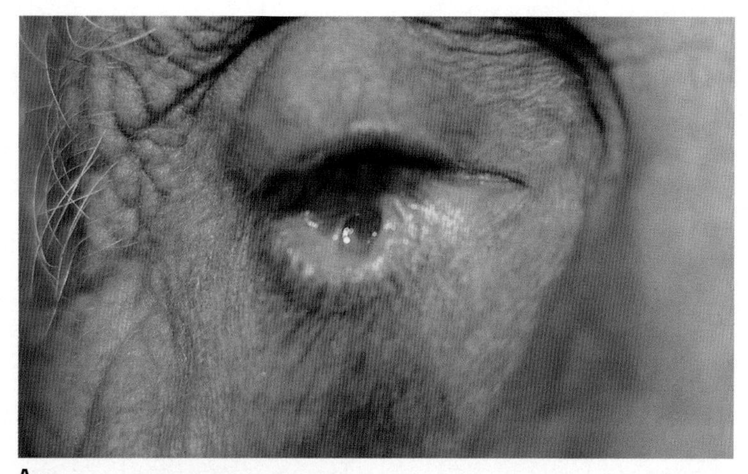

A

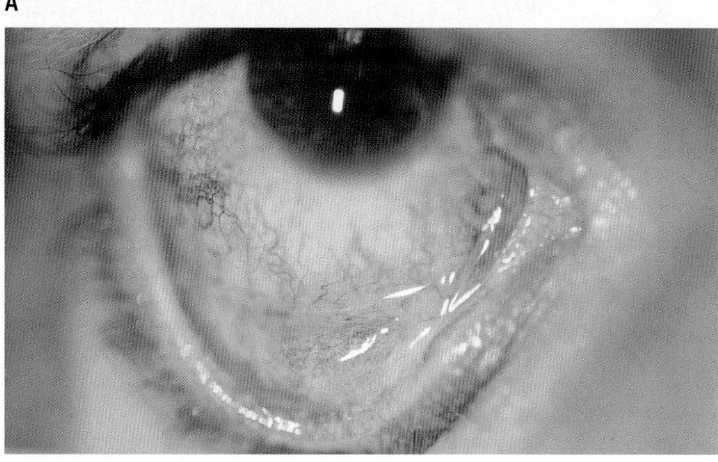

B

Figure 7-1 Ocular cicatricial pemphigoid **A.** *Scarring of the eyelid to the cornea in this advanced case.* **B.** *Earlier in the disease, the conjunctival scarring is less obvious and may even be overlooked if the conjunctiva in the fornices is not carefully examined. (Continued.)*

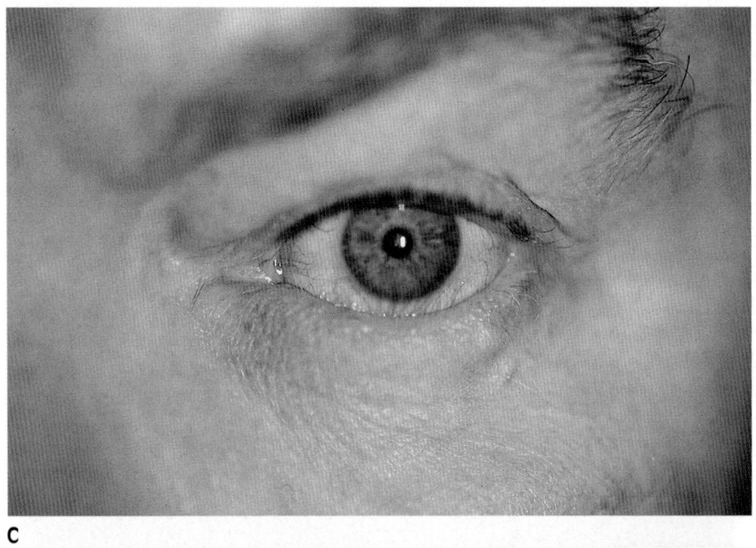

C

D

Figure 7-1 Ocular cicatricial pemphigoid (cont.) **C.** *The lower eyelid is entropic secondary to conjunctival scarring from pemphigoid.* **D.** *Oral ulcerations are often found in active ocular cicatricial pemphigoid and help solidify the diagnosis.*

Section II

LACRIMAL APPARATUS

Chapter 8

LACRIMAL OBSTRUCTIONS

CONGENITAL OBSTRUCTIONS

CONGENITAL NASOLACRIMAL DUCT OBSTRUCTION

Congenital nasolacrimal duct obstruction is seen in 2 to 6 percent of newborns but resolves in the first 3 to 4 weeks in most infants. The chronic purulent discharge is the main problem for caregivers but, with additional time, a large percent of these obstructions will resolve on their own.

Epidemiology and Etiology

Age Congenital.

Gender Equal in males and females.

Etiology Incomplete development of the distal lacrimal passage with a membranous block at the valve of Hasner.

History

Parents will note a chronic mucous discharge with matting of the eyelashes at 3 to 4 weeks of age in 2 to 6 percent of full-term infants in one or both eyes. Most obstructions will spontaneously resolve by the age of 6 to 12 months.

Examination

Diagnosis is based mainly on the history. Examination may reveal increased tear film and some crusting of the eyelashes. Mucous reflux with pressure over the lacrimal sac confirms the diagnosis but is not always present. Examination must rule out a dacryocystocele or any sign of infection (Fig. 8-1).

Differential Diagnosis

- Chronic conjunctivitis
- Punctal dysgenesis
- Entropion
- Trichiasis

Treatment

Timing of the treatment is controversial. Ninety percent of all congenital nasolacrimal duct obstructions will resolve by age 12 months. Many physicians will use conservative treatment until this time. This management consists of massage with topical antibiotics as needed to control the mucous discharge. Probing and irrigation under general anesthesia will successfully treat 90 percent of patients. Those patients not responsive to probing and irrigation may require intubation with silicone tubes with or without a balloon dacryoplasty. The rare patient will require a dacryocystorhinostomy.

Prognosis

Treatment is very successful. Waiting for spontaneous resolution while the child has chronic discharge is often difficult for the caregivers.

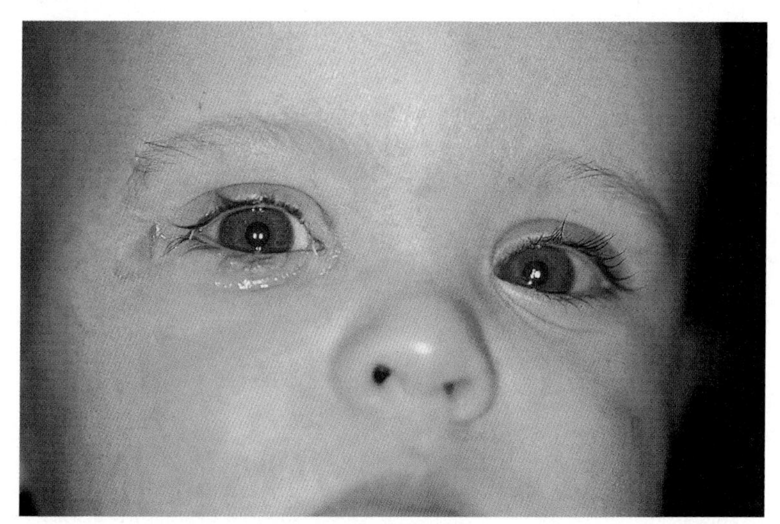

Figure 8-1 Congenital nasolacrimal duct obstruction *There is redness, crusting, and irritation of the right eyelids from the chronic discharge. The tear film is also increased. In many patients with congenital nasolacrimal duct obstruction, there will be no external signs and the diagnosis is based on the history the caregivers report.*

DACRYOCYSTOCELE

A dacryocystocele is a rare lesion noted at birth in the medial canthal area. It represents fluid and mucus trapped in the lacrimal sac. Dacryocystoceles will resolve but must be observed carefully because they can become infected.

Epidemiology and Etiology

Age Congenital.

Gender Equal in males and females.

Etiology Blockage of the lacrimal system distally, at the valve of Hasner, and proximally, at the valve of Rosenmuller, resulting in trapped amniotic fluid and/or mucus produced by the lacrimal sac goblet cells.

History

Cystic swelling of the medial canthus below the tendon noted at birth.

Examination

Prominent cystic mass below the medial canthal tendon (Fig. 8-2). If a mass is noted above the medial canthal tendon, another etiology must be considered.

Differential Diagnosis

- Hemangioma
- Meningoencephalocele
- Dacryocystitis

Treatment

Observation for the first 1 to 2 weeks with massage. Many will resolve on their own. Probing is required if there is any sign of infection or if there is not resolution after 2 weeks.

Prognosis

Excellent.

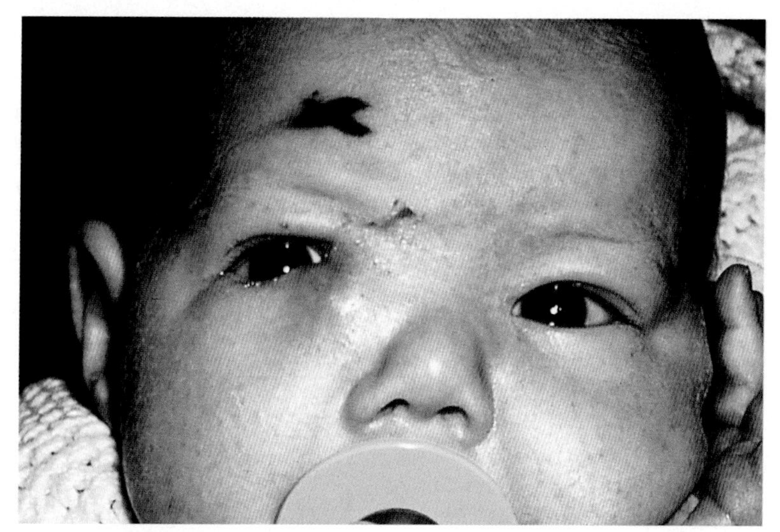

Figure 8-2 Dacryocystocele *The large, distended right lacrimal sac is easily seen and firm to palpation. This child underwent probing and irrigation, which resolved the obstruction.*

LACRIMAL FISTULA

A lacrimal fistula is an extra opening of the lacrimal system onto the skin usually inferior–nasal to the punctum. One third of fistulas will have an associated lacrimal obstruction with chronic mucous discharge. The other patients are often asymptomatic.

Epidemiology and Etiology

Age Typically congenital but acquired fistulas can occur at an age.

Gender Equal in males and females.

Etiology Abnormal embryonic development of the lacrimal system. Cases of acquired fistulas are related to dacryostenosis with dacryocystitis.

History

Often asymptomatic unless there is an associated dacryostenosis.

Examination

Small cutaneous opening inferior and nasal to the medial canthal angle. May or may not have tears exiting from it (Fig. 8-3).

Differential Diagnosis

- Must determine if there is associated dacryostenosis.

Treatment

If symptomatic, the epithelial lined fistula can be excised. If there is also an associated dacryostenosis, a dacryocystorhinostomy and excision of the fistula is indicated. Acquired fistulas will disappear when the dacryocystitis resolves.

Prognosis

Excellent.

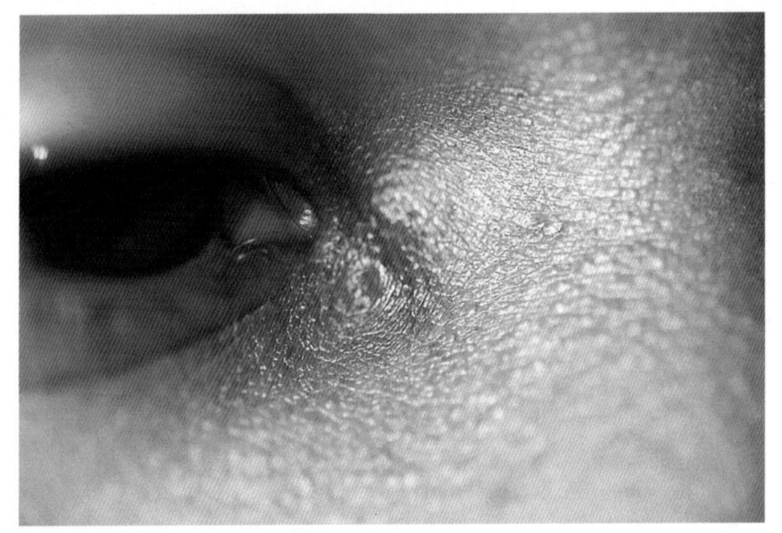

Figure 8-3 Congenital lacrimal fistula *Note the very small opening inferior-nasal to the puncta, which is connected to the lacrimal system.*

ACQUIRED OBSTRUCTIONS

ACQUIRED NASOLACRIMAL DUCT OBSTRUCTION

Acquired nasolacrimal duct obstruction becomes more common as patients age. The obstruction most commonly occurs in the nasolacrimal duct. Patients may present with tearing or an infection. Many patients may have an obstruction and be without symptoms.

Epidemiology and Etiology

Age Older patients.

Gender Females most commonly.

Etiology Involutional changes in the lacrimal duct/sac is the most common cause. Naso-orbital trauma or surgery, sinusitis, and dacryocystitis are also causes.

History

Continual tearing, which may have been preceded by intermittent episodes of tearing. The process is most commonly unilateral but may be bilateral.

Examination

Increased tear film on slit lamp examination with abnormal dye disappearance test. Definitive diagnosis made with irrigation of the lacrimal system, which will demonstrate obstruction of flow (Fig. 8-4).

Differential Diagnosis

Other causes of tearing such as:

- Keratitis sicca
- Blepharitis
- Ectropion
- Punctal abnormalities

Special Tests

Dacryocystography may help define lacrimal stenosis in difficult cases and in partial obstructions.

Treatment

Symptomatic complete obstruction requires a dacryocystorhinostomy. Partial obstructions can be treated with balloon dacryoplasty.

Prognosis

Dacryocystorhinostomy is successful 90 percent of the time or more often. Balloon dacryoplasty is 70 to 80 percent successful but is less invasive.

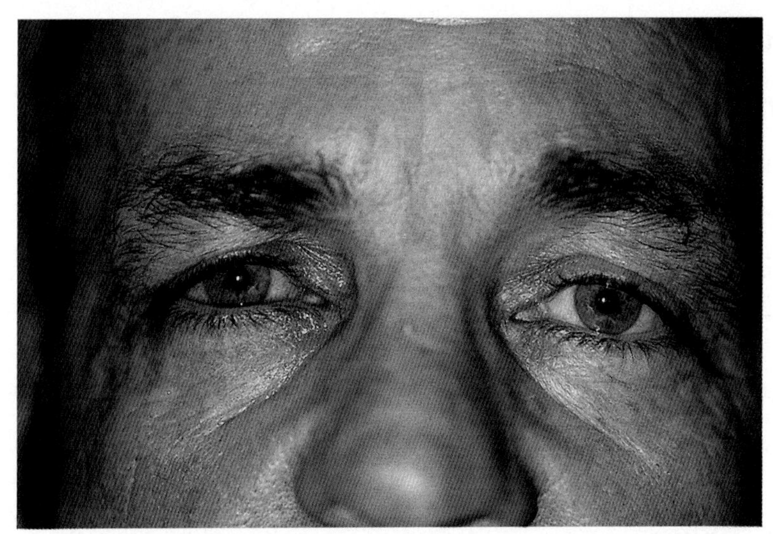

Figure 8-4 Acquired nasolacrimal duct obstruction *There are often no external signs of acquired nasolacrimal duct obstruction. There are excess tears running down the cheek and slight injection of the right eye. If there is some dacryocystitis associated with the blockage the eye may be red.*

CANALICULAR OBSTRUCTION

Epidemiology and Etiology

Age Any.

Gender More common in females.

Etiology Trauma, external conjunctival infections (EKC, herpes), canaliculitis, systemic chemotherapy.

History

Onset of tearing may be gradual or acute.

Examination

Increased tear film, normal eyelid position, and evidence of canalicular obstruction on probing of the canaliculi (Fig. 8-5).

Special Considerations

There may be an additional more distal obstruction in the lacrimal sac and duct in some of these cases.

Differential Diagnosis

- Keratitis sicca
- Blepharitis
- Ectropion
- Other lacrimal system abnormalities

Treatment

Silicone intubation with or without a dacryocystorhinostomy.

Prognosis

Canalicular obstructions have a poorer prognosis than more distal obstructions. Success is in the range of 50 percent, depending on the etiology.

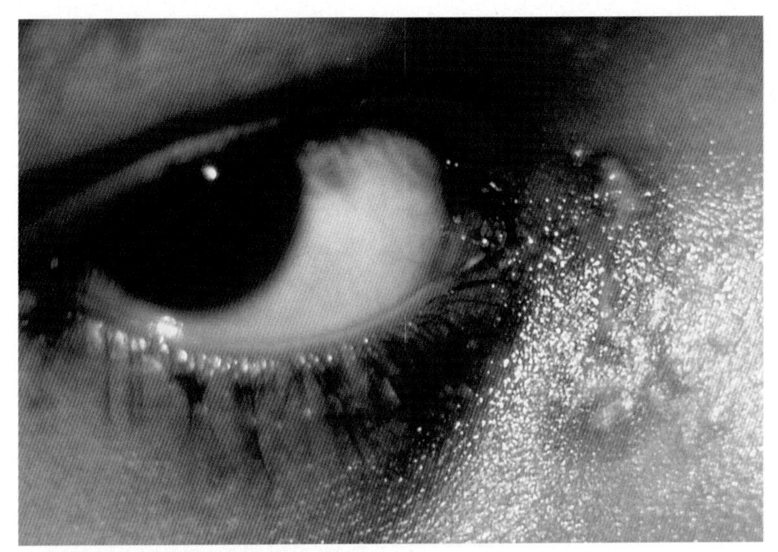

Figure 8-5 Canalicular obstruction *External signs of herpes simplex are the only sign of the canalicular obstruction. Probing demonstrates canalicular scarring as a result of herpes simplex.*

Chapter 9

LACRIMAL INFECTIONS

DACRYOCYSTITIS

Epidemiology and Etiology

Age Most common in older adults but can be seen at any age.

Gender More common in females.

Etiology Nasolacrimal obstruction from various causes with stasis of fluid in the lacrimal sac and eventual infection.

History

May have acute onset of pain and swelling over the lacrimal sac. Others may give the history of chronic tearing with chronic mucous discharge and a tender lump over the lacrimal sac. There may be a prolonged history of a chronic conjunctivitis.

Examination

Tenderness over the lacrimal sac is the most common finding. The lacrimal sac may be enlarged with significant swelling or it may be relatively small (Fig. 9-1A). Similarly, the amount of periorbital swelling varies with the severity of the infection. Orbital cellulitis must be considered if the infection is severe (Fig. 9-1B). Patients with a low-grade chronic infection may have mucus/pus expressible through the canaliculi with pressure over the lacrimal sac. The conjunctiva may be injected. Probing and irrigation should not be done in the setting of an infection.

Special Considerations

If a patient complains of blood expressed from the lacrimal system, a lacrimal sac tumor must be considered and imaging done. Infections can give bloody discharge as well.

Differential Diagnosis

- Lacrimal sac tumor

Laboratory Tests

Culture and sensitivity of any material expressed or drained from the lacrimal sac.

Imaging

CT or MRI scanning may be needed if a lacrimal sac tumor is suspected.

Treatment

Treatment of the acute infection is the first priority. Systemic antibiotics and warm compresses are the treatment of choice. If there is a formed

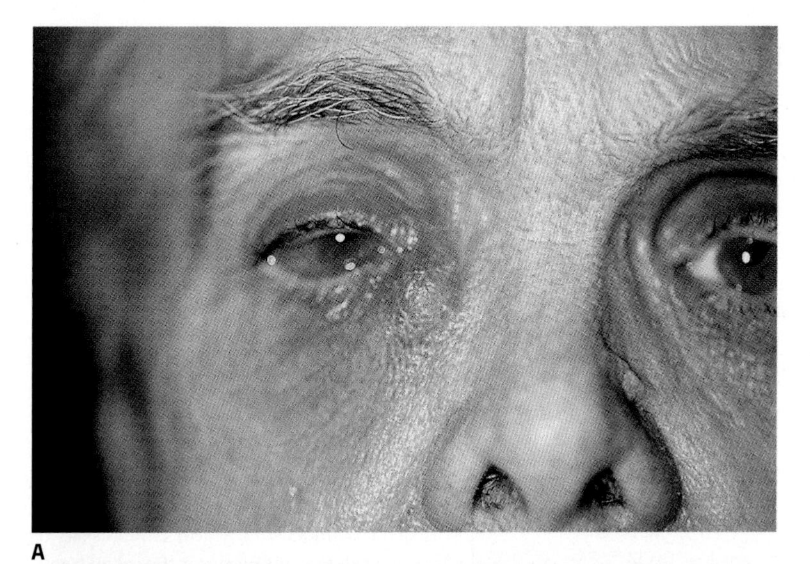

A

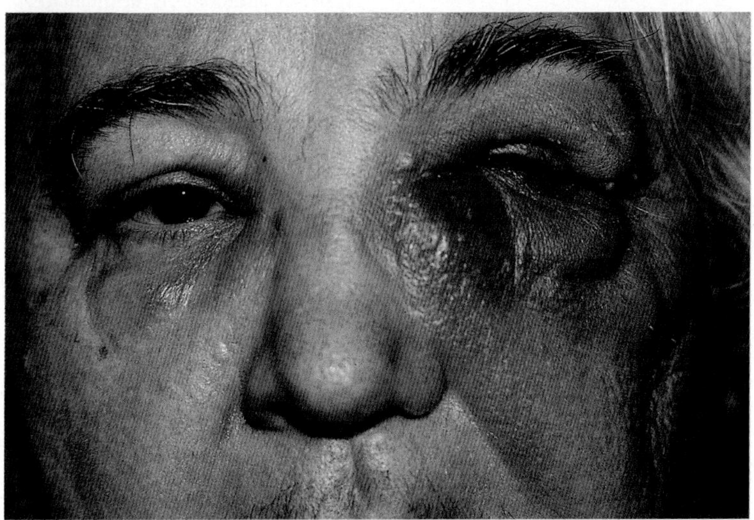

B

Figure 9-1 Dacryocystitis **A.** *This 68-year-old male has a formed lacrimal sac mass that is tender with a surrounding mild cellulitis.* **B.** *A more severe dacryocystitis with surrounding cellulitis.*

abscess of the sac, incision and drainage is indicated. Ultimately, when the infection has resolved, most patients will require a dacryocystorhinostomy. Rare patients will have an open lacrimal system after the infection is gone and will not require a dacryocystorhinostomy. Patients who have had a dacryocystitis and have an obstructed lacrimal system have an increased risk of recurrent dacryocystitis.

Prognosis

Excellent unless the patient is immunocompromised.

CANALICULITIS

Canaliculitis is a rare infection involving the proximal lacrimal system. The infection can be bacterial or fungal and is usually indolent. Making the diagnosis of canaliculitis can be difficult because it often presents as a chronic conjunctivitis and not until late does the lacrimal infection become apparent.

Epidemiology and Etiology

Age Usually older adults.

Etiology Some abnormality of the lacrimal system leads to concretion formation and a chronic infection.

History

Chronic mucous discharge, tearing, and conjunctivitis unresponsive to topical antibiotics.

Examination

The diagnosis can be difficult to confirm unless it is suspected. An erythematous, pouting, dilated punctum, which is often tender to palpation and very tender to probing, is often present. There may be a follicular conjunctivitis and a chronic mucous discharge. Pressure over the canaliculus may express pus or concretions (Fig. 9-2).

Differential Diagnosis

- Chronic conjunctivitis
- Migrated punctal plug

Laboratory Tests

Culture and sensitivity of material in canaliculus is helpful in determining treatment.

Treatment

Treatment with warm compresses, topical, and systemic antibiotics is the initial treatment. Most patients will have concretions in the canaliculus and the process will recur until the concretions are removed with incision and drainage of the canaliculus.

Prognosis

Good once recognized. A second obstruction lower in the lacrimal system may result in a recurrence.

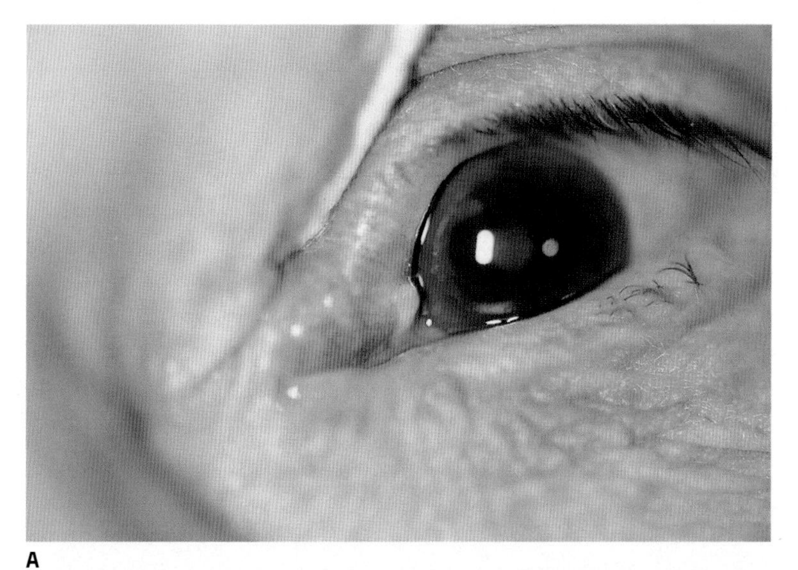

A

B

Figure 9-2 Canaliculitis **A.** *A red, tender upper canaliculus with expression of pus with pressure over the canaliculus.* **B.** *The lacrimal stones found on opening the canaliculus.*

Chapter 10

LACRIMAL SAC TUMORS

Lacrimal sac tumors are rare and the etiology is widely varied from benign to malignant. Any dacryostenosis or dacryocystitis has the potential to be a lacrimal sac tumor. When the lacrimal obstruction is accompanied by bloody discharge, the suspicion of tumor needs to be raised.

Epidemiology and Etiology

Age Adults.

Etiology Squamous cell papillomas and carcinomas are the most common cause. Etiologies include:

- Lymphoma
- Benign squamous cell papilloma
- Benign transitional cell papilloma
- Transitional cell carcinoma
- Squamous cell carcinoma

History

Patients present with chronic or acute dacryocystitis or a mass in the area of the lacrimal sac. A history of bloody discharge in the setting of dacryocystitis should alert the examiner to a possible tumor. Classically, the mass may be above the medial canthal tendon but early in the course may present like a dacryocystitis.

Examination

Findings vary from being identical to dacryocystitis to a palpable mass in the lacrimal sac area. The tumor may be found during dacryocystorhinostomy when there was no evidence of a tumor preoperatively. If a tumor is suspected, nasal examination by an otolaryngologist may help define its extent, along with CT and/or MRI scanning (Fig. 10-1).

Differential Diagnosis

- Dacryocystitis

Laboratory Tests

Biopsy of the lacrimal sac for any abnormal appearing lacrimal sac. Dacryocystogram may be helpful.

Imaging

CT or MRI scanning is needed if a lacrimal sac tumor is suspected. It may not be able to differentiate a tumor from an enlarged sac secondary to infection but will show a large erosive mass.

Treatment

Complete excision of any benign or malignant tumor is important. Frozen section control is required to try to assure complete excision. Benign papillomas may recur with malignant transformation. Lymphomas are sensitive to irradiation. Careful long-term follow up is important for any lacrimal sac tumor.

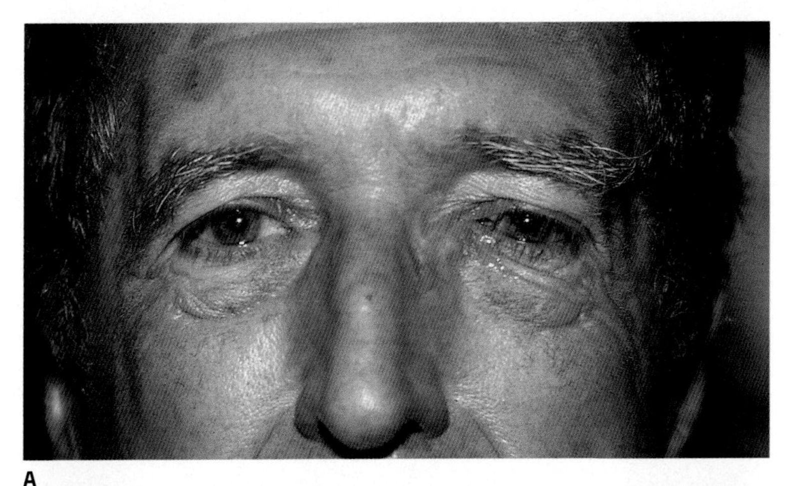

A

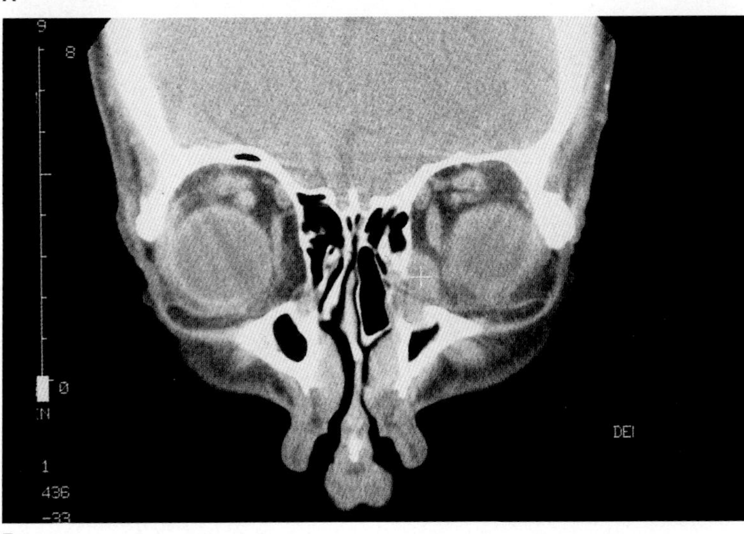

B

Figure 10-1 Lacrimal sac tumor **A.** *The patient has fullness of the left lacrimal sac area and bloody discharge.* **B.** *An axial CT scan showing a mass in the lacrimal sac fossa, which was a lymphoma on biopsy.*

Prognosis

Recurrence is not uncommon. Fifty percent of transitional and squamous cell carcinomas will recur and 50 percent of these recurrences will be fatal.

Section III

THE ORBIT

Chapter 11

ORBITAL INFECTIONS

ORBITAL CELLULITIS

Orbital cellulitis is a real ophthalmic emergency that needs prompt recognition and treatment. The infection can progress rapidly over a few hours in severe cases with potential life-threatening complications.

Epidemiology and Etiology

Age All ages.

Gender Equal incidence in males and females.

Etiology Sinusitis is the most common cause but other causes include skin infections or skin wounds, dental infections, and dacryocystitis.

History

One to three days of progressive swelling around the eye. The process may be preceded by an upper respiratory infection. The patient may have a history of sinus infections.

Examination

Erythema, swelling, chemosis, restricted motility, pain on eye movement, and proptosis characterize orbital cellulitis. These symptoms are progressive over 24 to 48 hours. As the infection advances, vision can be affected. Patients may or may not have a fever and leukocytosis. It is very important to make the distinction between the signs of orbital cellulitis and preseptal cellulitis where there is just swelling and redness of the eyelids (Fig. 11-1).

Imaging

CT scanning is not required to make the diagnosis of orbital cellulitis but is needed to look for the source of infection (e.g., sinusitis, orbital abscess) and to rule out other processes such as an orbital tumor. A CT scan will show sinusitis, which can require drainage. Orbital foreign bodies or an orbital abscess can require additional surgery.

Special Considerations

Aggressive and prompt treatment of orbital cellulitis is required to prevent posterior extension of the infection, which can result in cavernous sinus thrombosis.

Differential Diagnosis

- Preseptal cellulitis
- Orbital pseudotumor
- Orbital abscess
- Phycomycosis
- Metastatic orbital tumor

Laboratory Tests

CBC: white count may be normal.
Blood cultures are of questionable value.

Treatment

Immediate broad-spectrum intravenous antibiotics, orbital imaging, and careful monitoring for improvement in the first 24 to 48 hours.

Prognosis

Good. Rare complications from development of an abscess or cavernous sinus thrombosis.

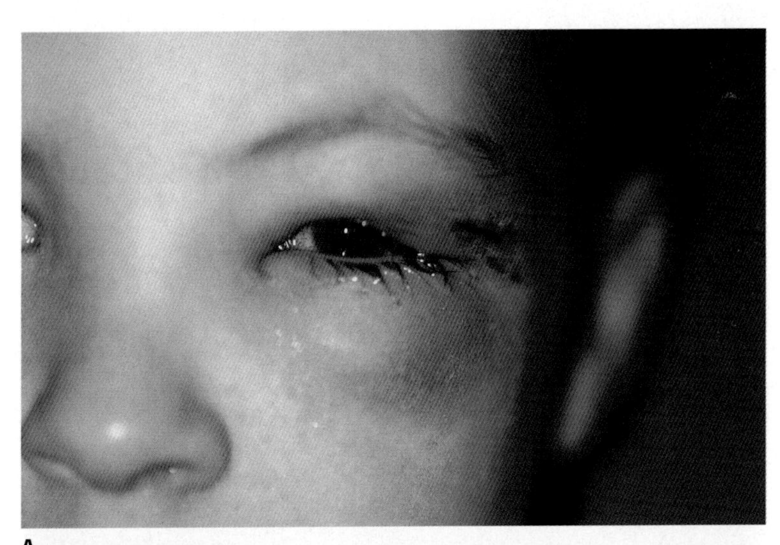

A

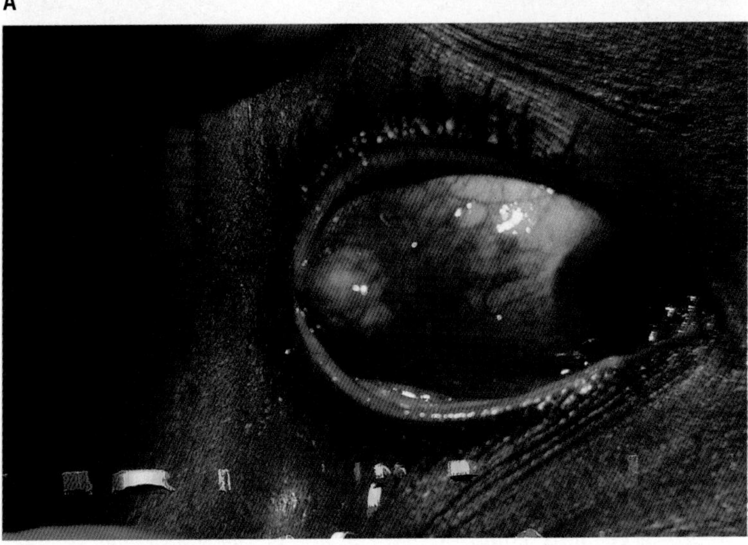

B

Figure 11-1 Preseptal cellulitis **A.** *Child with a scratch on the lateral left upper eyelid that resulted in preseptal cellulitis 2 days later. Ocular motility is normal. The patient responded to antibiotics within 48 hours.* **B.** *Early cellulitis related to a subconjunctival abscess that required drainage and oral and topical antibiotics. (Continued.)*

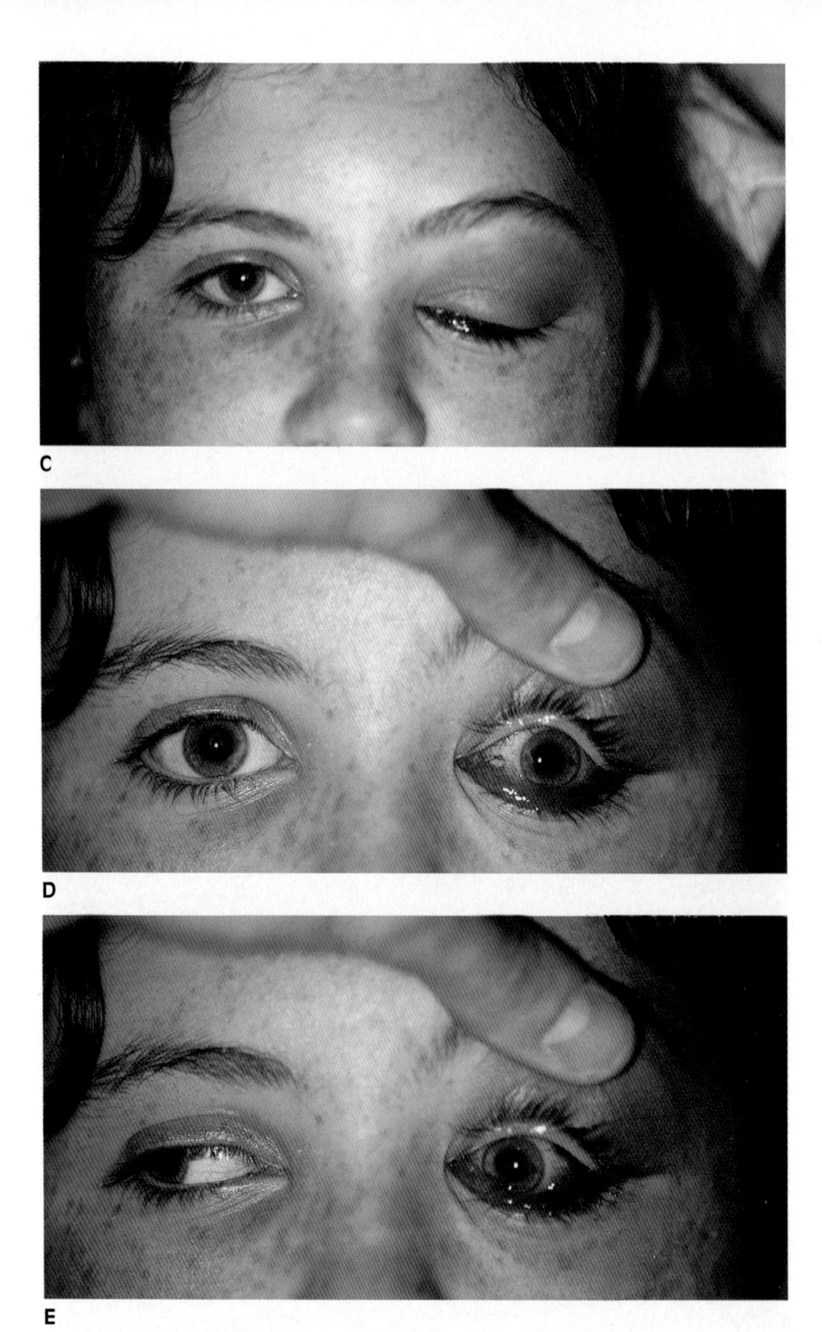

Figure 11-1 Orbital cellulitis (cont.) **C** *to* **F.** *Patient with 2 days of swelling of the left eye with orbital cellulitis. The eye is swollen shut but, with lifting, the eyelid ocular motility is limited and there is chemosis. The patient responded with improvement in 48 hours on intravenous antibiotics. (Continued.)*

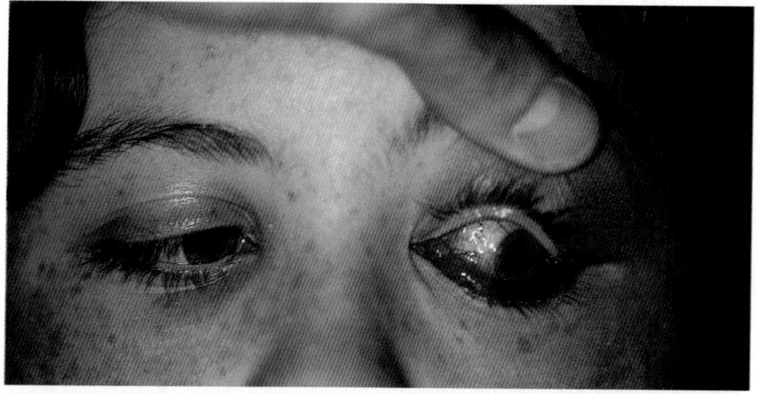

F

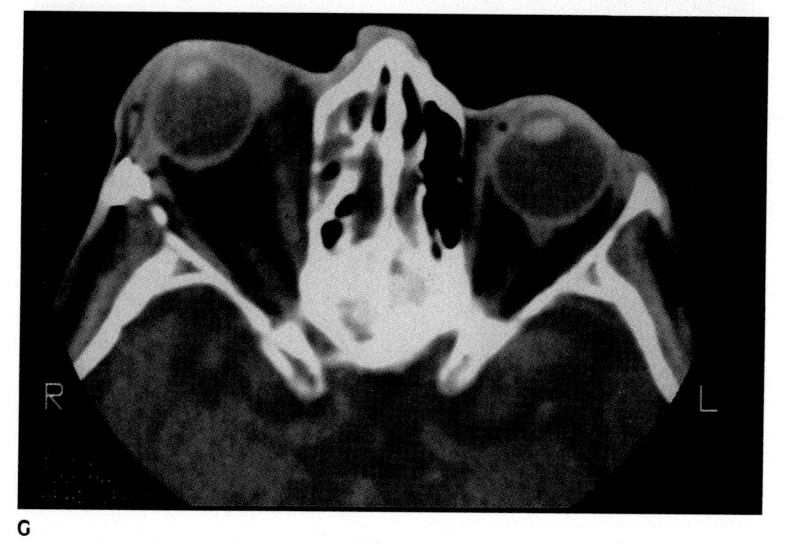

G

Figure 11-1 Orbital cellulitis (cont.) **G.** *CT scan shows proptosis and sinusitis and is consistent with the clinical diagnosis of orbital cellulitis.*

ORBITAL ABSCESS

An orbital abscess is a rare complication of sinusitis and orbital cellulitis. Orbital cellulitis that does not improve on broad-spectrum IV antibiotics needs careful imaging to look for an orbital abscess.

Epidemiology and Etiology

Age Any.

Gender Equal.

Etiology Sinus disease is the most common source of a subperiosteal abscess. Rarely, an orbital foreign body can be the cause and must be suspected if the abscess is intraorbital.

History

Orbital cellulitis with no sign of improvement on appropriate antibiotics.

Examination

Signs are those of orbital cellulitis that do not improve on appropriate intravenous antibiotics. The globe may be displaced away from the abscess. The abscess is diagnosed on CT scanning (Fig. 11-2).

Imaging

CT scanning will demonstrate a subperiosteal opacity usually adjacent to an infected sinus. Rarely, the abscess may be intraconal.

Differential Diagnosis

- Orbital cellulitis
- Phycomycosis
- Cavernous sinus thrombosis
- Orbital pseudotumor

Laboratory Tests

CBC; culturing of the abscess contents.

Treatment

Most patients will require immediate surgical drainage of the abscess and treatment with broad-spectrum IV antibiotics. Some abscesses have been treated with IV antibiotics alone and close observation in children under age 9 years.

Prognosis

Prompt and aggressive treatment usually allows successful treatment. An orbital abscess does have the potential to result in visual loss, motility problems, or even severe CNS morbidity.

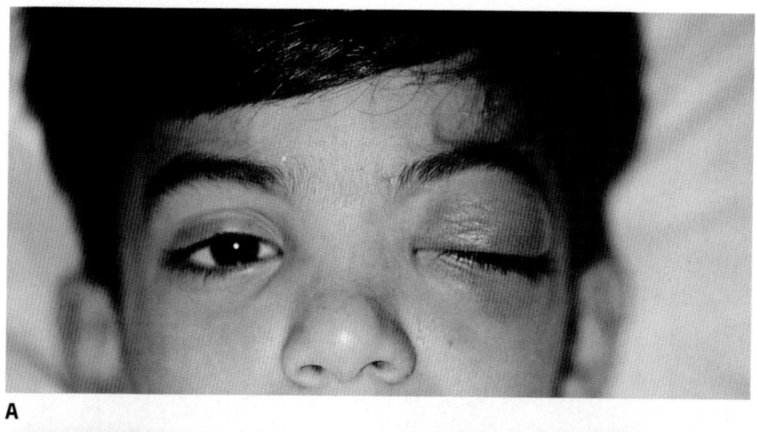
A

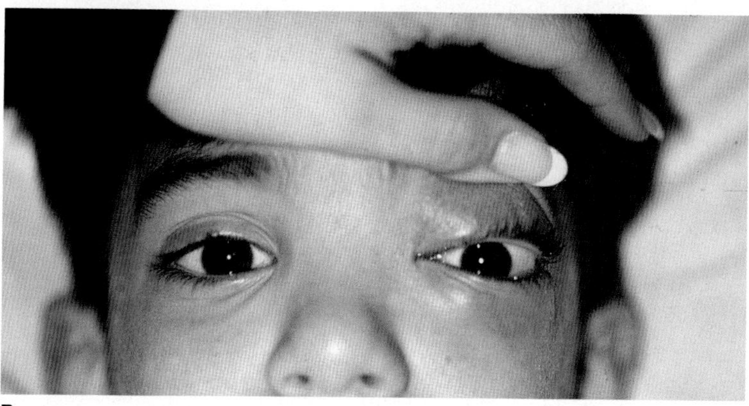
B

Figure 11-2 Orbital abscess **A.** *A patient with a 2- to 3-day history of swelling of the left eye.* **B.** *There is 5 mm of proptosis and limited motility. (Continued.)*

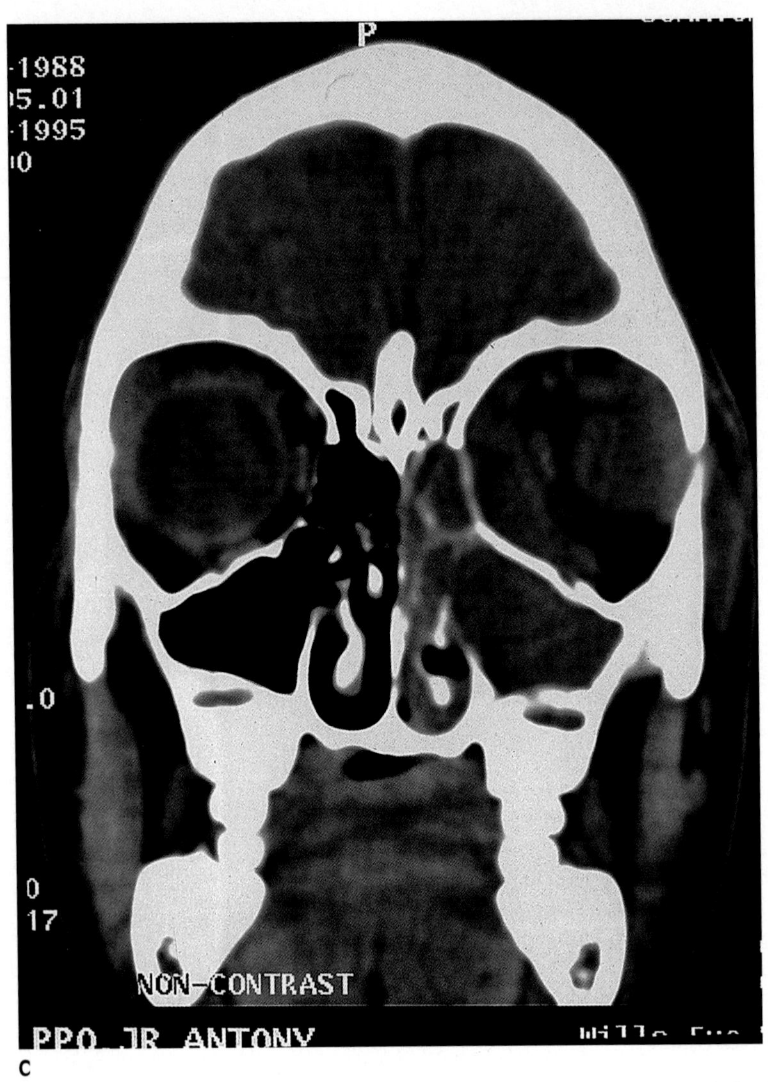

C

Figure 11-2 Orbital abscess (cont.) **C.** *CT scan shows pan sinusitis with a medial orbital abscess that required surgical drainage. (Continued.)*

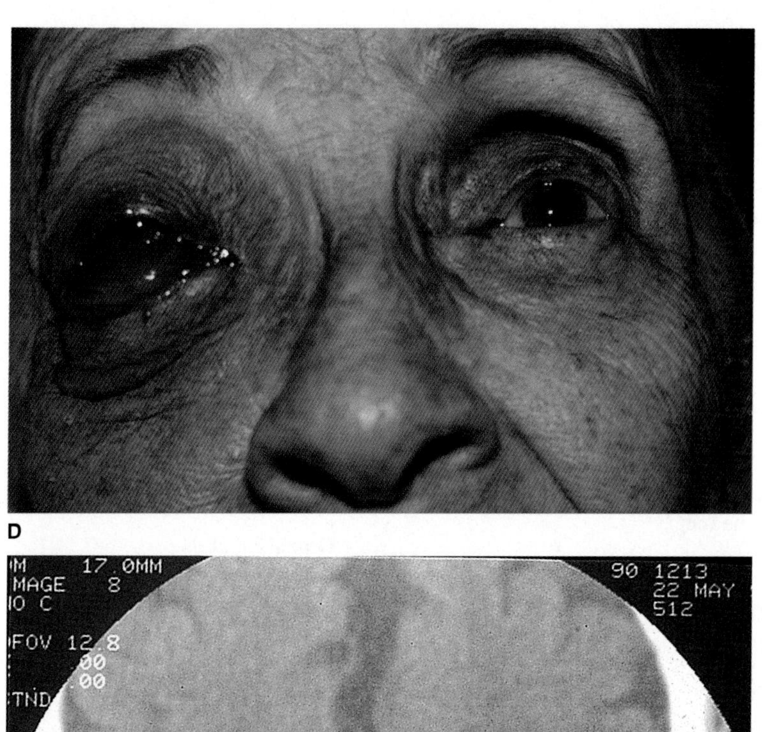

D

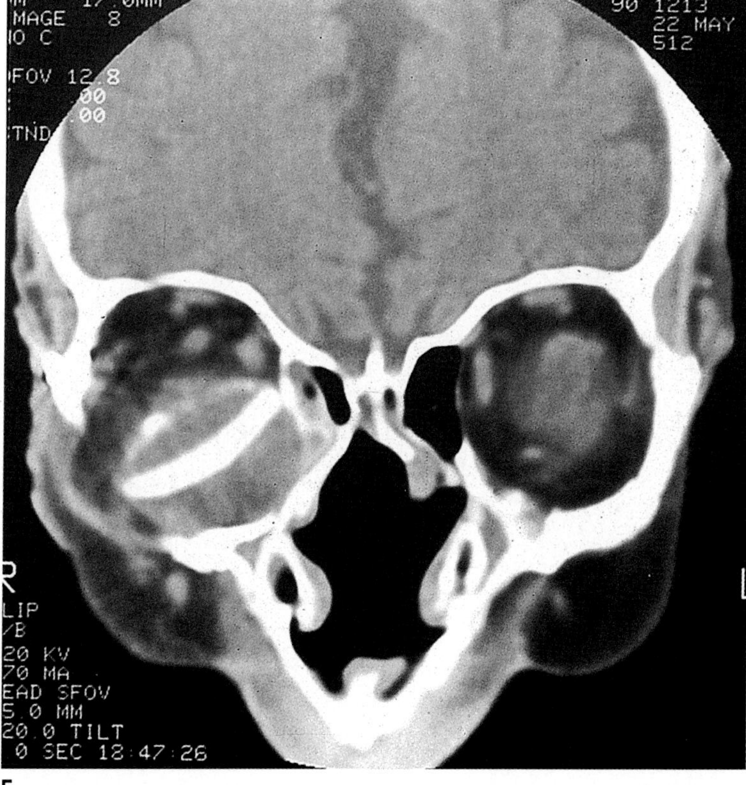

E

Figure 11-2 Orbital abscess (cont.) **D.** *A patient with weeks of a red irritated eye.* **E.** *CT scan shows an abscess around an old orbital floor implant.*

PHYCOMYCOSIS (MUCORMYCOSIS)

Phycomycosis is a rare, often fatal fungal infection that occurs in very sick, immunocompromised patients, most commonly in poorly controlled diabetics. This infection starts in the nasopharynx or sinuses and secondarily invades the orbit. Aggressive treatment has improved the survival in this often fatal condition.

Epidemiology and Etiology

Age Adults.

Gender Equal male and female occurrence.

Etiology Fungi invade the orbit from the sinuses or nose. The fungi invade blood vessel walls and produce thrombosis, ischemia, and allow spread of the fungi.

History

Patients often have a history of severe sinus pain and progressive orbital swelling. The patients who develop this infection are immunocompromised in some way. The most common underlying condition is severe diabetes with poor control but others include malignancy, chemotherapy, and chronic steroid use.

Examination

Proptosis is the most common finding with an orbital apex syndrome. Black escar in the nasal cavity is a late finding and is not a reliable diagnostic sign. Patients are very sick systemically (Fig. 11-3A).

Imaging

CT scanning will show evidence of sinus disease, which at times can be very mild (Fig. 11-3B). An MRI with gadolinium should be done to look for evidence of extension into the cavernous sinus.

Pathology

Diagnosis is made on biopsy. Nonseptate, large branching hyphae that stain on H&E staining, unlike most fungi, are found.

Differential Diagnosis

- Orbital cellulitis
- Orbital pseudotumor
- Cavernous sinus thrombosis

Laboratory Tests

Evaluation for diabetic control, leukocyte count.

Pathophysiology

Opportunistic fungal infection that grows in an immunocompromised host.

Treatment

Control systemic disease; intravenous amphotericin B; and surgical debridement of necrotic tissue, which rarely involves orbital exenteration.

Prognosis

Poor. Depending on state of the patient's systemic disease, this condition can often be fatal. Even if the disease is controlled, vision is often lost in the affected eye.

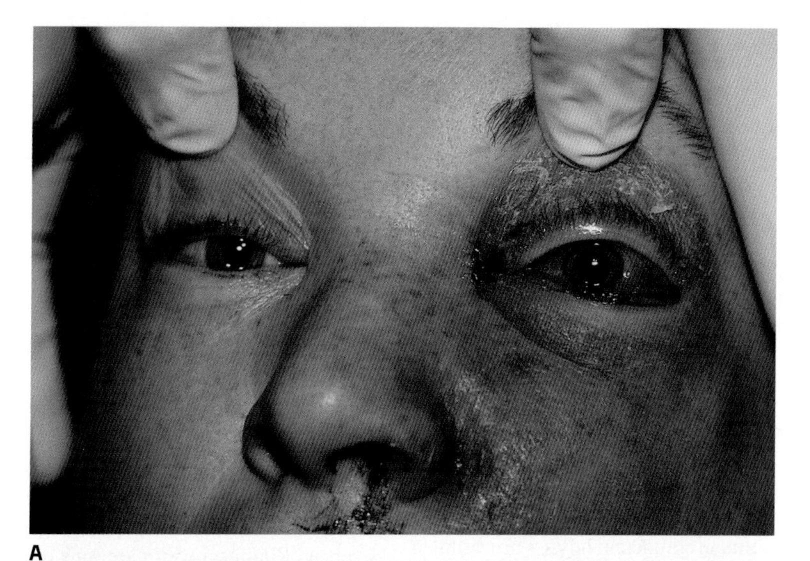

A

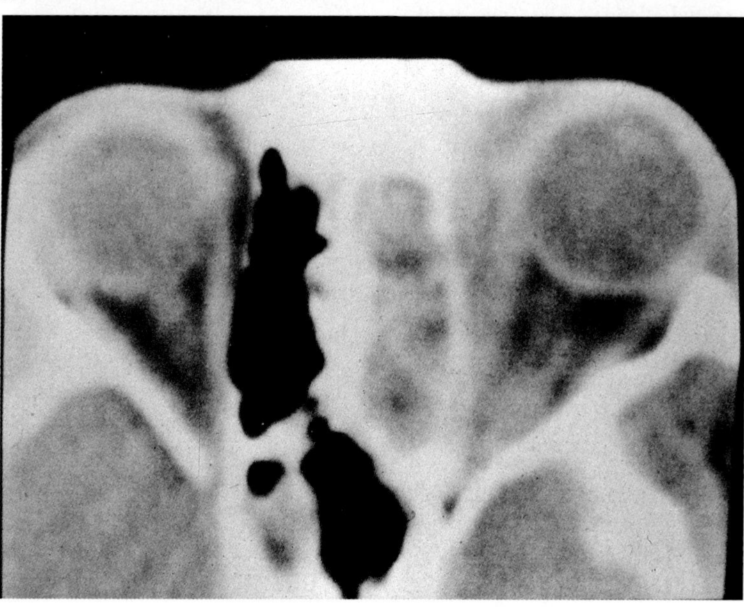

B

Figure 11-3 Phycomycosis **A.** *A patient with poorly controlled diabetes with a 1-week history of sinusitis. The patient has a frozen globe and a central retinal artery occlusion. There is a dusky erythema of the cheek.* **B.** *CT scan shows diffuse sinus disease with orbital involvement. Biopsy of the sinus revealed fungus consistent with phycomycosis.*

ASPERGILLOSIS

Aspergillosis occurs in two forms. One form, very similar to phycomycosis, occurs in immunocompromised patients and has a poor prognosis. The second form occurs in healthy patients with chronic sinus disease and allergies and has a good prognosis.

Epidemiology and Etiology

Age Adults.

Gender Equal male and female incidence.

Etiology An opportunistic infection that grows in the sinuses and secondarily invades the orbit. It can occur in two forms. One form acts like phycomycosis and thus occurs in immunocompromised hosts. The second, "allergic" form occurs in immune competent hosts with chronic sinus disease and allergies. The sinus is filled with mucin and fungus and may have bone erosion.

History

Aspergillosis occurring in immunocompromised hosts presents similar to phycomycosis. The allergic form will present as chronic sinus problems but will invade the orbit with time in 17 percent of patients, resulting in orbital signs depending on the sinus involved.

Examination

Findings on examination are dependent on the form of infection. The presentation of aspergillosis in the immunocompromised host is the same as that of phycomycosis and is only differentiated on biopsy. The allergic form will only present with orbital findings in the minority of cases. The signs vary from displacement of the globe to an orbital apex syndrome, depending on the location of the infection and exact direction of invasion (Fig. 11-4).

Imaging

CT scan will show sinus disease with secondary orbital invasion. MRI can be helpful in defining extent of the disease in the orbit and looking for possible CNS extension. The allergic form shows the sinus filled with mottled area of increased attenuation on nonenhanced CT scan. There may be areas of bone remodeling and even erosion. MRI imaging shows a signal void on T_2 images.

Pathology

Diagnosis is made by biopsy. Septate branching hyphae of uniform width are seen on Gomori's methenamine silver staining.

Differential Diagnosis

- Sinusitis with mucocele
- Phycomycosis
- Metastatic orbital tumor

Laboratory Tests

Immunocompromised patients will have associated blood finding such as ketoacidosis, leukopenia, and so forth, depending on the etiology of the immune deficiency. Patients with allergic form may have a peripheral blood eosinophilia, elevated total immunoglobulin E, and positive allergy skin testing for fungus.

Treatment

Immunocompromised patients with aspergillosis are treated the same as phycomycosis (see previous discussion). Cleaning out the mucin and fungus from the affected sinus and orbit definitively treats the allergic form.

Prognosis

Poor in the immunocompromised form. Good in the allergic form with appropriate treatment.

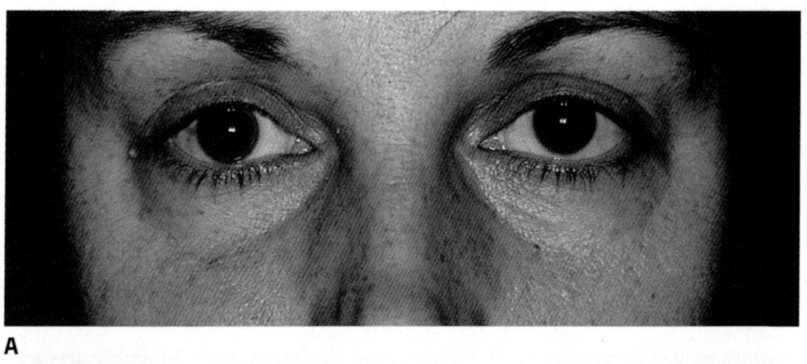

A

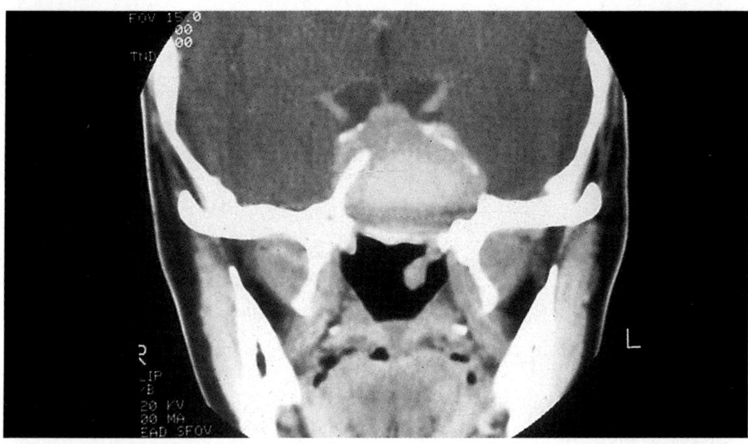

B

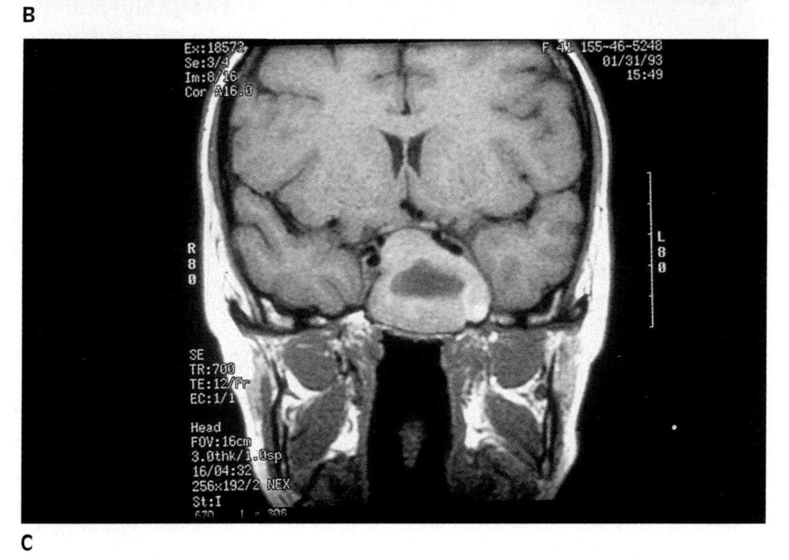

C

Figure 11-4 Aspergillosis **A.** *A 45-year-old patient with loss of vision in the left eye and very mild proptosis on the left. There are no other orbital signs.* **B.** *CT scan shows a large mass of the sphenoid sinus with erosion into the cavernous sinus.* **C.** *On MRI imaging, the central area of signal void is classic for aspergillosis. This mass was simply cleaned out via transnasal sinus surgery and the vision returned to normal.*

Chapter 12

ORBITAL INFLAMMATION

THYROID-RELATED OPHTHALMOPATHY

Thyroid-related ophthalmopathy (TRO) is the most common cause of proptosis in adults. The disease can range from mild eyelid retraction to severe proptosis with optic nerve compression and corneal exposure. Early in the disease course TRO can be difficult to diagnose but later the ocular signs become classic.

Epidemiology and Etiology

Age Rare in children, mainly adults.

Gender Women affected 5 to 8 times more often than men.

Etiology Poorly understood autoimmune inflammatory process that affects the orbital tissues.

History

Initial onset of nonspecific ocular irritation followed by eyelid retraction, lid lag, eyelid swelling, and bulging of the eyes. Patients will note symptoms to be worse in the morning and improve over the day. Many patients will have the history of a systemic thyroid imbalance but up to 30 percent may be euthyroid at the onset of symptoms.

Examination

The earliest signs of TRO are very nonspecific and it can be difficult to make the diagnosis at this time. Eyelid retraction and eyelid lag are also early signs that will help confirm the diagnosis. As the disease progresses, chemosis, proptosis, and motility restriction with diplopia will become apparent. Late signs are decreased vision from optic nerve compression and severe corneal exposure (Fig. 12-1A to F).

Imaging

CT scan will show enlargement of the rectus muscles with tendon sparing. The inferior rectus is the most commonly involved muscle followed by medial rectus and superior rectus. The lateral rectus is rarely involved. CT scan is not needed to make the diagnosis of TRO, as this is a clinical diagnosis. CT scanning is helpful to confirm unusual cases, evaluate optic nerve compression, and before surgery or irradiation (Fig. 12-1G and H).

Special Considerations

The course and severity of disease is widely variable. Patients may have a few months of mild inflammation without any sequelae, whereas others can have severe inflammation that can lead to severe proptosis, double vision, and visual loss over a few months or years.

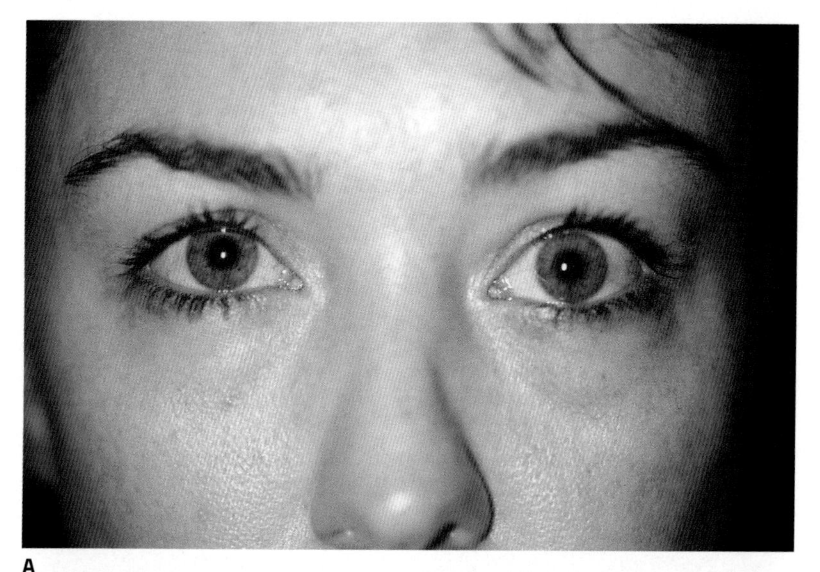

A

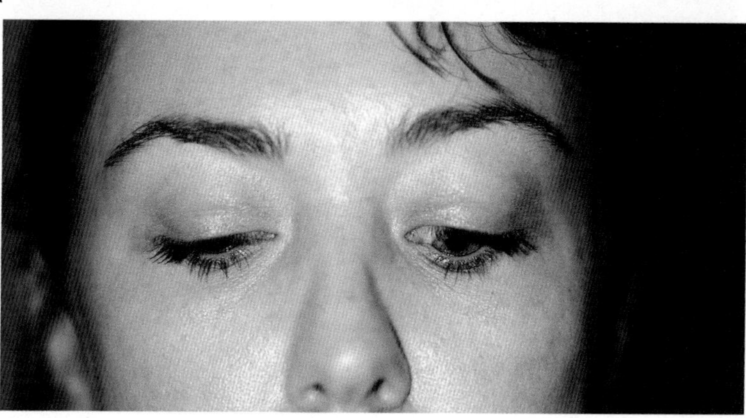

B

Figure 12-1 Thyroid-related ophthalmopathy **A.** *A patient with very early thyroid-related ophthalmopathy with slight lid retraction on the left.* **B.** *In down gaze, there is eyelid lag.* *(Continued.)*

Differential Diagnosis

- Orbital pseudotumor
- Orbital cellulitis
- Orbital lymphoma

Laboratory Tests

Thyroid stimulating hormone.

Pathophysiology

Chronic inflammatory process leads to deposition of glycosaminoglycans in the muscles and orbital fat with eventual scarring and dysfunction of these tissues.

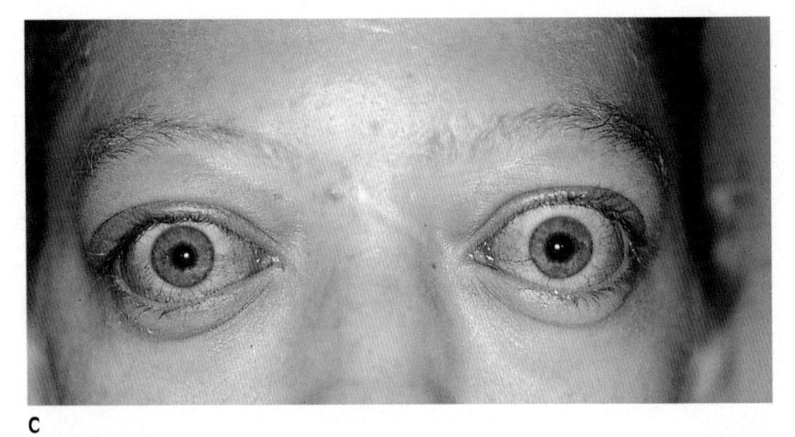

C

Figure 12-1 Thyroid-related ophthalmopathy (cont.) **C.** *A 20-year-old patient with severe proptosis, eyelid retraction, and corneal exposure. (Continued.)*

Treatment

Limiting the inflammation will limit the scarring and severity of the disease. Systemic steroids will decrease inflammation but because of the side effects from long-term use, they are usually limited to use as a temporary, short-term treatment. Orbital irradiation appears to be effective at stopping the progression of the disease but not very effective at reversing any of the changes that have occurred. Any patient with significant, active disease is a potential candidate for irradiation. Once the inflammatory phase is over, surgical correction of residual proptosis, diplopia, and eyelid deformities can be considered. This is done via a combination of orbital decompression and eye muscle and eyelid surgery. Patients presenting with severe inflammation and an optic neuropathy or corneal decompensation can require an urgent orbital decompression.

Prognosis

Good but some patients may require multiple surgical procedures over years as part of the treatment.

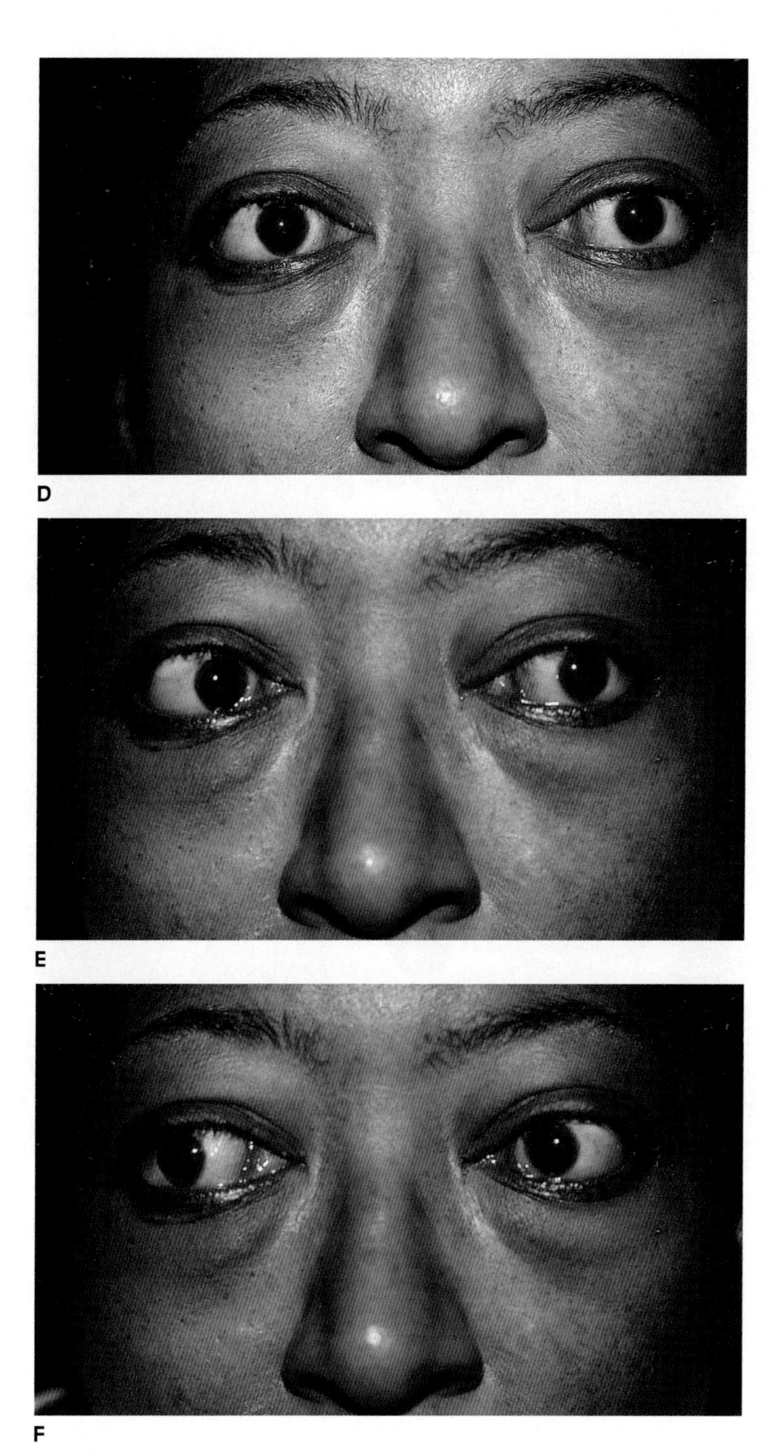

Figure 12-1 Thyroid-related ophthalmopathy (cont.) **D** *to* **F.** *A 45-year-old patient with progressive swelling of the eyes with double vision and recent decreased vision. There is proptosis, chemosis, and limitation of motility. Vision was 20/80 from optic nerve compression. (Continued.)*

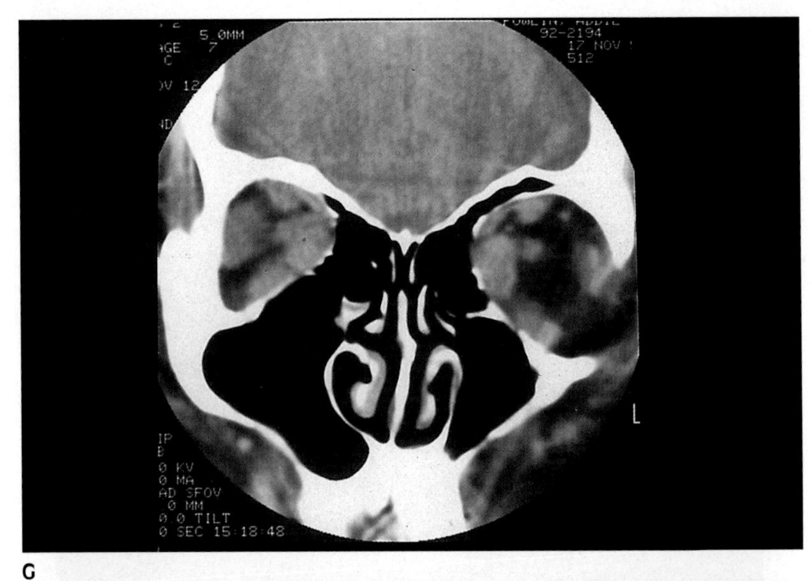

G

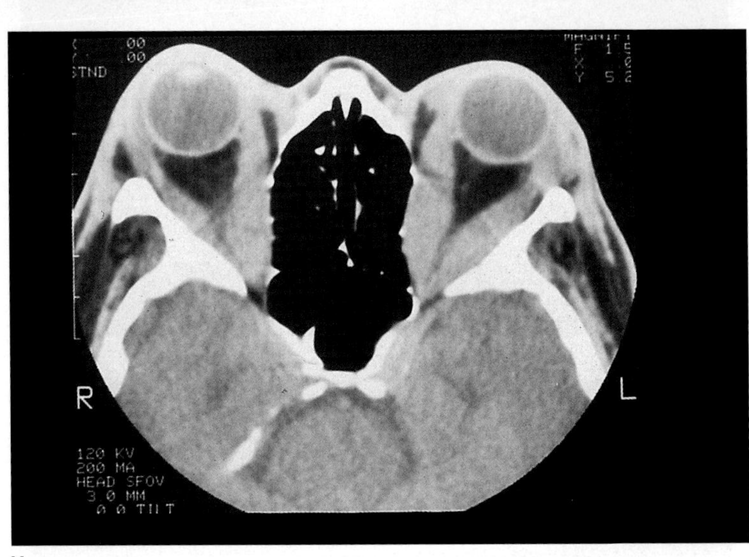

H

Figure 12-1 Thyroid-related ophthalmopathy (cont.) **G** *and* **H.** *CT scan shows enlargement of all rectus muscles with crowding at the orbital apex. The patient required an orbital decompression and her vision returned to normal. (Continued.)*

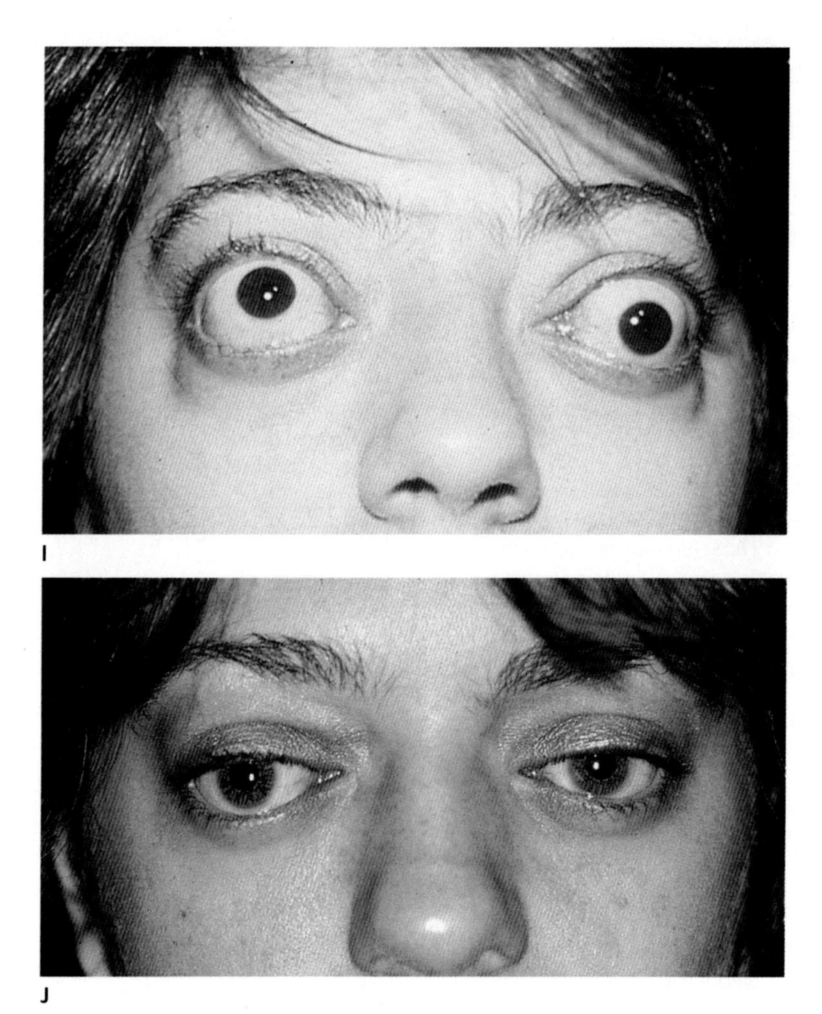

Figure 12-1 Thyroid-related ophthalmopathy (cont.) **I.** *A patient with severe thyroid-related ophthalmopathy.* **J.** *After 3 years and multiple surgeries, there is significant improvement.*

IDIOPATHIC ORBITAL INFLAMMATION (ORBITAL PSEUDOTUMOR)

Epidemiology and Etiology

Age Children and adults.

Gender Equal incidence in males and females.

Etiology This inflammatory process is by definition unrelated to any systemic abnormality and the cause remains unknown.

History

Acute onset of orbital pain often associated with proptosis, erythema, swelling, and restricted eye movements. The symptoms depend on the exact location of the process but pain is common to all presentations. Adults more commonly have unilateral disease but in children this can be a bilateral process.

Examination

The acute inflammatory process can occur anteriorly and present with acute erythema and swelling of the lids and globe. It may present as a myositis with restricted motility and pain with eye movement, as a scleritis, a dacryoadenitis, or in the orbital apex with few external signs but significant pain, dysmotility, and decreased vision. The presentation is variable depending on the tissues affected. Patients with orbital pseudotumor can have a fever and a leukocytosis (Fig. 12-2).

Imaging

CT scanning will show thickening of the affected tissues such as enlarged muscles, thickened sclera, enlarged lacrimal gland, or an infiltrate in the orbital fat.

Special Considerations

Rarely, there may be very few inflammatory signs and a more chronic fibrotic process that is termed sclerosing inflammatory orbital pseudotumor. This condition is not very responsive to treatment as treatment is geared toward eliminating inflammation and there is very little in this process. Systemic conditions, such as sarcoidosis, may cause a very similar picture.

Differential Diagnosis

- Orbital cellulitis
- Thyroid-related ophthalmopathy
- Lymphoma
- Ruptured dermoid cyst
- Metastatic disease

Laboratory Tests

Patients may have a leukocytosis, peripheral blood eosinophilia, elevated ESR, and a positive ANA. None of these are diagnostic.

Pathophysiology

A pleomorphic cellular inflammatory response occurs and if not treated or not responsive to treatment there will be a resultant fibrotic response that will progress with time and result in chronic scarring.

Treatment

Systemic steroids are the mainstay of treatment. There should be an improvement in symptoms in 24 to 48 hours. The longer the process has been present, the longer it can take for a clinical response. Once there is a good clinical response, the steroids are tapered over 4 to 6 weeks. Patients without response to steroids or with multiple recurrences of the inflammation require an orbital biopsy to confirm the diagnosis. If confirmed, they are then candidates for orbital irradiation.

Prognosis

Excellent prognosis in most acute cases. There may be recurrences. Cases that are chronic with less inflammatory response are less responsive to treatment and can be progressive.

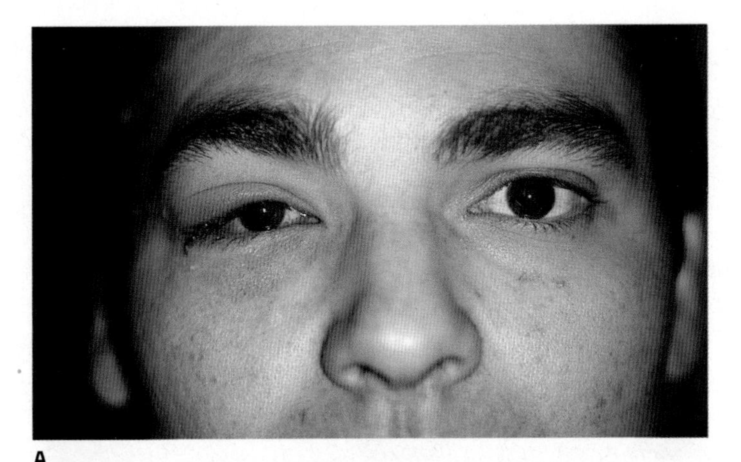

A

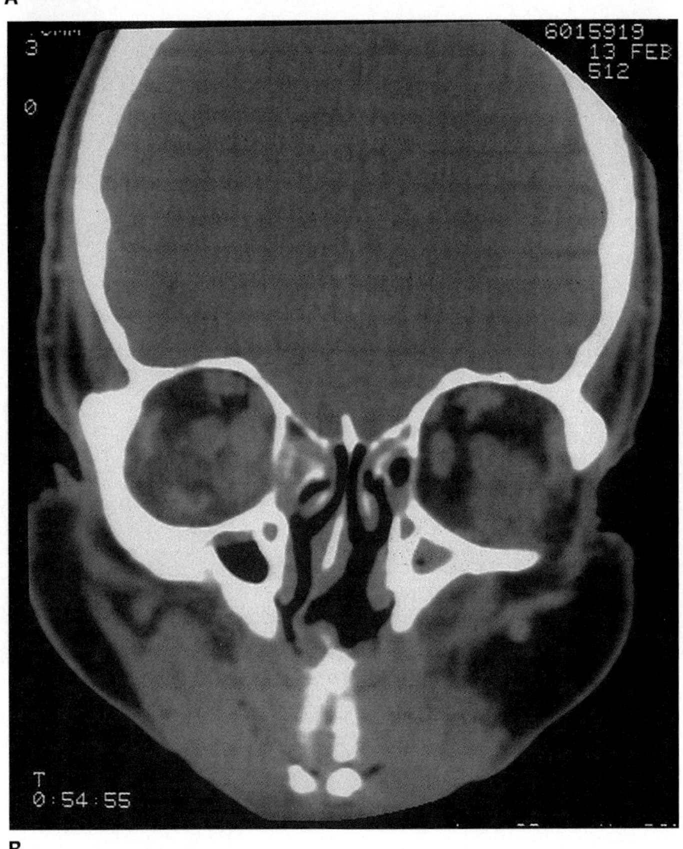

B

Figure 12-2 Orbital pseudotumor **A.** *A 33-year-old male with a 5-day history of swelling, erythema, and pain that is worse with eye movement. The eye is red with orbital swelling and tenderness to palpation. Eye movements are limited by pain.* **B.** *Diffuse infiltration of the orbit and slight enlargement of the medial rectus. The clinical presentation along with the CT scan are consistent with orbital pseudotumor. The patient responded within 24 hours to oral prednisone. (Continued.)*

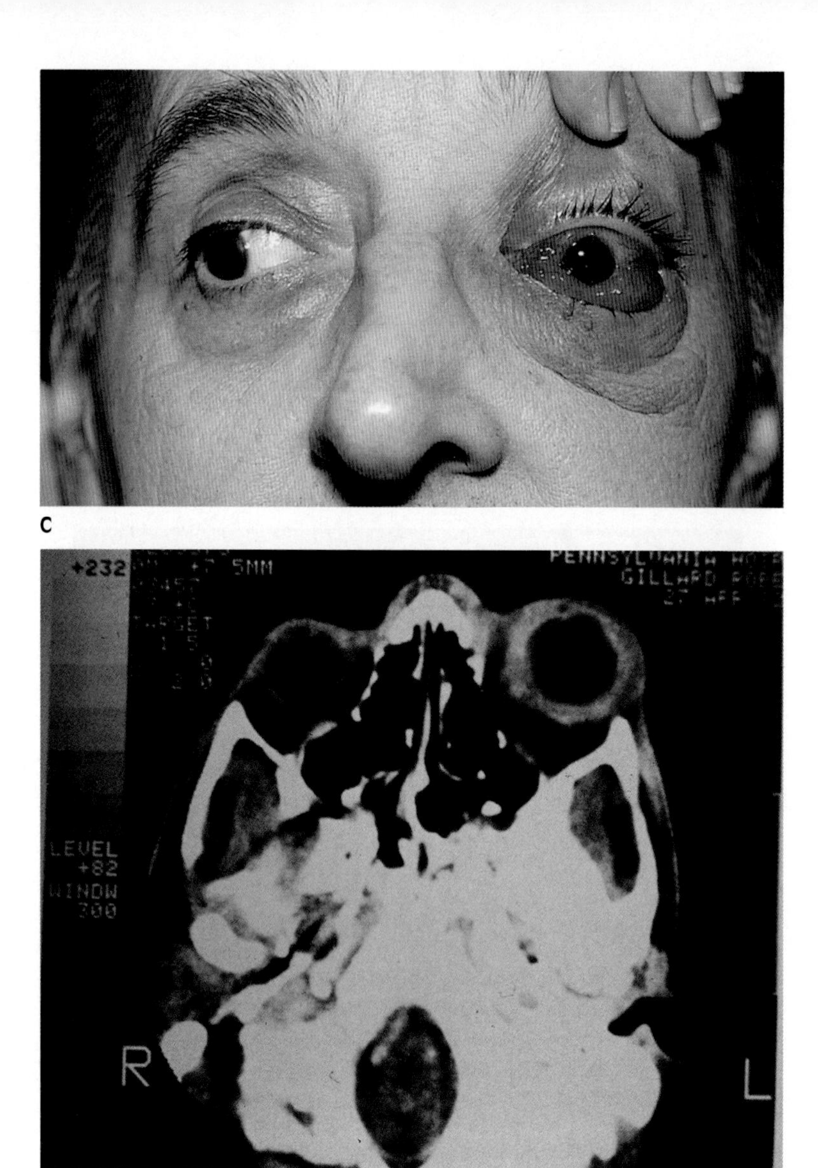

Figure 12-2 Orbital pseudotumor (cont.) **C.** *This is a scleritis with some anterior orbital swelling.* **D.** *Diffuse scleral thickening on left side. (Continued.)*

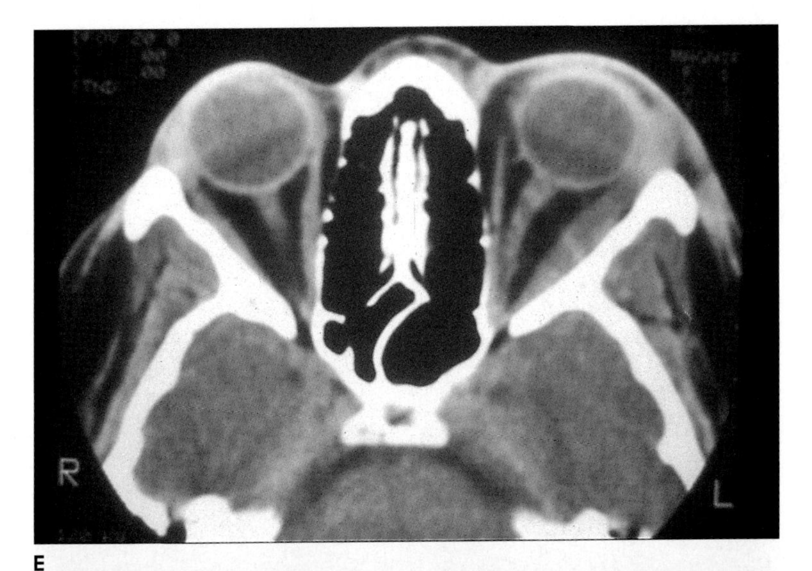

E

F

Figure 12-2 Orbital pseudotumor (cont.) **E.** *CT shows a diffuse enlargement of the lateral rectus muscle consistent with a myositis. The patient had limited adduction and abduction as well as pain with eye movement.* **F.** *CT scan showing inflammation at the orbital apex. On examination, the eye may be white and quiet with minimal proptosis. There is often decreased vision and motility dysfunction consistent with an orbital apex syndrome.*

SARCOIDOSIS

Sarcoidosis can occur in the orbit in multiple forms and with varying amounts of inflammation. Most commonly, it presents with lacrimal gland enlargement with very mild inflammatory signs. Sarcoidosis may have a much more acute swelling and can affect the sclera, extraocular muscles, or other orbital tissues.

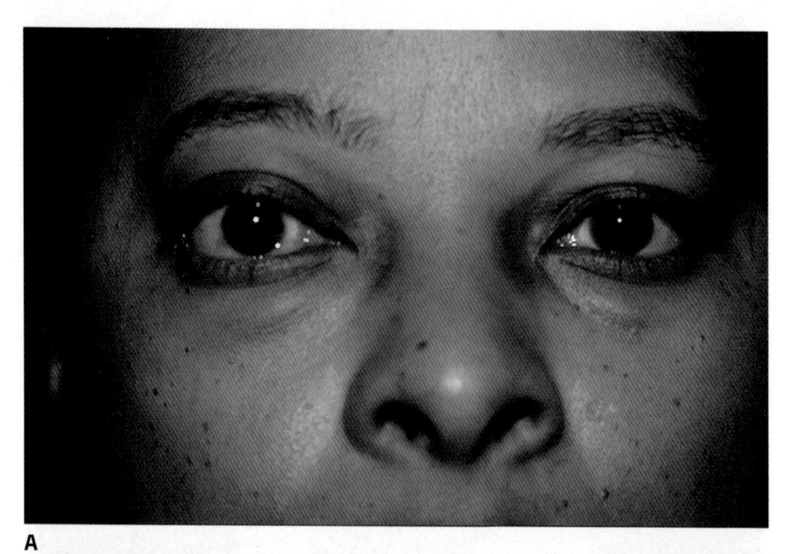

A

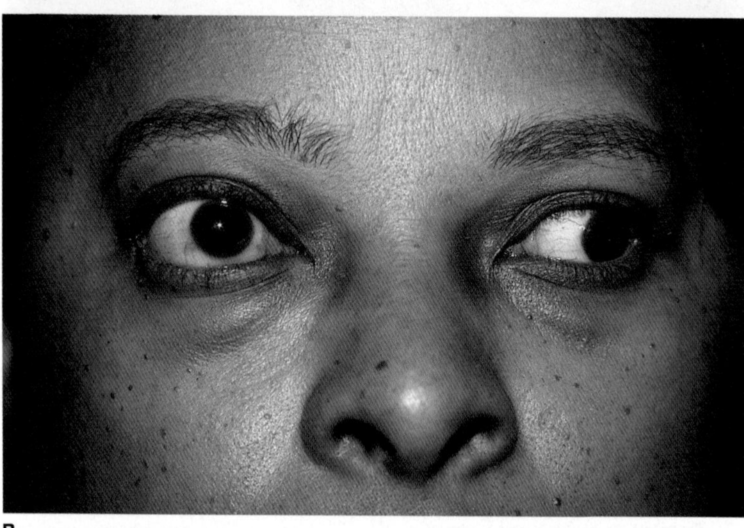

B

Figure 12-3 Orbital sarcoidosis **A.** *and* **B.** *A patient with proptosis and double vision with some mild aching of the right eye. Motility shows poor adduction of the right eye. (Continued.)*

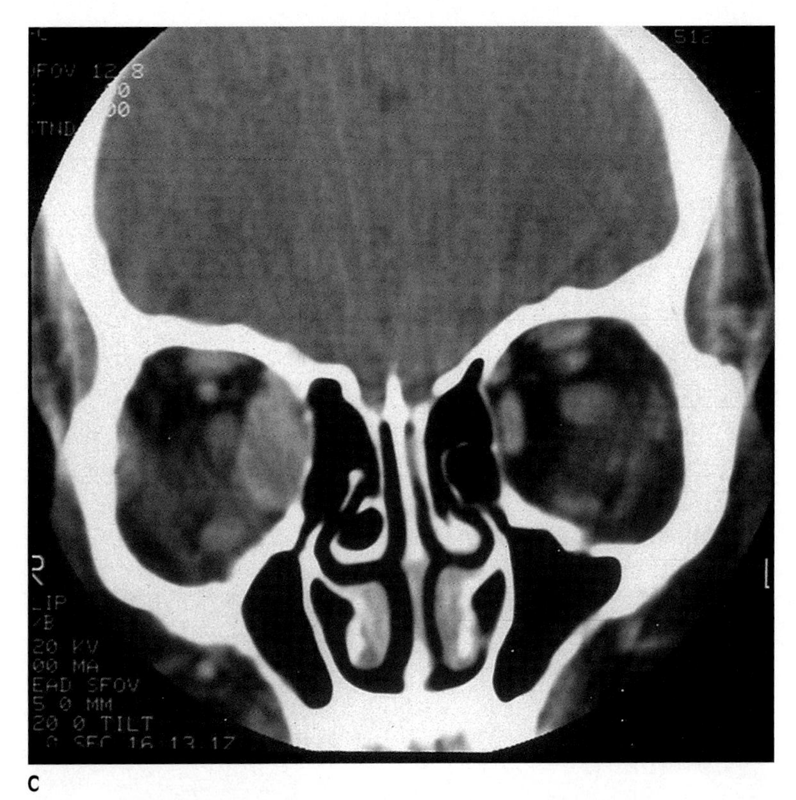

C

Figure 12-3 Orbital sarcoidosis (cont.) **C.** *CT scan shows an enlarged medial rectus muscle. This myositis responded to oral prednisone but recurred. Biopsy showed sarcoidosis. (Continued.)*

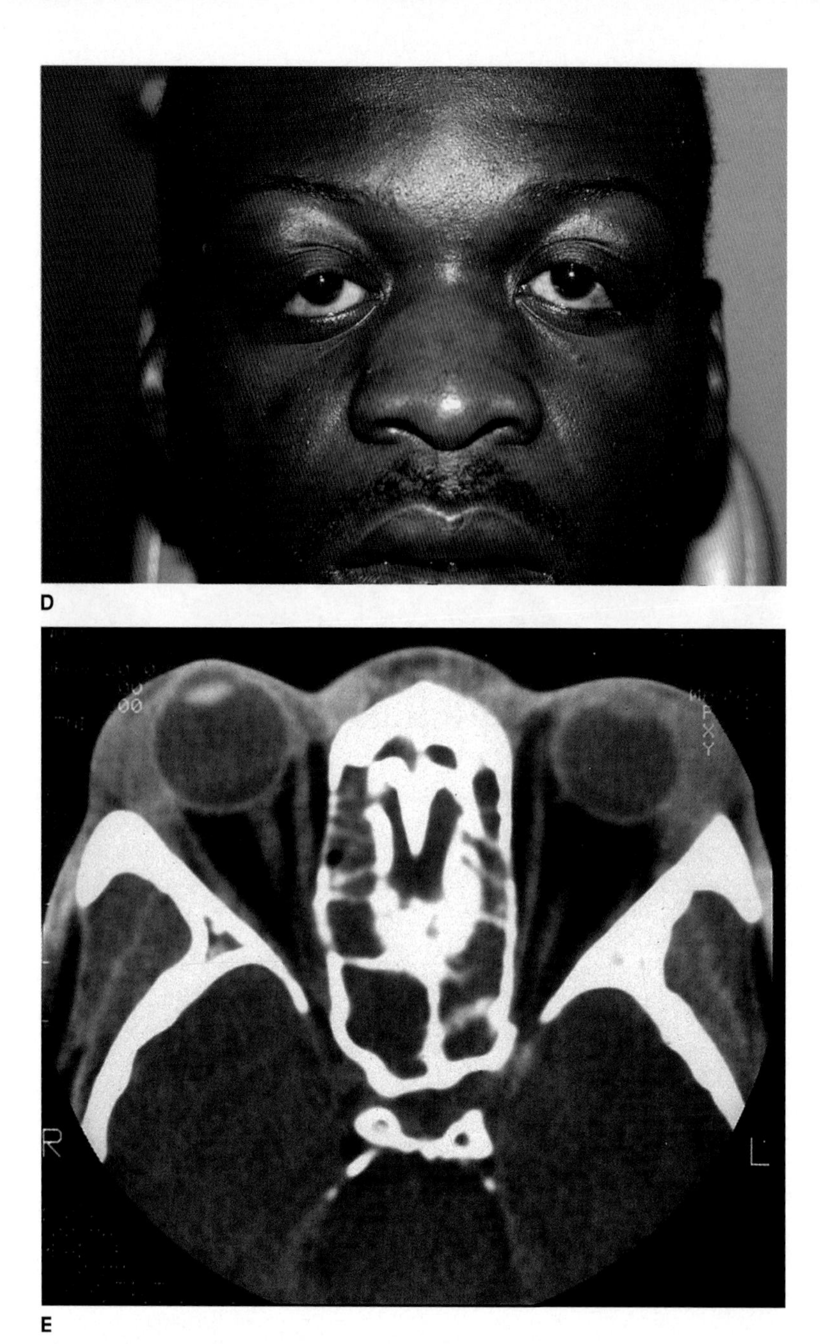

Figure 12-3 Orbital sarcoidosis (cont.) **D.** *Bilateral lacrimal gland enlargement on the external photograph.* **E** *and* **F.** *Axial and coronal CT scan shows enlarged lacrimal glands. Biopsy showed sarcoidosis. (Continued.)*

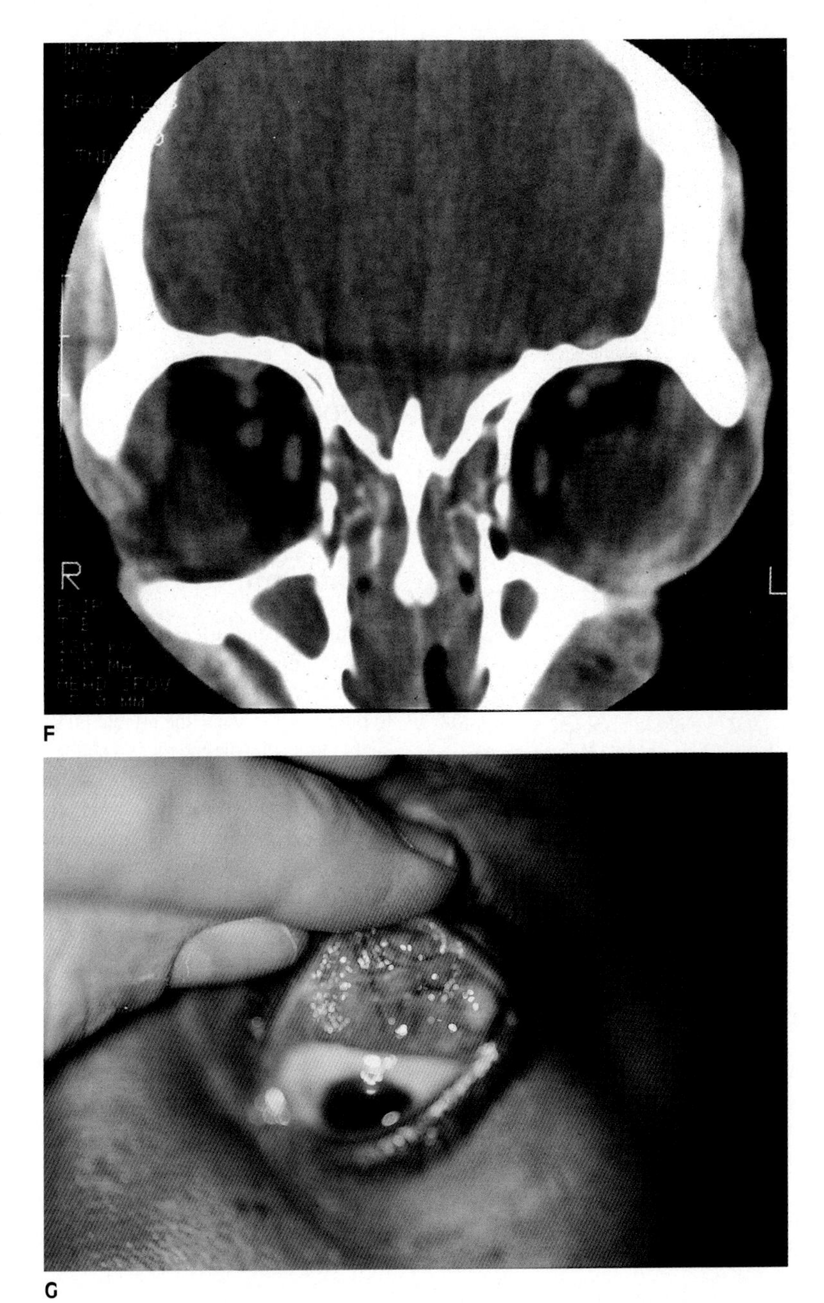

G

Figure 12-3 Orbital sarcoidosis (cont.) **G.** *Infiltration of the eyelid and anterior lacrimal tissue by sarcoidosis. Under the eyelid, the infiltration is yellow-brown with prominent blood vessels.*

SARCOIDOSIS (cont.)

Epidemiology and Etiology

Age Any age but most common in adulthood.

Gender Equal.

Etiology Multisystem inflammatory disease that occurs primarily in individuals of African and Scandinavian descent.

History

Most commonly presents with lacrimal gland enlargement with varying amount of inflammatory signs.

Examination

Bilateral lacrimal gland enlargement is the most common presentation. Extraocular muscles, the optic nerve, and eyelid skin are less commonly affected. Inflammation in adjacent sinuses may secondarily affect the orbit. The entire eye must be evaluated for signs of sarcoidosis causing uveitis (anterior or posterior), iris nodules, or retinal vascular changes. Conjunctival granulomas as well as sarcoid skin lesions can help confirm the diagnosis (Fig. 12-3).

Imaging

CT scanning will show enlargement of the lacrimal gland, muscle, or other affected structure. Chest x-ray or a chest CT is needed to evaluate the lungs for possible pulmonary sarcoidosis.

Special Considerations

Most patients with sarcoidosis will have systemic disease with pulmonary findings. Some patients will have the disease isolated to the orbit without systemic findings.

Differential Diagnosis

- Idiopathic orbital pseudotumor
- Dacryoadenititis

Laboratory Tests

Angiotensin converting enzyme (ACE) may be helpful in establishing the diagnosis.

Treatment

A biopsy of the affected tissue is usually required to confirm the diagnosis of sarcoidosis. When present, a conjunctival nodule is simple to biopsy. Otherwise, the affected tissue is biopsied. Once the diagnosis is established, careful systemic evaluation is needed to look for sarcoid. Treatment is most commonly systemic prednisone although other immunosuppressive agents have been used. Treatment is usually aimed at disease control whether it is for control of orbital inflammation or to control pulmonary disease.

Prognosis

Most patients do well but rare patients can have significant systemic manifestations. The orbital disease can be chronic and recurrent.

WEGENER'S GRANULOMATOSIS

Wegener's granulomatosis can involve the eye and orbit as a secondary extension from the sinuses or it can present involving the eye itself with scleritis, keratitis, uveitis, and so forth. The systemic disease can be life-threatening and the ocular involvement can cause blindness and loss of the eye.

Epidemiology and Etiology

Age Mainly adults.

Gender Equal occurrence in males and females.

Etiology A systemic necrotizing granulomatous vasculitis that classically affects the upper and lower respiratory tract, and can affect the small vessels of any major organ system.

History

Diagnosis may or may not already be made when the patient presents with eye findings. Most commonly, there is bony erosion via extension of the disease into the orbit from the sinus cavity. Patients can also have a necrotizing scleritis, which can be severe.

Examination

Findings include scleritis, which may be anterior or posterior and is often necrotizing. Proptosis with or without orbital inflammation may be present (Fig 12-4A).

Imaging

CT scans show bone erosion from sinus extension of the disease (Fig 12-4B,C).

Differential Diagnosis

- Malignant tumor of the sinus

Laboratory Tests

Antineutrophil cytoplasmic antibodies (ANCA) are often present with Wegener's disease.

Pathology

Vasculitis, granulomatous inflammation, and tissue necrosis are found on pathologic evaluation.

Treatment

Immunosuppressive medication, specifically corticosteroids and cyclophosphamide, is the treatment of choice.

Prognosis

Variable. The disease can be progressive and fatal.

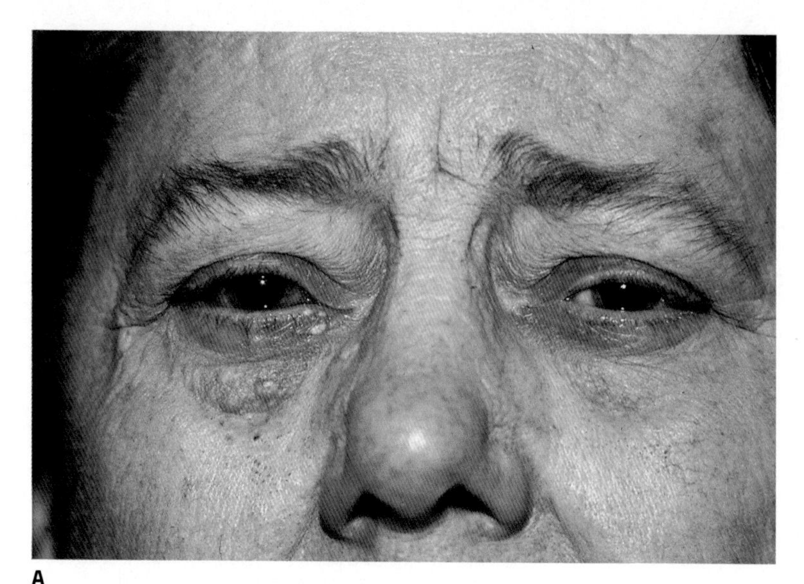

A

Figure 12-4 Wegener's granulomatosis **A.** *A patient with orbital pseudotumorlike picture. (Continued.)*

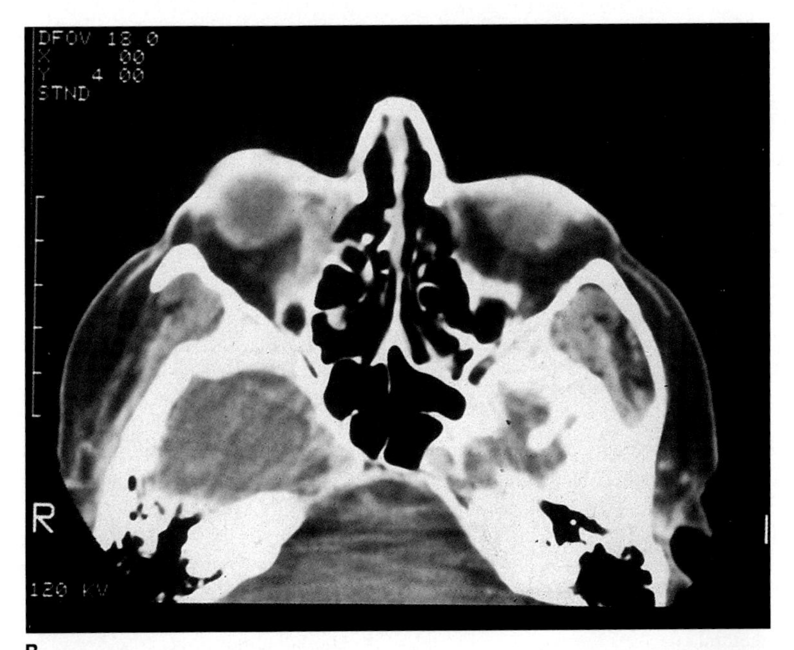

B

C

Figure 12-4 Wegener's granulomatosis (cont.) **B** *and* **C.** *CT scans show infiltration along the inferior–medial orbit and into the sinus. Poor response to prednisone and a positive ANCA led to a biopsy, which was consistent with Wegener's granulomatosis.*

Chapter 13

CONGENITAL ORBITAL ANOMALIES

MICROPHTHALMOS

Microphthalmos is a defect in the eye development. The eye is small and there are usually structural defects. The microphthalmos can be mild or the eye can be so small that it cannot easily be seen at all.

Epidemiology and Etiology

Age Congenital.

Gender Equal occurrence in males and females.

Etiology Developmental defect with failure of the choroidal fissure to close as an embryo. This results in a small eye with structural abnormalities (Fig. 13-1).

Examination

The eye may be small to virtually nonexistent. There are structural abnormalities within the eye and the eye usually has poor or no vision. There may be an accompanying cyst, which may be quite large. This condition is usually unilateral, rarely bilateral.

Differential Diagnosis

- Anophthalmos

Treatment

Treatment is aimed at stimulating the orbit to grow and mature normally. If the eye is only slightly small or if there is a large cyst, orbital growth may continue as normal. However, if the eye is very small, expanding conformers should be used to try to stimulate orbital growth. Dermis fat grafts are used sometimes.

Prognosis

These patients often have some orbital asymmetry even with aggressive treatment. The cosmetic result is generally acceptable.

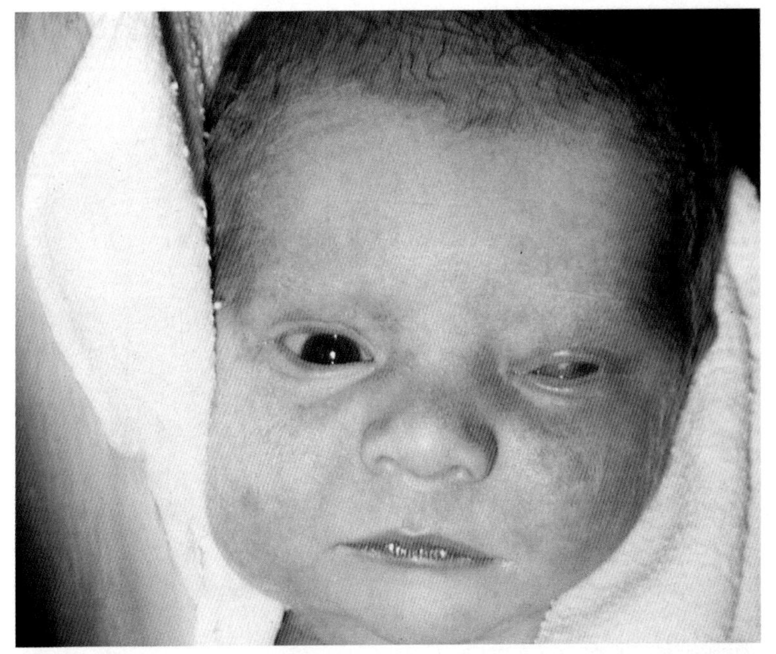

A

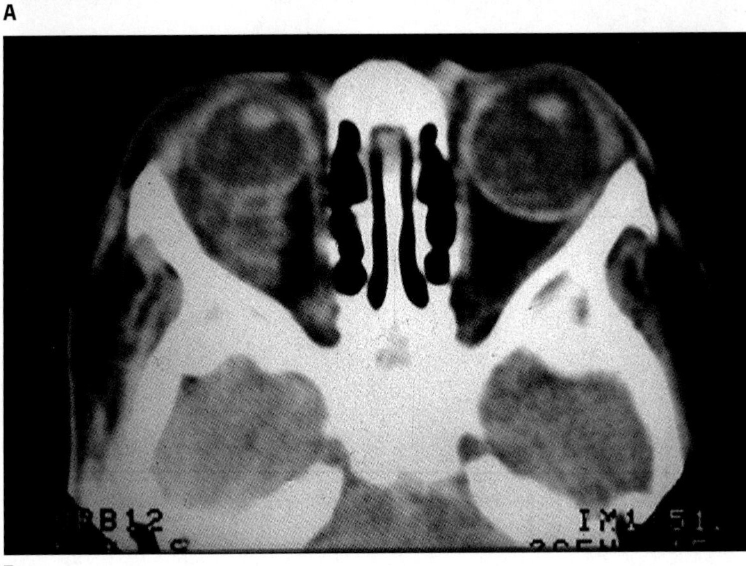

B

Figure 13-1 Microphthalmos **A.** *A child with microphthalmos with cyst.* **B.** *CT scan shows a small eye and attached cyst. (Continued.)*

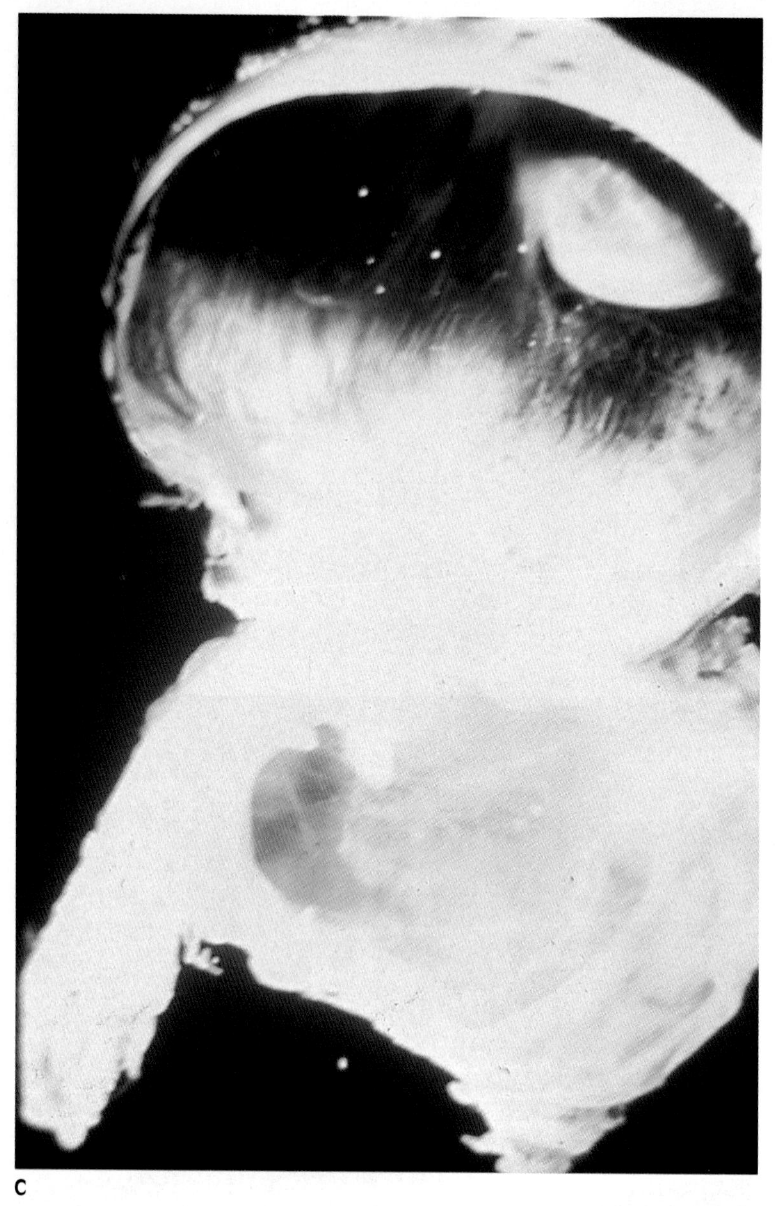

C

Figure 13-1 Microphthalmos (cont.) **C.** *Pathologic specimen shows the cystic outpouching coming from the abnormally developed eye.*

Chapter 14

ORBITAL NEOPLASMS

CONGENITAL ORBITAL TUMORS

DERMOID CYSTS

Dermoid cysts are relatively common, benign, orbital tumors in children. Classically, they are present at birth, are located superior temporally at the orbital rim, and enlarge with time.

Epidemiology and Etiology

Age Congenital and enlarge with age.

Gender Equally seen in males and females.

Etiology Epidermal elements are left during embryonic development in deeper tissues. These epidermal elements then form a cyst that enlarges with time.

History

More superficial dermoids are often noted in the first 1 to 2 years of life as they grow and become more noticeable. The dermoids that are deeper, such as in the orbit, may not become symptomatic until adulthood when they have become large, start to leak, or rupture from trauma.

Examination

The classic location for a superficial dermoid cyst is at the lateral brow over the frontozygomatic suture. Less commonly, they can be superior medial or even in the lower lid. They are smooth, painless masses that slowly enlarge. They can be freely mobile or fixed to the bony suture. Deeper dermoids can be in the superior and/or lateral orbit. "Dumbbell" dermoids occur in the temporal fossa and have a component in the orbit and a part in the temporal fossa. Deeper dermoids present with proptosis or with symptoms of orbital inflammation as the dermoid cyst either leaks or ruptures (Fig. 14-1).

Imaging

CT scan: nonenhancing cystic mass.
MRI: hypointense on T_1; hyperintense on T_2.

Differential Diagnosis

- When located superficially and temporally, there are very few lesions this can be confused with. Imaging usually helps make the diagnosis if located deep in the orbit.

Pathology

The cyst is lined by keratinizing epidermis with dermal appendages such as hair follicles and sebaceous glands. The cyst is filled with keratin and oil.

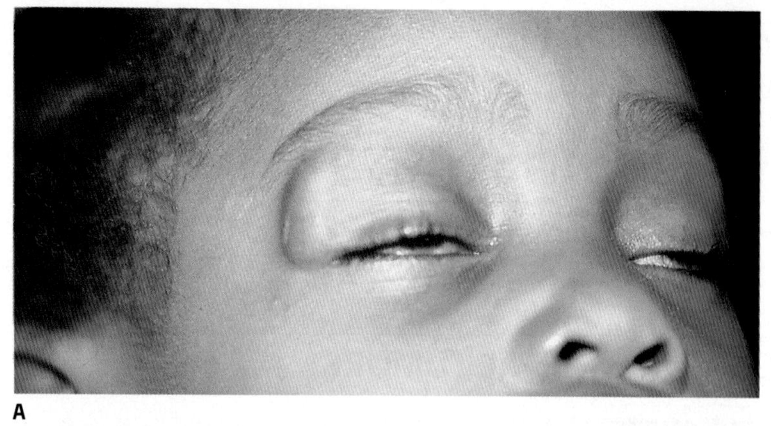

A

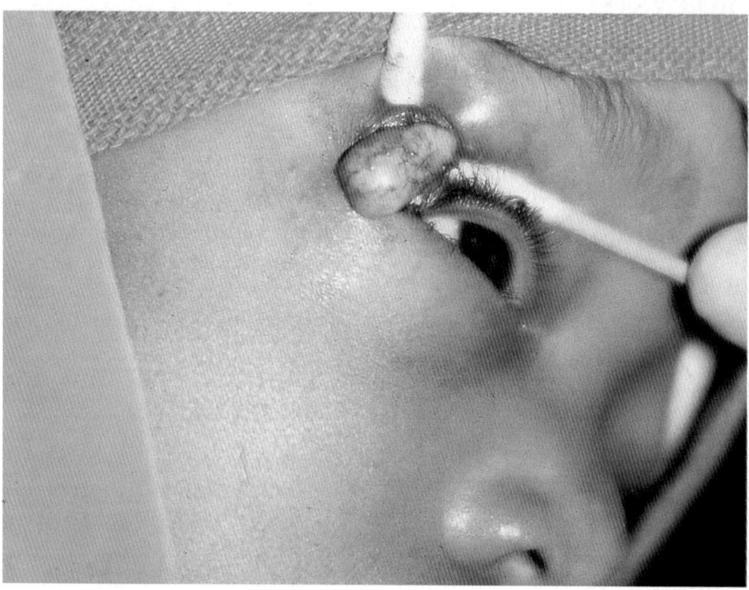

B

Figure 14-1 Dermoid cyst **A.** *Soft, mobile mass along the superior temporal rim in a 1-year-old patient. This has been present since birth.* **B.** *Excision of the dermoid through a lid crease incision. (Continued.)*

Treatment

Complete surgical excision with an intact capsule is the surgery of choice. This procedure should be done when the potential for cyst rupture becomes a risk. This most often occurs when the child begins to walk and be more active.

Prognosis

Excellent for superficial dermoids. Good for deep dermoids as long as the entire cyst is removed.

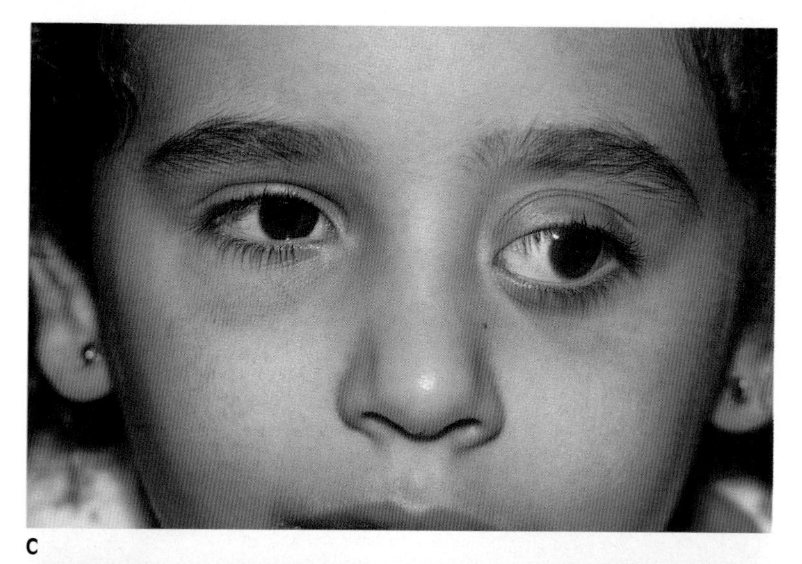

C

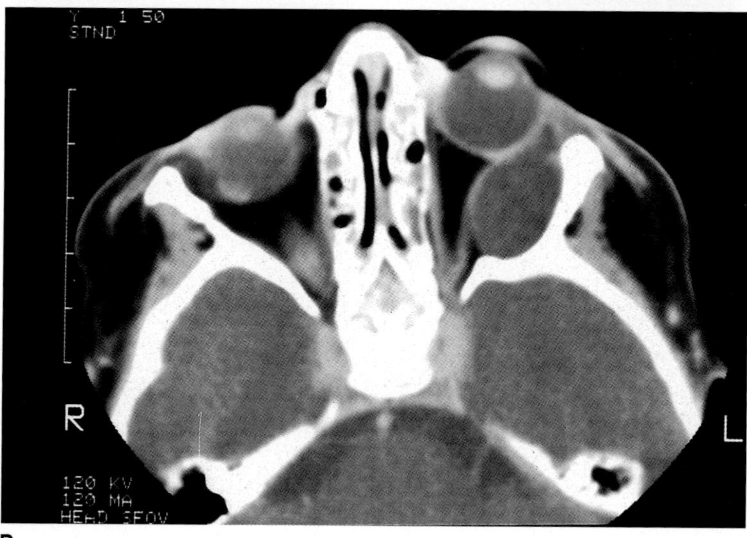

D

Figure 14-1 Dermoid cyst (cont.) **C.** *and* **D.** *Proptosis and globe displacement caused by a deep orbital dermoid which was noted at age 5 years. The fossa formation caused by these lesions is seen on the CT scan. The deep orbital location means they are often not noticed until the child is older. This was completely excised and the patient did well without any further problems. (Continued.)*

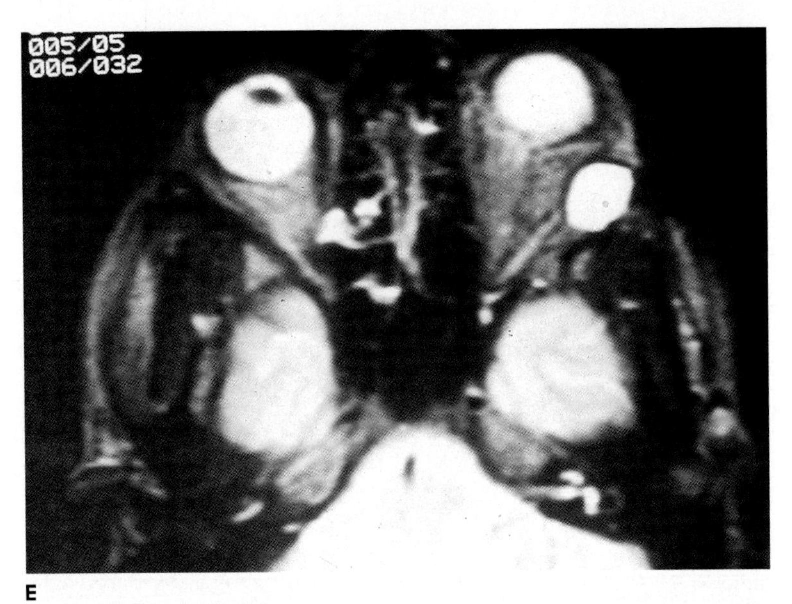

E

Figure 14-1 Dermoid cyst (cont.) **E.** *MRI of a dermoid cyst. On a T_2-weighted image the cyst is hyperintense to fat and muscle.*

LIPODERMOIDS

Lipodermoids are congenital solid tumors located temporally below the conjunctiva. These are sometimes not noted until later in life. They should be left alone in almost all cases.

Epidemiology and Etiology

Age Congenital.

Gender Equal occurrence in males and females.

Etiology Developmental anomaly.

History

Present at birth and generally does not change with time.

Examination

Yellowish, pink lesion over the lateral surface of the globe deep to the conjunctiva. They vary in size and often have hairs on the surface (Fig. 14-2).

Imaging

If large, CT scan will show a mass with fat density.

Differential Diagnosis

- Fat prolapse
- Lymphoma
- Prolapsed lacrimal gland

Pathology

Keratinizing squamous epithelium with adenexal structures. The underlying dermis usually contains fat and connective tissue.

Treatment

No treatment. Attempted excision can damage the adjacent lacrimal ducts and rectus or levator muscles. In rare cases when the lipodermoid is very large, the anterior portion can be debulked leaving the conjunctiva unresected.

Prognosis

Excellent if left alone.

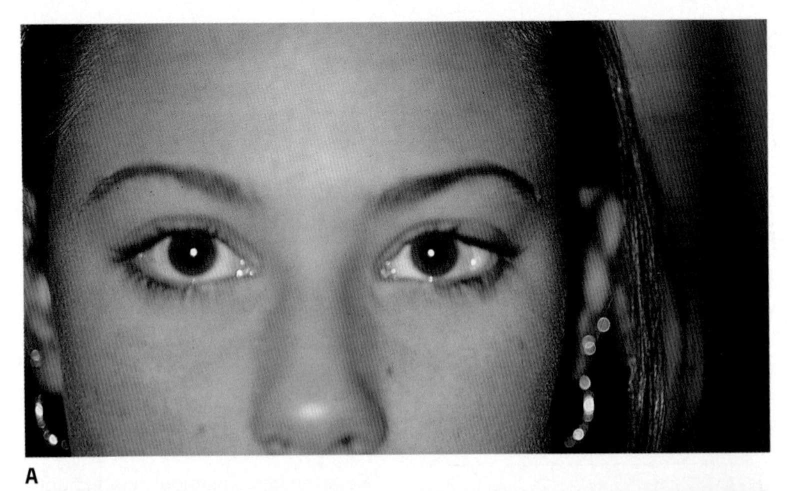

A

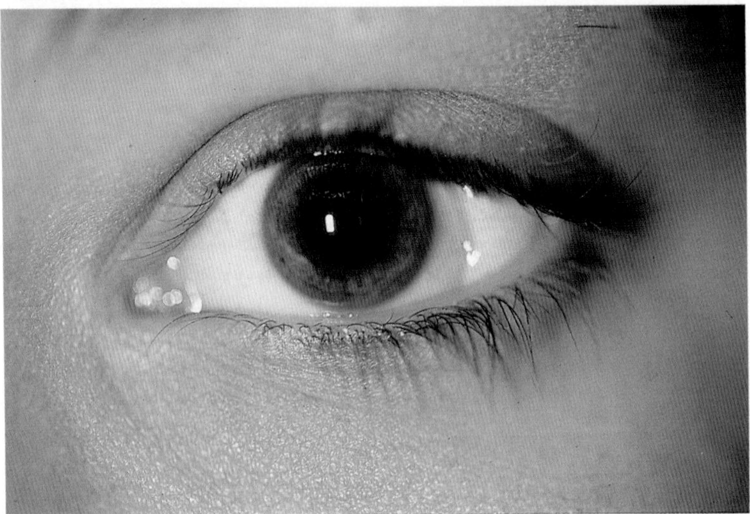

B

Figure 14-2 Lipodermoid **A.** *Classic location for a lipodermoid, which has been present since birth.* **B.** *Close inspection often shows hairs on the lesion. Despite the cosmetic appearance, these are best left alone.*

VASCULAR ORBITAL TUMORS

CAPILLARY HEMANGIOMAS

Capillary hemangiomas are benign tumors of the orbit that appear in the first few weeks of life and enlarge over the first 6 to 12 months. They then tend to shrink over time but the initial presentation can be dramatic.

Epidemiology and Etiology

Age Noted in the first year of life.

Gender Equally seen in males and females.

Etiology Abnormal growth of blood vessels with varying degrees of endothelial cell proliferation.

History

Lesions are often noted in first few weeks of life and they grow, sometimes rapidly, over weeks to months. They can present deeper in the orbit with proptosis or more superficially as an expanding mass. The hemangioma will then involute over months to years. Seventy five percent of lesions will resolve over 4 years.

Examination

The lesion appearance is dependent on the location. The more common superficial lesions produce an elevated, dimpled, strawberry-colored lesion. Deeper lesions may give a bluish discoloration. Deep orbital lesions may only give symptoms of an expanding orbital mass. Differentiation between rhabdomyosarcoma and deep capillary hemangioma can only be made with biopsy (Fig. 14-3).

Imaging

CT scan reveals a mass that can be well or poorly marginated with enhancement with contrast. MRI is hypointense on T_1 and hyperintense on T_2. The lesion enhances with gadolinium.

Differential Diagnosis

- Rhabdomyosarcoma

Pathology

Proliferation of endothelial cells organized into a network of basement membrane lined vascular channels.

Treatment

These lesions will regress so hemangiomas are observed for regression unless they cause visual obstruction or astigmatism leading to amblyopia. In this case, treatment is required. Orbital lesions causing severe proptosis may also require treatment. Orbital biopsy is required if the lesion cannot be differentiated from a rhabdomyosarcoma. Treatment options include intralesional steroid injection, systemic steroids, or, in select cases, surgical excision.

Prognosis

Good.

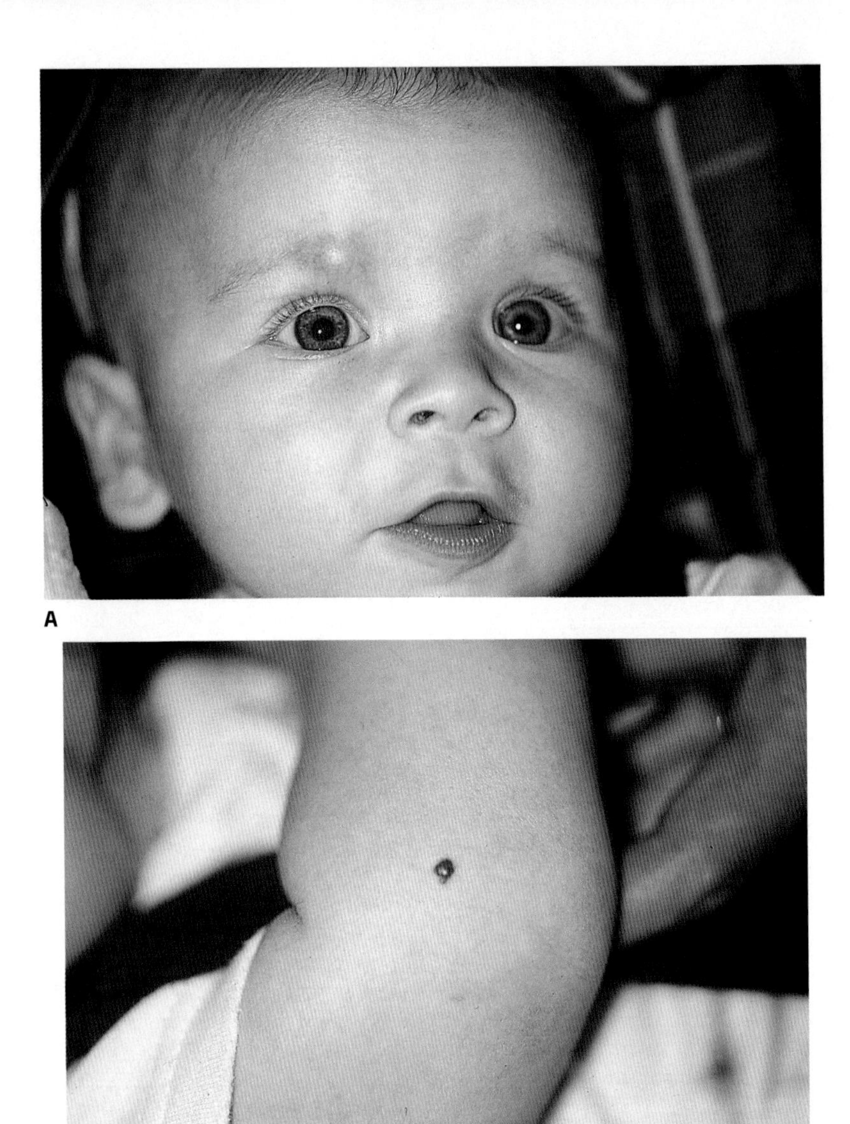

Figure 14-3 Capillary hemangioma **A.** *Subcutaneous capillary hemangioma of the right eyebrow that increased in size over 6 months. The lesion becomes more prominent and red with crying. This lesion resolved over 3 years.* **B.** *A small hemangioma on the child's arm. (Continued.)*

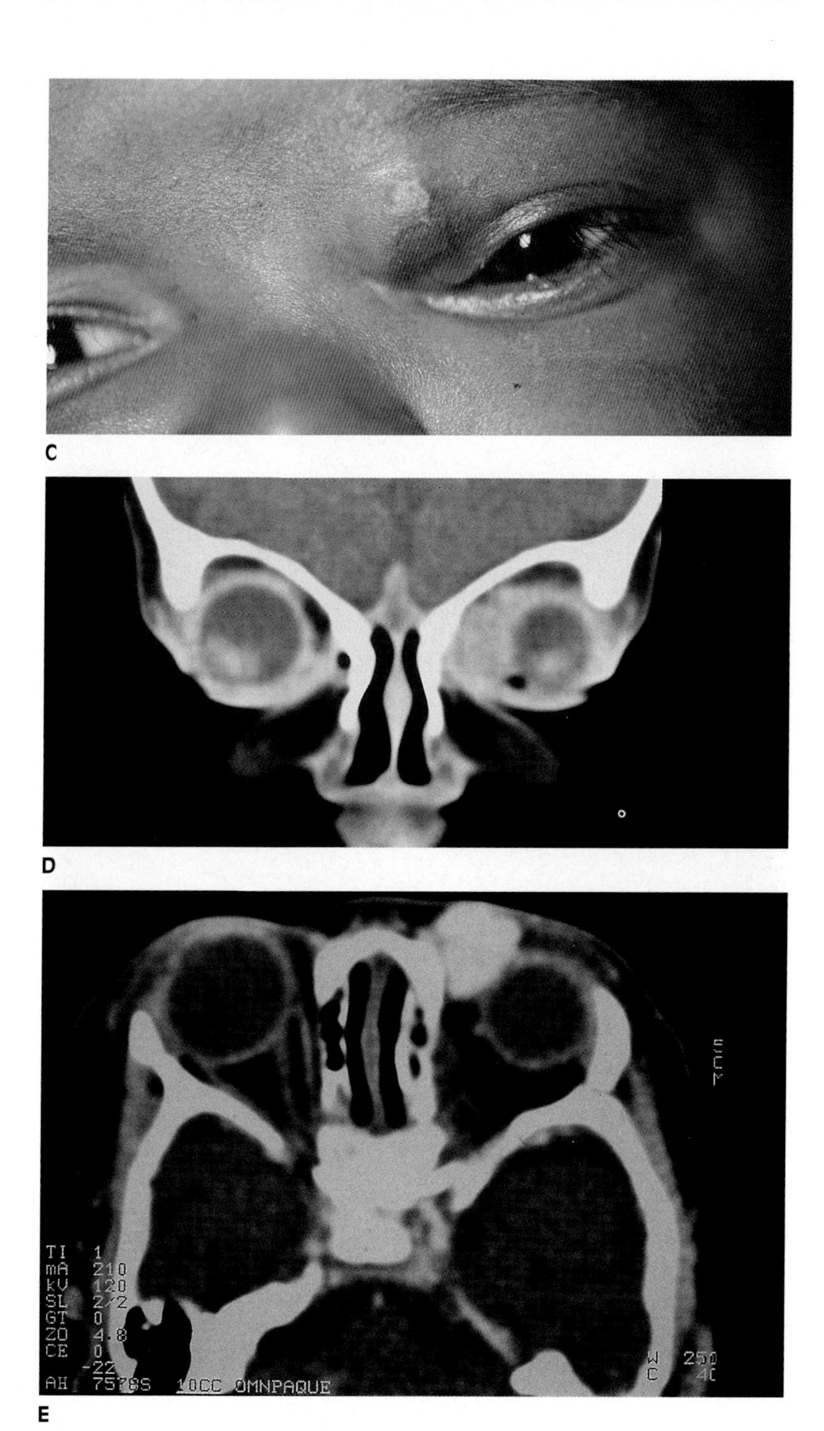

Figure 14-3 Capillary hemangioma (cont.) **C.** *Superficial orbital hemangioma that had increased in size and was causing amblyopia from 7 diopters of induced astigmatism.* **D.** *and* **E.** *CT scan shows this anterior orbital mass, which is well circumscribed and enhances with contrast. This was excised because of the astigmatism and amblyopia. (Continued.)*

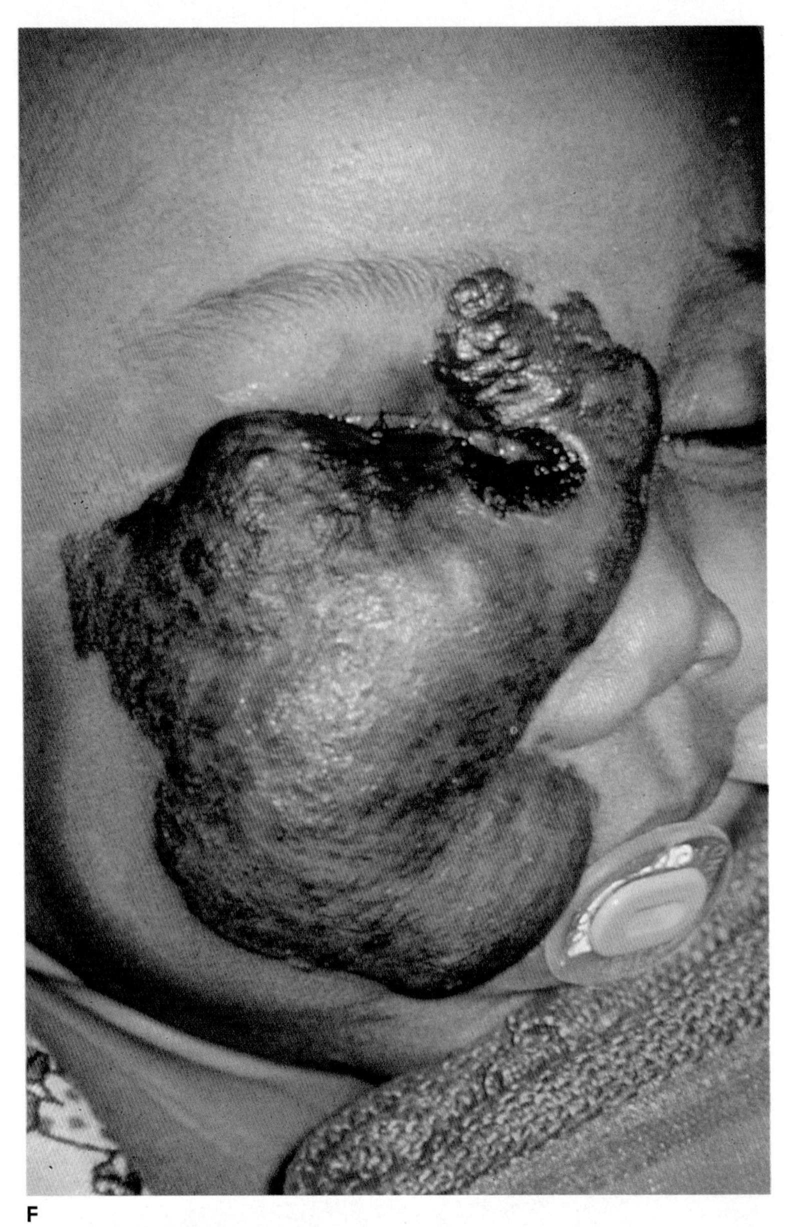

F

Figure 14-3 Capillary hemangioma (cont.) **F.** *Large cutaneous capillary hemangioma with visual obstruction. (Continued.)*

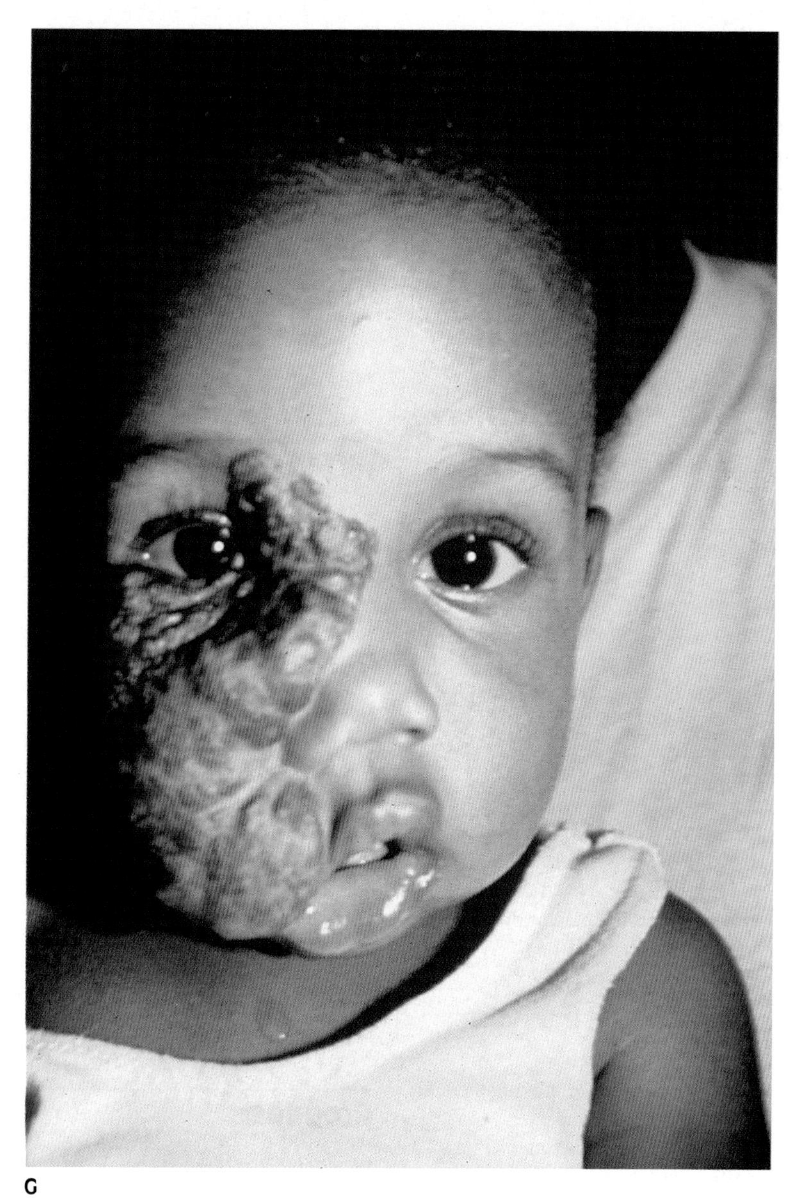

G

Figure 14-3 Capillary hemangioma (cont.) **G.** *This lesion responded well to a series of intralesional steroid injections.*

CAVERNOUS HEMANGIOMAS

Cavernous hemangiomas can present as asymptomatic, very insidious onset proptosis. More commonly, these lesions present without any symptoms and are found on imaging done for unrelated reasons. They are slowly growing masses that are generally easy to remove depending on their location.

Epidemiology and Etiology

Age Adults.

Gender Most commonly middle-aged women.

Etiology Unknown.

History

Very slow growth usually means the patient is unsure of the onset or duration of the lesion. Most commonly, the presentation is proptosis but rarely there can be symptoms of visual loss.

Examination

Axial proptosis is the common presentation. If the lesion is at the apex or is very large, it can cause optic nerve compromise or strabismus. Lesions can rarely cause orbital pain or the appearance of a choroidal mass (Fig. 14-4).

Imaging

CT scan shows an encapsulated, homogeneous, round mass with variable enhancement.
MRI: isointense on T_1 and hyperintense on T_2. Marked enhancement with gadolinium.

Special Considerations

Rarely, lesions may grow rapidly during pregnancy.

Differential Diagnosis

- Hemangiopericytoma
- Schwannoma
- Fibrous histiocytoma

Pathology

Encapsulated tumor consisting of large endothelial lined channels with abundant, loosely distributed smooth muscle in the vascular walls and smooth muscle.

Treatment

Surgical excision is the treatment of choice. These lesions are easily removed once exposed. They do not regress and slowly enlarge so observation only delays surgery.

Prognosis

Excellent.

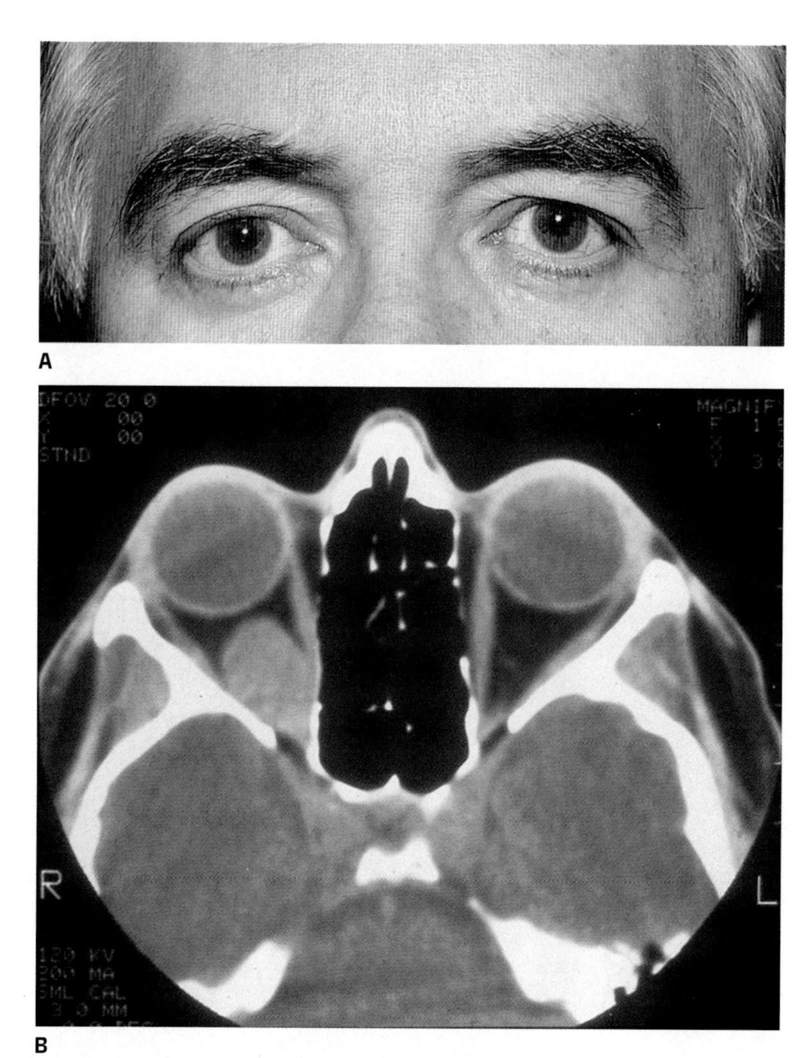

Figure 14-4 Cavernous hemangioma **A.** *A patient with proptosis of the right eye of unknown duration and no other visual or orbital complaints.* **B.** *CT scan shows a well-circumscribed intraconal orbital mass. (Continued.)*

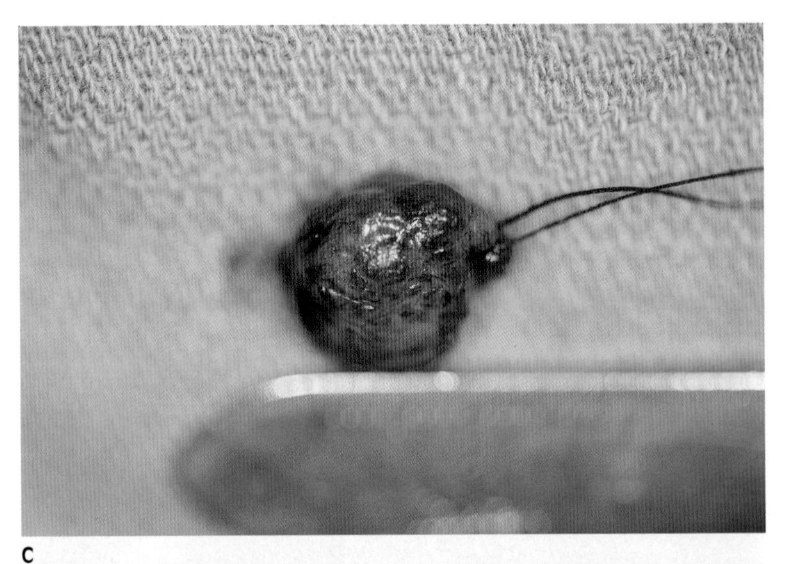

C

D

Figure 14-4 Cavernous hemangioma (cont.) **C.** *The mass was excised and was a cavernous hemangioma.* **D.** *MRI of a cavernous hemangioma. The T_1-weighted image shows the lesion isointense to muscle and hypointense to fat. (Continued.)*

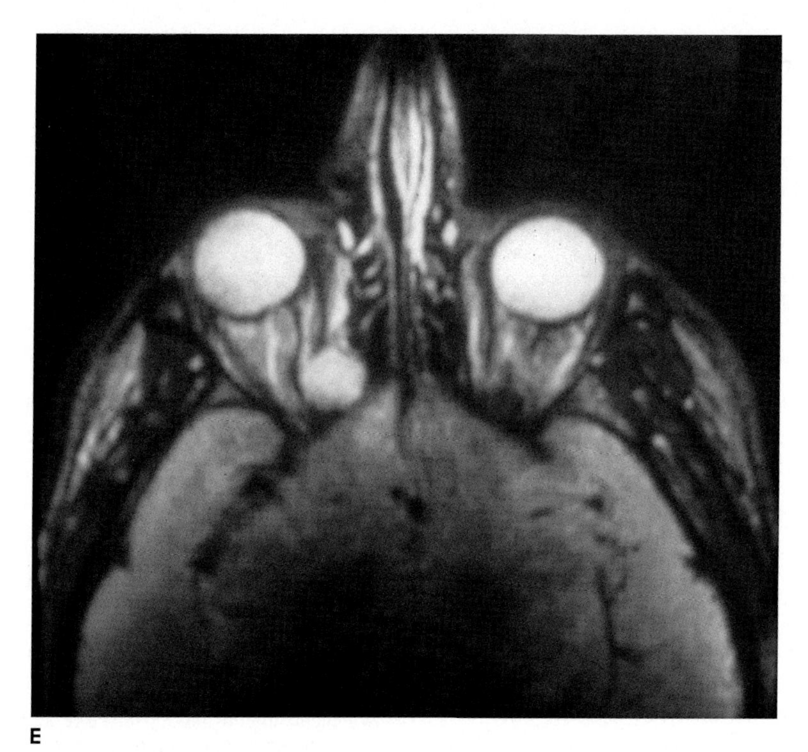

E

Figure 14-4 Cavernous hemangioma (cont.) **E.** *On the T_2-weighted image, the lesion is hyperintense to fat and muscle.*

LYMPHANGIOMAS

Lymphangiomas are rare vascular hamartomas that can behave in many different ways depending on location and growth patterns. This condition can vary from mild rather asymptomatic lesions, to progressively growing, infiltrative lesions, to acute proptosis and visual loss from bleeding into these lesions.

Epidemiology and Etiology

Age Usually noted in the first decade of life.

Gender More common in females.

Etiology Congenital lesion.

History

These lesions are often noted associated with a spontaneous bleed of the lesion although they likely were present for years prior. They can grow slowly and then have a sudden hemorrhage. Lymphangiomas can manifest as pain, subconjunctival hemorrhage, or as proptosis. Less commonly, the cysts of these lesions are noted subconjunctivally. These lesions enlarge with upper respiratory infections.

Examination

The findings on examination are dependent on the location of the lesion. The most common presentation is associated with sudden bleeding into the lymphangioma. If the bleed is superficial then a subconjunctival bleed is seen and the cysts of the lymphangioma are often found. If the hemorrhage is in the orbit, the findings may only be proptosis. Careful evaluation for evidence of a lymphangioma superficially should be done in these cases. Imaging will aid in the diagnosis if the lesion is entirely orbital. (Fig 14-5A to C).

Imaging

CT scan: poorly circumscribed, heterogeneous mass.

MRI: Hyperintense on T_1; very hyperintense on T_2, with possible area of fluid and blood (Fig. 14-5D and E).

Special Considerations

Surgery performed on a lymphangioma increases the chances of spontaneous bleeds within the lesion. Surgery should only be done if absolutely necessary.

Differential Diagnosis

- Diagnosis can usually be made with MRI.

Pathology

Nonencapsulated mass with large serum-filled spaces lined by flat endothelial cells. The interstitium has scattered lymphoid follicles.

Treatment

Observation unless the spontaneous bleeding causes visual loss, corneal exposure, or severe cosmetic disfigurement. Generally, with time the blood will resorb. When an orbital hemorrhage causes visual loss, drainage of the hemorrhage should be performed. Debulking of the lesion or orbital decompression are other treatment options. Lymphangiomas are infiltrative so excision is very difficult and there is usually significant bleeding associated with excision, which is only done as a last resort.

Prognosis

Variable depending on the growth of the lymphangioma. Progressive lesions have a high incidence of visual disability and poor cosmetic result.

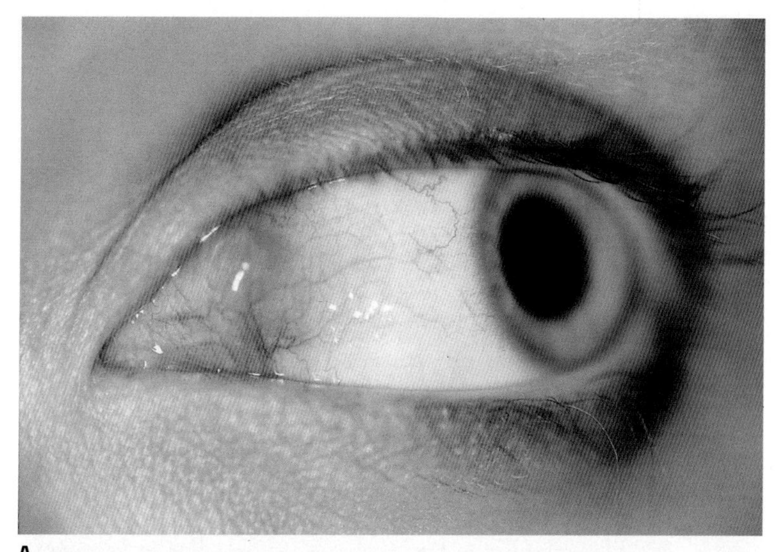

A

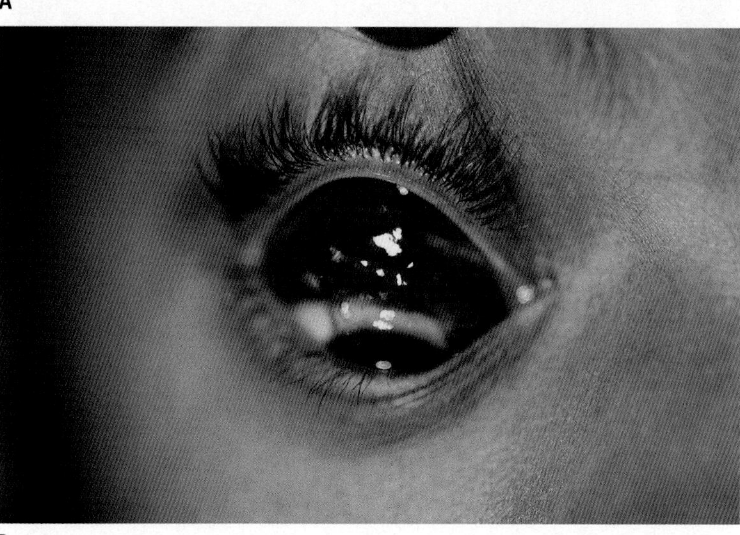

B

Figure 14-5 Lymphangioma **A.** *Patient with sudden onset of orbital discomfort and proptosis. Medially, a small area of hemorrhage is noted with subconjunctival cysts consistent with a lymphangioma.* **B.** *More obvious hemorrhage was noted along with the onset of deep orbital pain. Multiple cysts can be seen in the hemorrhage. Imaging was consistent with a lymphangioma. (Continued.)*

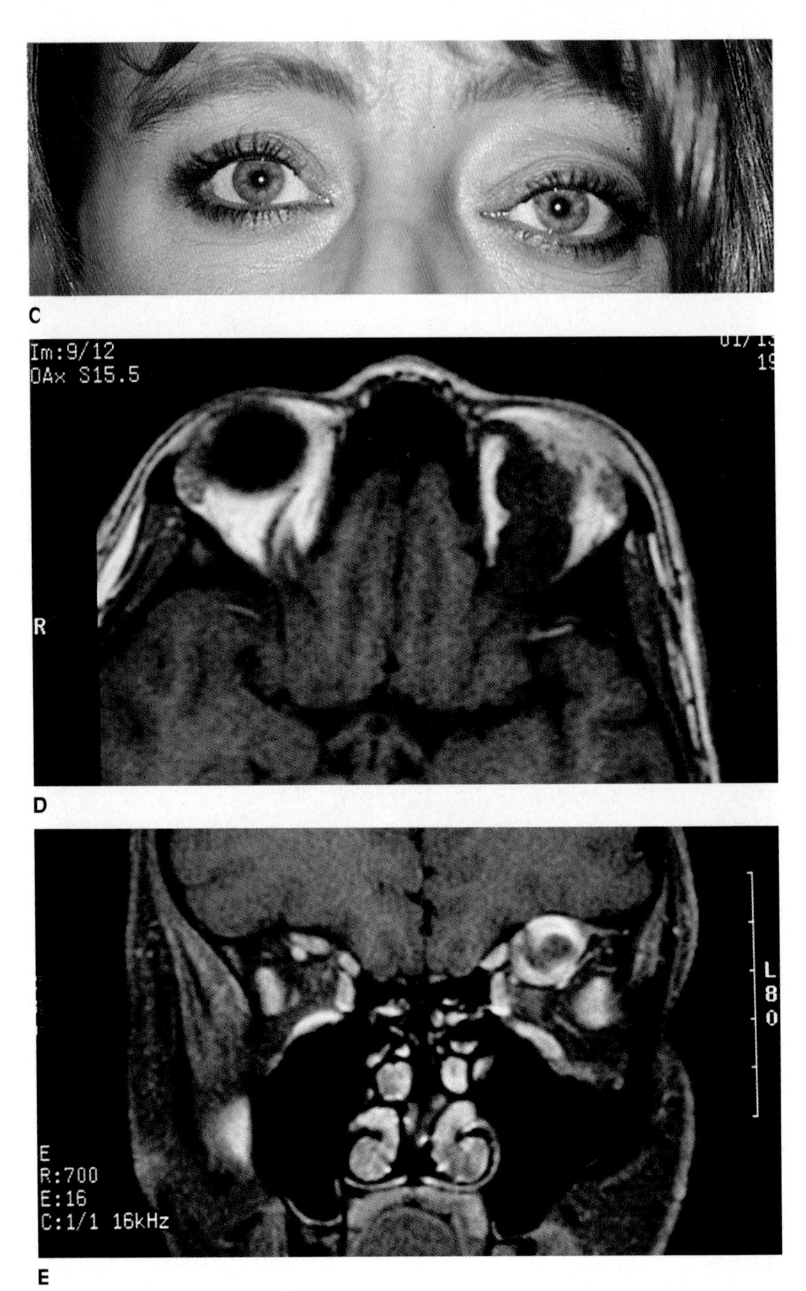

Figure 14-5 Lymphangioma (cont.) **C, D,** *and* **E.** *Proptosis of the left eye with recurrent episodes of orbital pain. The pain was usually associated with an increase in the proptosis. MRI shows a superior orbital mass with area of fresh and old blood consistent with a lymphangioma.*

HEMANGIOPERICYTOMA

Hemangiopericytoma is a rare lesion that can mimic a cavernous hemangioma but has more rapid growth and is more likely to cause symptoms. These can recur and have a chance of metastasis.

Epidemiology and Etiology

Age Middle age.

Gender Equally seen in males and females.

Etiology Tumor originates from the pericyte. This is a rare orbital tumor.

History

Insidious onset of proptosis and mass effect but usually more rapid onset than a cavernous hemangioma.

Examination

Proptosis is often the only finding. These lesions appear more often in the superior orbit but intraconal location is also common (Fig. 14-6).

Imaging

CT scan: well circumscribed, encapsulated mass.
MRI: isointense on T_1; hyperintense on T_2. Enhances with gadolinium.

Special Considerations

These lesions have the potential for recurrence locally whether the pathology is benign or malignant. Malignant lesions can recur and can also metastasize.

Differential Diagnosis

- Cavernous hemangioma
- Fibrous histiocytoma
- Schwannoma

Pathology

Uniform spindle-cell tumor with a sinusoidal vascular pattern; can be divided into benign, intermediate, and malignant forms.

Treatment

Complete excision in the capsule is the best treatment. Recurrence, if malignant, may require exenteration.

Prognosis

Variable. Patients must be followed for at least 10 years for local recurrence or metastasis.

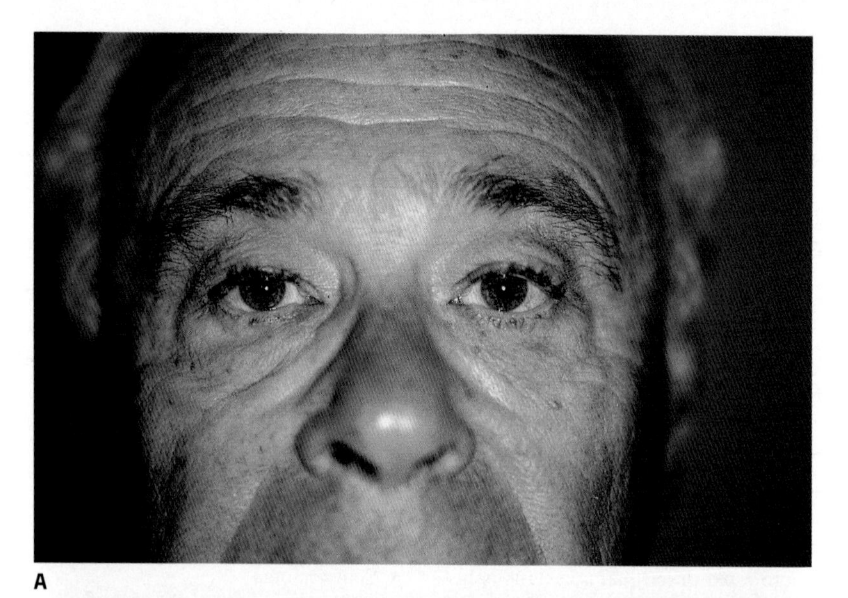

A

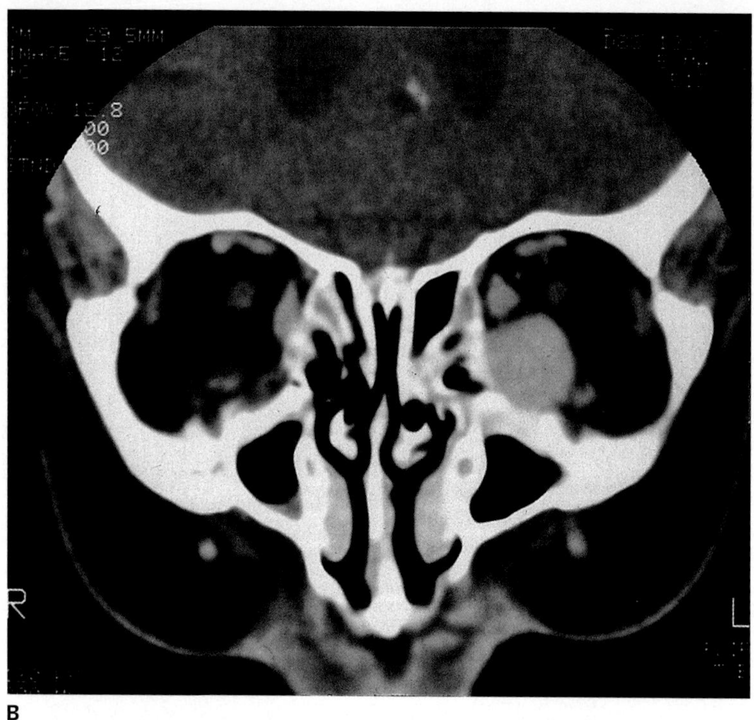

B

Figure 14-6 Hemangiopericytoma **A.** *and* **B.** *A 55-year-old male presents with increasing proptosis over 6 months and diplopia. There is axial proptosis on the left and a well circumscribed mass on CT scan. Pathologic examination revealed a hemangiopericytoma.*

ORBITAL VARICES

Orbital varices will present in the 20s and 30s with a history of years of intermittent proptosis. These lesions can be superficial and noticeable or deep with only proptosis as a sign of the lesion. Most lesions should be left alone unless there is extreme orbital pressure with functional deficit or a severe cosmetic disfigurement.

Epidemiology and Etiology

Age Usually noted in the first through third decades of life.

Gender Equally seen in males and females.

Etiology Dilatation of preexisting venous channels.

History

Patients with nondistensible varices present with recurrent episodes of thrombosis and hemorrhage in the lesion. This leads to proptosis, pain, motility restriction, and even decreased vision. These symptoms resolve as the hemorrhage resolves. The distensible varicies present with pain, proptosis, and pressure symptoms associated with straining, bending forward, or Valsalva. The changes in the orbit and lids associated with this venous distension are also noted.

Examination

Distensible varicies are diagnosed easily by having the patients bring their head into a dependent position and note the filling of the varix. Nondistensible varicies are more difficult to diagnose. The patient will present with symptoms of an acute hemorrhage into the lesion as noted previously. There is generally no external hemorrhage present or any sign of a varix in this type (Fig. 14-7A, B, E, and F).

Imaging

CT scan may appear relatively normal or with just a small diffuse mass on axial cuts. In the dependent position (coronal cuts), the mass will enlarge as the varix fills with blood. Nondistendible varicies will show a diffuse mass that enhances with contrast (Fig. 14-7C and D).

Differential Diagnosis

- Lymphangioma is the main differential and differentiation from the nondistensible varix is not always possible.

Pathology

Well-defined venous channels.

Treatment

Conservative observation in most cases. If a nondistensible varix bleeds and visual or exposure symptoms require intervention, drainage of the blood clot is usually the treatment of choice.

Prognosis

Variable. Progressive lesions can be disfiguring and successful treatment is difficult.

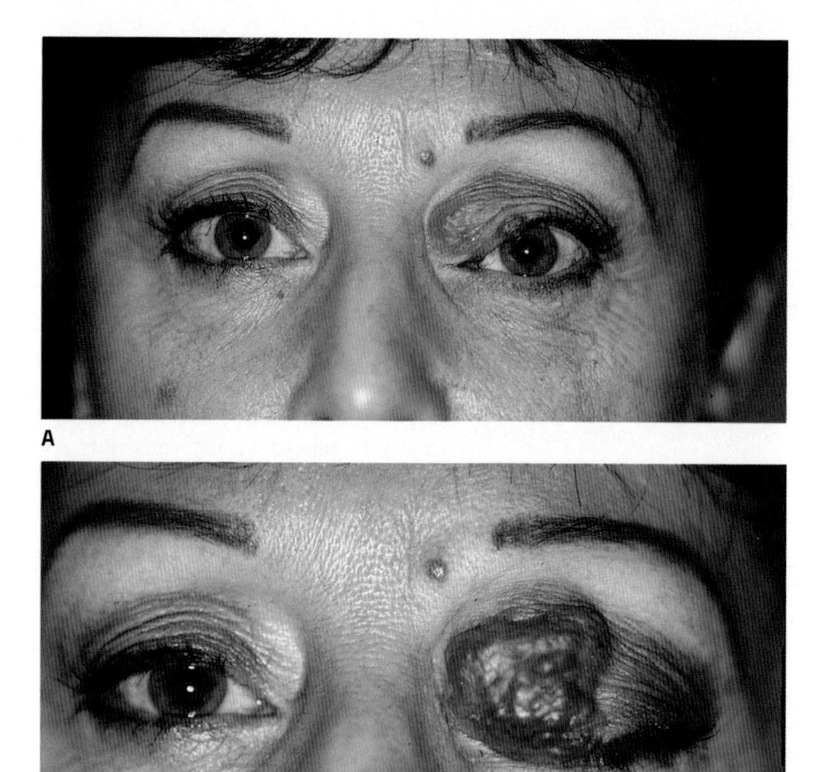

Figure 14-7 Distensible orbital varix **A.** *A 55-year-old female with a distensible varix in her superior medial orbit.* **B.** *Valsalva results in massive enlargement and closure of the eye.* *(Continued.)*

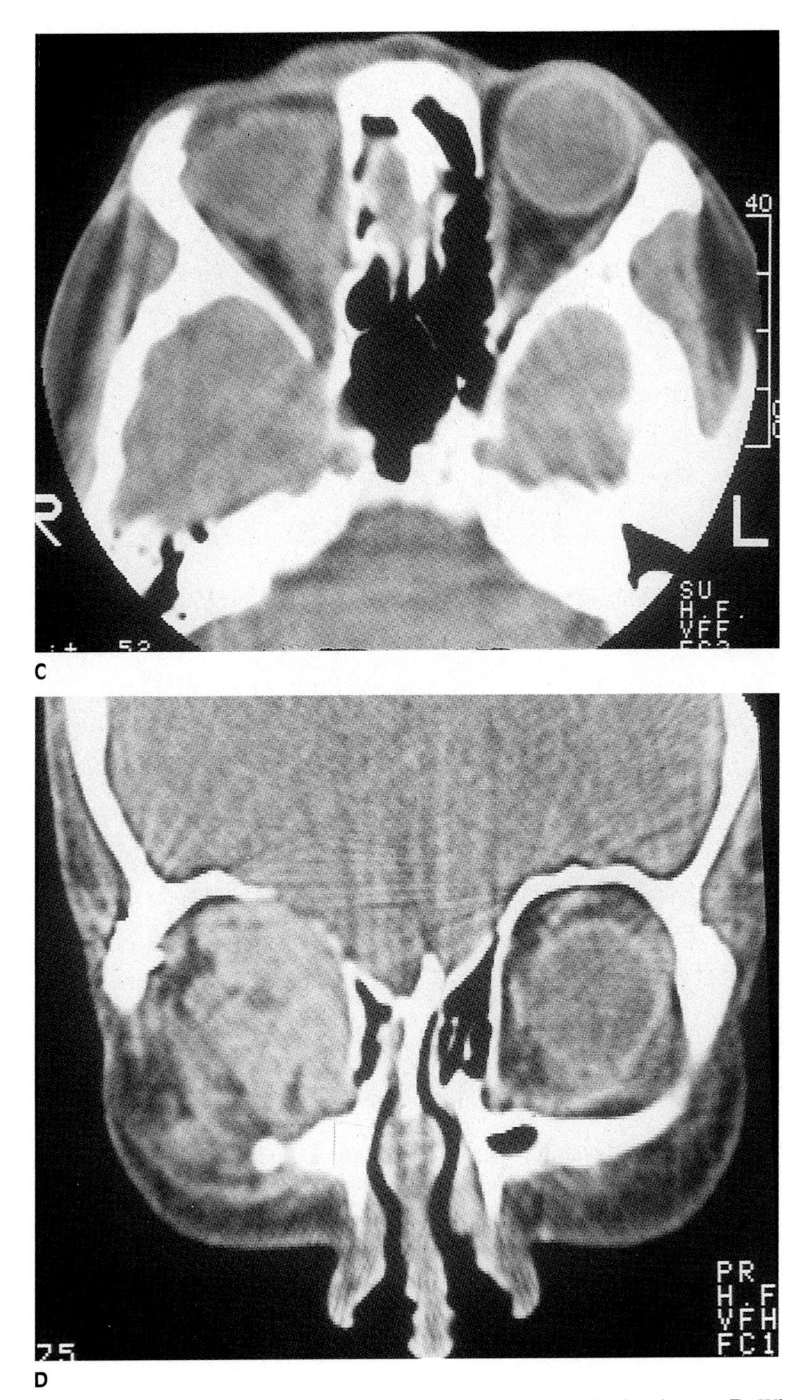

Figure 14-7 Orbital varix (cont.) **C.** *CT scan showing the medial orbital varix.* **D.** *When the head is placed in a dependent position for the coronal CT, the varix fills with blood, accounting for the enlargement of the lesion on the coronal cuts. (Continued.)*

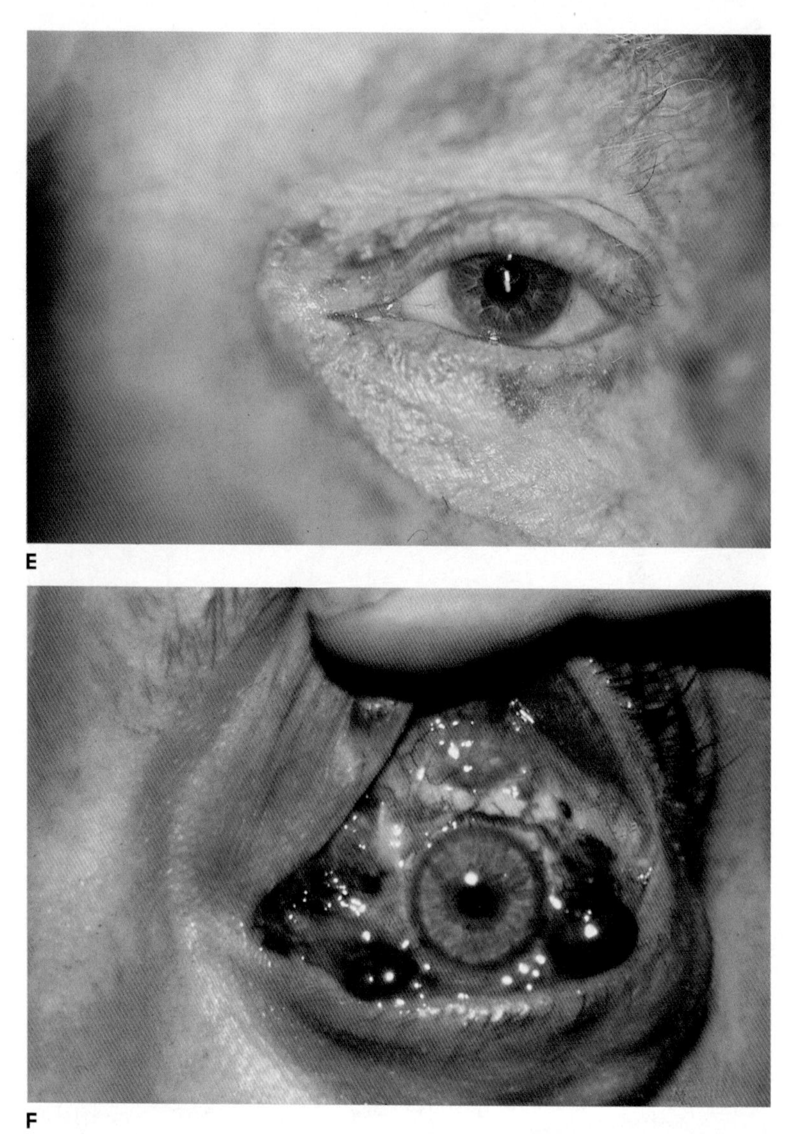

Figure 14-7 Coronal varix (cont.) **E.** *Nondistensible varix may be deep in the orbit with only a small anterior component.* **F.** *Diffuse orbital involvement with multiple varices.*

ARTERIOVENOUS MALFORMATIONS

Arteriovenous malformations (AVM) present with variable severity. All cases involve the connection of an arterial flow into a venous drainage area such as the cavernous sinus. There may be subtle swelling and redness of the eye and orbit or the presentation may be severe proptosis, exposure, and intraocular vascular congestion.

Epidemiology and Etiology

Age Older adults, except after trauma, which can occur at any age.

Gender Equally seen in males and females.

Etiology Trauma (basal skull fracture) results in high-flow fistulas. Degenerative vascular process in patients with hypertension and atherosclerosis results in a low-flow fistula.

History

Abrupt onset of proptosis, chemosis, arterialization of the conjunctival vessels in one eye. This occurs in a high-flow AVM. High-flow AVMs will have more severe symptoms but often have the history of head trauma. Low-flow AVMs are in older patients, are slower in onset, and the symptoms are less dramatic.

Examination

Proptosis, chemosis, dysmotility, arterialization of the conjunctival vessels (corkscrew pattern), and elevated intraocular pressure are seen in AVMs. In high-flow states, the retinal vessels are affected with venous congestion (Fig. 14-8A and B).

Imaging

CT scan and MRI show an enlarged superior ophthalmic vein and there may be enlargement of the extraocular muscles (Fig. 14-8D and E). Orbital Doppler shows reversal of flow in the superior ophthalmic vein and is diagnostic of an AVM (Fig. 14-8C).

Differential Diagnosis

- Orbital pseudotumor
- Orbital cellulitis
- Thyroid-related ophthalmopathy
- Chronic conjunctivitis

Treatment

Low-flow AVMs will often resolve spontaneously. The signs may worsen as the fistula closes off. High-flow lesions often require attempted selective embolization to close the fistula. This may also be needed in low-flow lesions that result in uncontrolled glaucoma, diplopia, or vascular occlusion.

Prognosis

Variable. Many low-flow AVMs will close on their own. Treatment for AVMs is successful but does have a risk of visual loss.

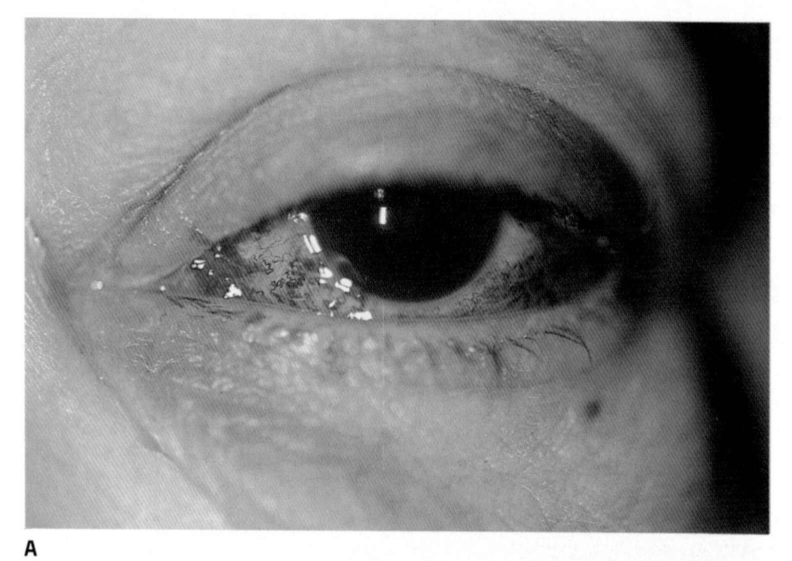

A

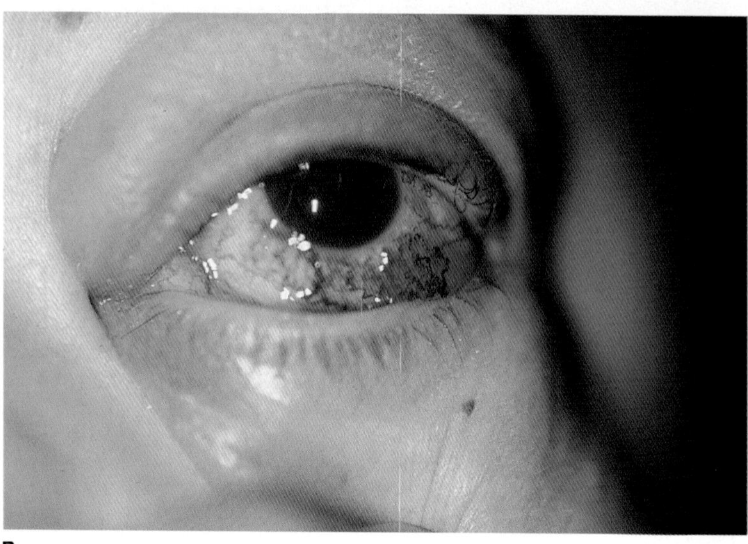

B

Figure 14-8 Arteriovenous malformation **A.** *and* **B.** *A patient with a 3- to 4-week history of swelling and redness of the left eye. Motility is limited as noted in attempted upgaze. (Continued.)*

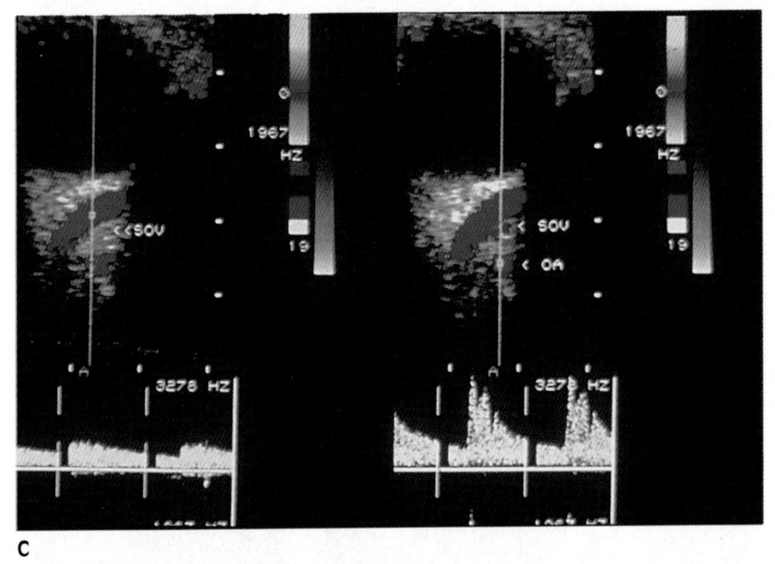

C

Figure 14-8 Arteriovenous malformation (cont.) **C.** *Color Doppler imaging shows arterialization of the superior ophthalmic vein, which is diagnostic of an arteriovenous malformation. (Continued.)*

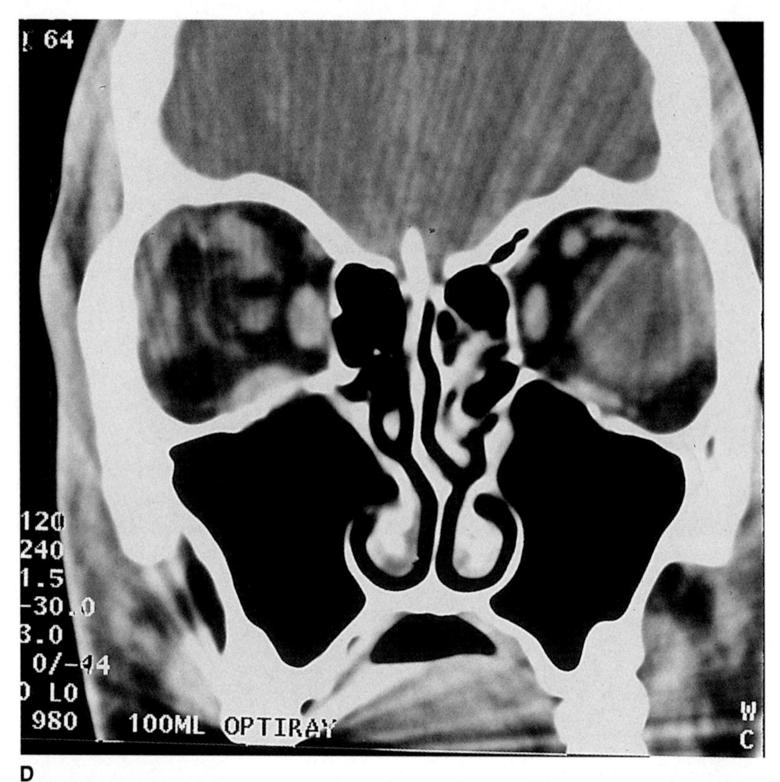

D

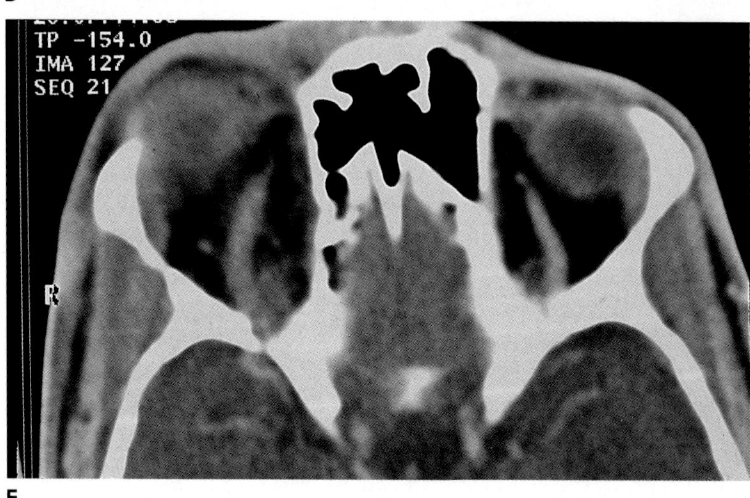

E

Figure 14-8 Arteriovenous malformation (cont.) **D.** *and* **E.** *CT scan shows enlarged superior ophthalmic vein and engorged rectus muscles, which is usually seen with an AVM.*

NEURAL TUMORS

OPTIC NERVE GLIOMAS

Optic nerve glioma is a glial tumor that most commonly presents in children and includes painless proptosis and visual loss. These can initally involve the optic chiasm or grow to involve it. Treatment remains controversial.

Epidemiology and Etiology

Age Predominantly in children during the first decade of life. Malignant gliomas occur in middle-aged males.

Gender Equal occurrence in males and females.

Etiology Unknown.

History

In children gliomas present with gradual, painless, unilateral, axial, proptosis with loss of vision and an afferent pupillary defect. The malignant form in adults presents with symptoms of optic neuritis but rapidly progress to blindness and death.

Examination

Axial proptosis with visual loss, afferent pupillary defect, optic atrophy, or nerve swelling are all findings. There are no inflammatory signs or pain. Diagnosis is usually made on the basis of orbital imaging (Fig. 14-9). The malignant form in adults may show inflammatory signs along with signs of an optic neuropathy and proptosis.

Imaging

CT scan demonstrates fusiform enlargement of the optic nerve. MRI is the imaging of choice to evaluate the extent and growth of an optic nerve glioma. T_1 imaging is iso- to hypointense, whereas T_2 imaging shows prolonged relaxation times.

Special Considerations

Neurofibromatosis is associated with 25 to 50 percent of optic nerve gliomas.

Differential Diagnosis

- Optic nerve meningioma; the differential diagnosis is more related to how extensive the tumor is and not what it is.

Pathology

These are intradural lesions that are juvenile pilocytic astrocytomas.

Treatment

Controversial and must be individualized. Most gliomas can be observed, as these are usually very slow growing lesions. If there is significant growth, surgical excision is the best treatment. If the tumor is unresectable, radiation is considered.

Prognosis

Variable. Some gliomas grow aggressively; others can remain stable for years.

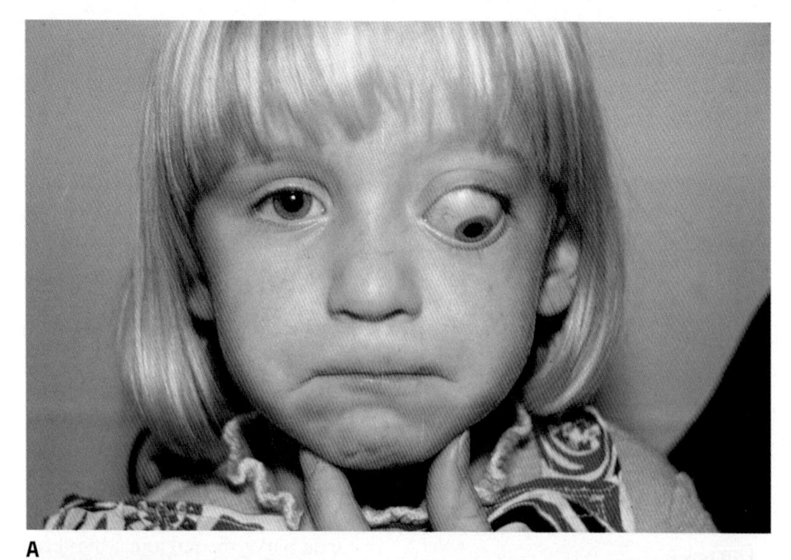

A

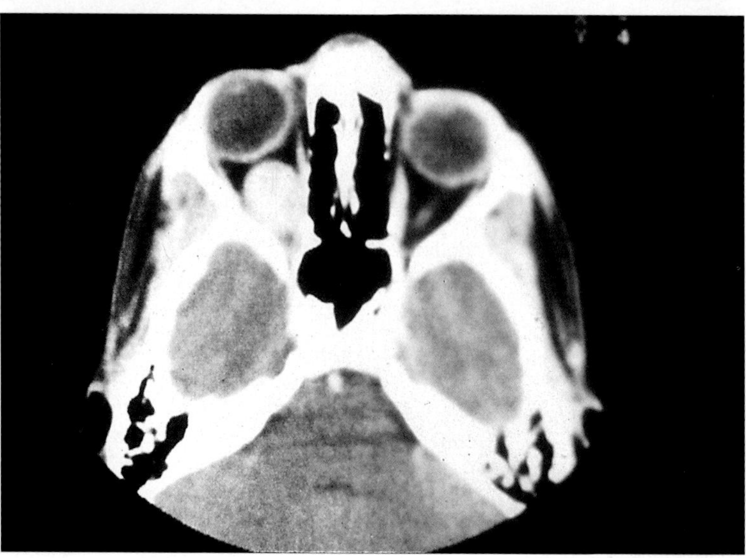

B

Figure 14-9 Optic nerve glioma **A.** *A 6-year-old female with painless proptosis and visual loss.* **B.** *CT scan shows fusiform enlargement of the optic nerve consistent with an optic nerve glioma.*

NEUROFIBROMAS

Neurofibromas are composed of proliferating Schwann cells within their nerve sheath. There are multiple forms of neurofibromas. Plexiform neurofibromas are often associated with neurofibromatosis.

Epidemiology and Etiology

Age Plexiform neurofibromas are usually seen in the first decade. Isolated lesions occur in the third through fifth decades.

Gender Equal occurrence in males and females.

Etiology Plexiform neurofibromas are the most common neurofibroma to involve the orbit and are associated with neurofibromatosis type 1.

History

Patients will often already have the diagnosis of neurofibromatosis and will develop thickening and hypertrophy of the affected nerve. They may present with thickening of eyelid or periorbital skin, or with proptosis. Isolated neurofibromas are not usually associated with neurofibromatosis.

Examination

Findings will vary depending on the nerve or nerves that are involved. The involved nerves grow as a tortuous, ropy tangle of nerves. This growth is usually slow but progressive and results in thickening of involved periorbital and orbital tissues, proptosis, and orbital bony abnormalities. These bony changes include orbital enlargement, abnormalities of the sphenoid wing, and hypoplasia of the ethmoid and maxillary sinuses (Fig. 14-10). Isolated neurofibromas present with mass effect. Proptosis, diplopia, and decreased vision may occur.

Imaging

CT and MRI show a diffuse infiltrating lesion in plexiform neurofibromas. An isolated neurofibroma will be well-circumscribed with characteristics similar to a schwannoma.

Special Considerations

Any patient with a plexiform neurofibroma must be carefully evaluated for neurofibromatosis if they are not known to have the disease. Solitary neurofibromas are rare orbital tumors that can be excised and are unlikely to be associated with neurofibromatosis. These tend to occur in middle age.

Differential Diagnosis

- Lymphangioma
- Orbital pseudotumor
- Isolated lesions must consider schwannoma, cavernous hemangioma, fibrous histiocytoma

Pathology

Proliferating, intertwining bundles of Schwann cells, axons, and endoneural fibroblasts within the nerve sheaths.

Treatment

Observation with surgical debulking only as a last resort. These tumors cannot be completely excised and recur and regrow with time. Rare, isolated lesions can be completely excised.

Prognosis

Generally poor cosmetic and functional results because of the progressive nature of these infiltrative tumors. Isolated lesions have a good prognosis.

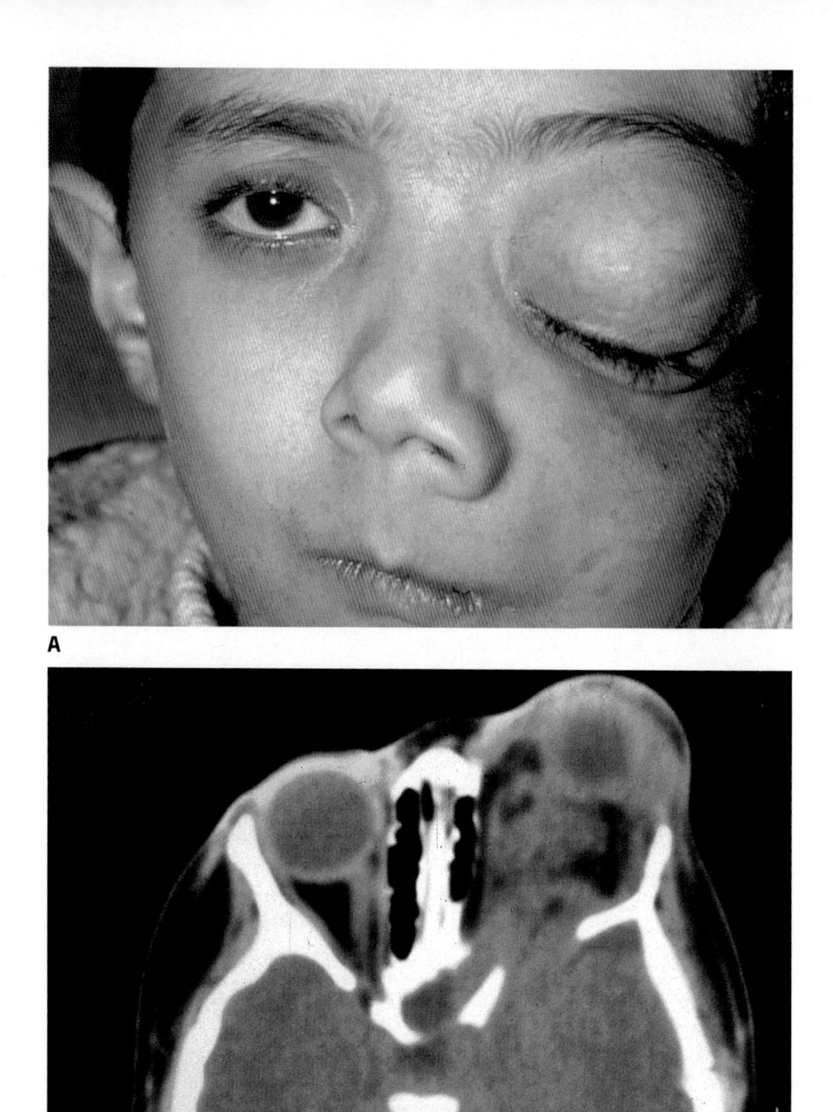

Figure 14-10 Neurofibroma **A.** *Severe proptosis, complete ptosis, and orbital infiltration by a plexiform neurofibroma.* **B.** *CT scan shows orbital infiltration as well as absence of part of the sphenoid bone of the orbit. All is consistent with neurofibromatosis.*

MENINGIOMAS

Meningiomas are invasive tumors that arise intracranially and secondarily invade the orbit. They are usually slowly progressive tumors that are very difficult to completely excise because of their infiltrative nature.

Epidemiology and Etiology

Age Bimodal peak in the second and fifth decades.

Gender More common in women.

Etiology These tumors arise from arachnoid villi. Most commonly, these tumors start as intracranial tumors and extend into the orbit secondarily. A primary orbital form arises from the optic nerve sheath arachnoid tissue.

History

Meningiomas will have a gradual onset of symptoms as they slowly extend from their intracranial origin into the orbit. Ophthalmic manifestations are dependent on the location of the tumor. Most common orbital presentation is tumors arising near the pterion that present as a temporal fossa mass and proptosis that can often be suddenly noticed but have been present for years. Optic nerve meningiomas present with slow, painless, progressive visual loss.

Examination

Findings on examination depend on the location of the meningioma. If located in the temporal fossa, findings include temporal fossa fullness, proptosis, eyelid edema, and chemosis. If the meningioma arises near the sella and optic nerve, early findings will be visual loss with optic nerve edema or atrophy (Fig. 14-11A and B).

Optic nerve meningiomas present with decreased vision, an afferent pupillary defect, proptosis, and possible ophthalmoplegia. The optic nerve may be normal, swollen, atrophic, or have shunt vessels (Fig. 14-11C–F).

Imaging

CT scan: hyperostosis, calcification, with adjacent soft tissue fullness.
MRI: useful to detect growth along the dura. Gadolinium enhancement and fat suppression techniques help define these lesions in the orbit.

Differential Diagnosis

- Optic nerve glioma
- Lymphangioma

Pathology

These tumors are composed of cells that can be round, polygonal, or spindle shaped. In addition, there are varying admixtures of blood vessels, fibroblasts, and psammoma bodies. The different patterns of meningiomas show varying mixtures of these components.

Treatment

Intracranial meningiomas that extend into the orbit are usually treated surgically. If well encapsulated, these can be completely excised with a neurosurgical and orbital approach. Meningiomas can be infiltrative and involvement of vital structures may prevent complete excision and allow for debulking only.

Treatment of optic nerve sheath meningiomas is required if there is aggressive growth, threat of intracranial spread, or visual loss. Surgical excision is the treatment of choice in most cases but vision will generally be lost. Radiotherapy has application for certain cases where vision may be spared.

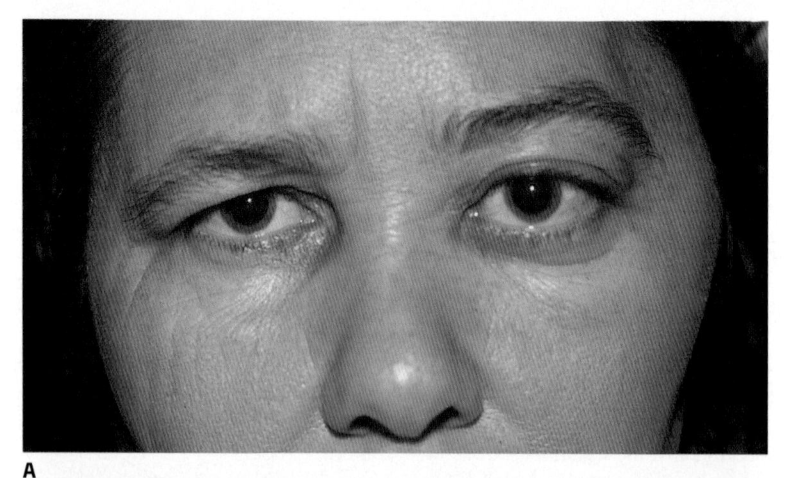

A

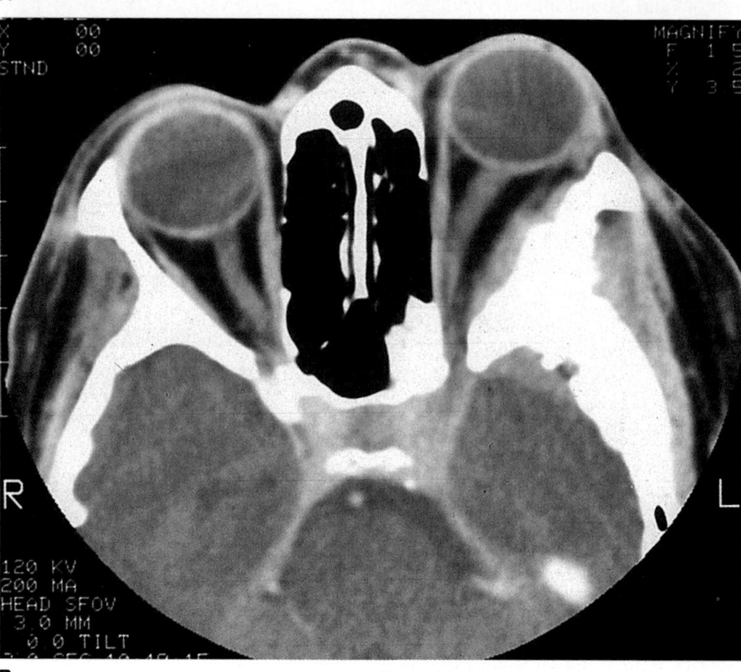

B

Figure 14-11 Meningioma **A.** *A patient with a left-sided proptosis of gradual progressive onset. Note the temporal fossa fullness.* **B.** *CT scan shows hyperostosis and an associated soft tissue mass, all consistent with a sphenoid wing meningioma. (Continued.)*

Prognosis

Tumors are generally progressive but very slowly. Often complete surgical excision is not possible once they are in the orbit and debulking is the best treatment. Later recurrence is possible.

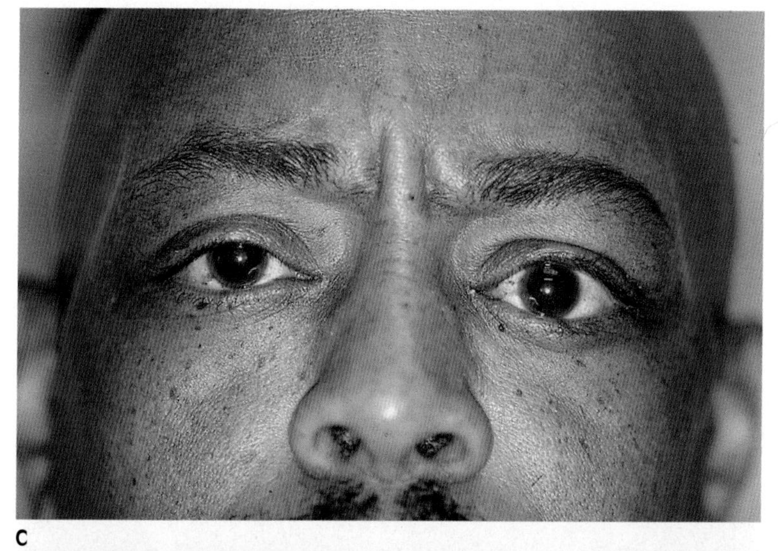

C

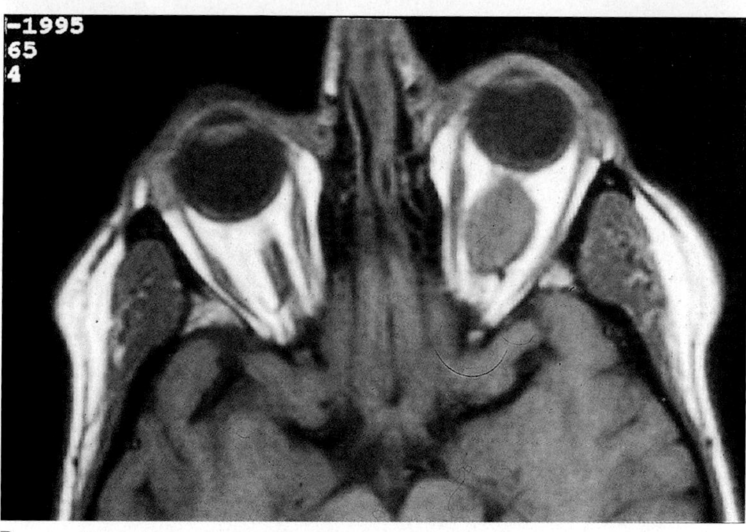

D

Figure 14-11 Optic nerve meningioma (cont.) **C.** *A patient with axial proptosis and visual loss.* **D.** *MRI scan shows a fusiform enlargement of the optic nerve and is consistent with a meningioma. (Continued.)*

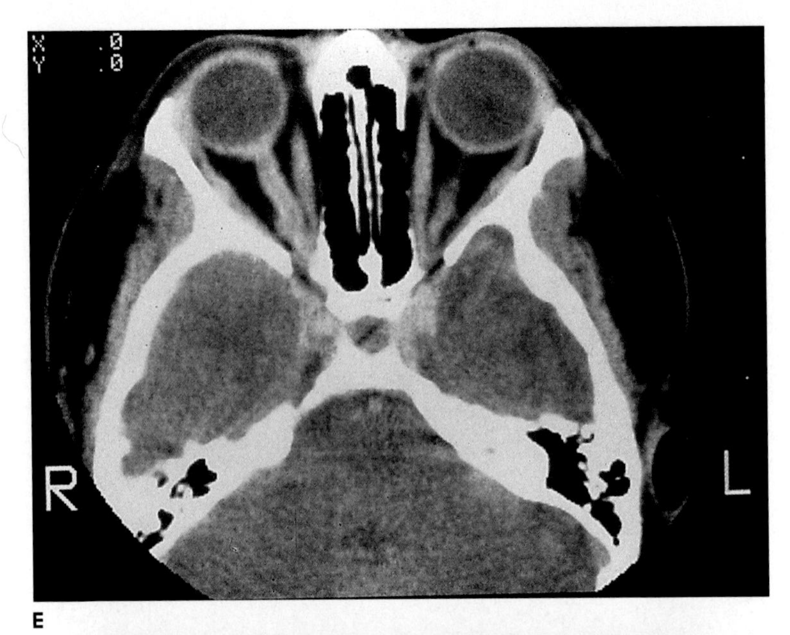

E

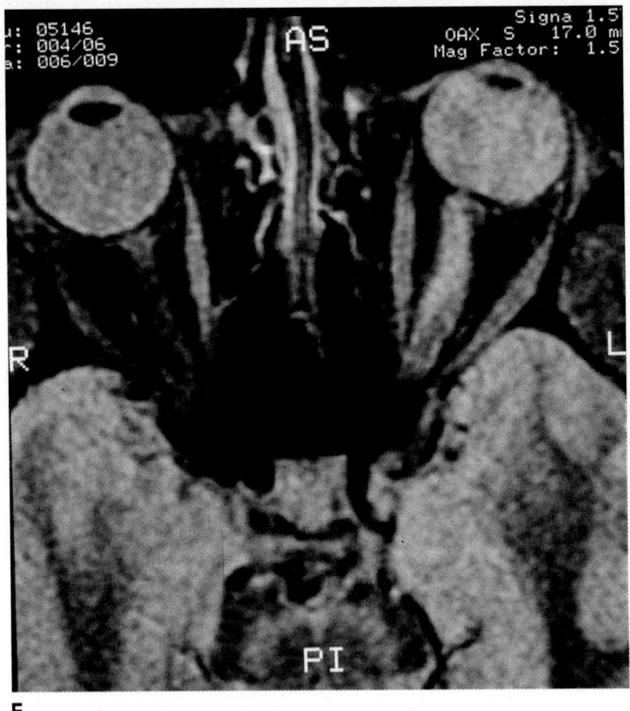

F

Figure 14-11 Optic nerve meningioma (cont.) **E.** *More commonly, there is diffuse thickening of the optic nerve. The thickened right optic nerve has a central lucency, termed the "railroad track" sign.* **F.** *The T_2-weighted image can be hypointense to hyperintense to fat and muscle as seen on the left side.*

SCHWANNOMAS

Schwannomas present as well-encapsulated, slowly growing masses that act very much like a cavernous hemangioma. These masses are usually easily excised and cause no subsequent problems.

Epidemiology and Etiology

Age 20 to 50 years of age.

Gender Equal occurrence in males and females.

Etiology Eccentric growths from peripheral nerves.

History

Slow, insidious onset of proptosis over years.

Examination

Proptosis with the direction dependent on the tumor position (most commonly intraconal). Less commonly, there may be eyelid swelling, diplopia, visual distortion (Fig. 14-12).

Imaging

CT and MRI scan show a well-circumscribed, round lesion.

Special Considerations

Eighteen percent of patients with schwannomas have neurofibromatosis.

Differential Diagnosis

- Capillary hemangioma
- Hemangiopericytoma
- Fibrous histiocytoma

Pathology

Proliferation of Schwann cells in a perineural capsule is seen. These may be in a tightly ordered arrangement (Antoni A) or loose arrangement (Antoni B).

Treatment

Surgical excision is the treatment of choice. Since they are outpouchings of a nerve, they can often be stripped off the nerve. Recurrence of the tumor, even if there is only partial resection, is very rare.

Prognosis

Excellent.

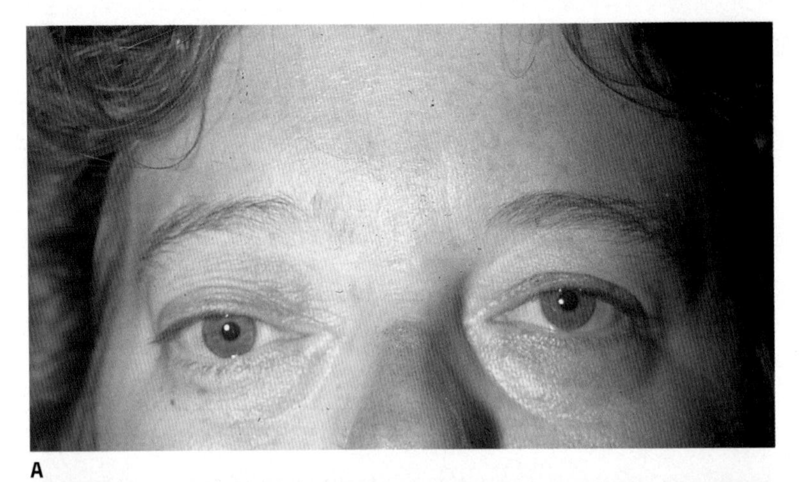

A

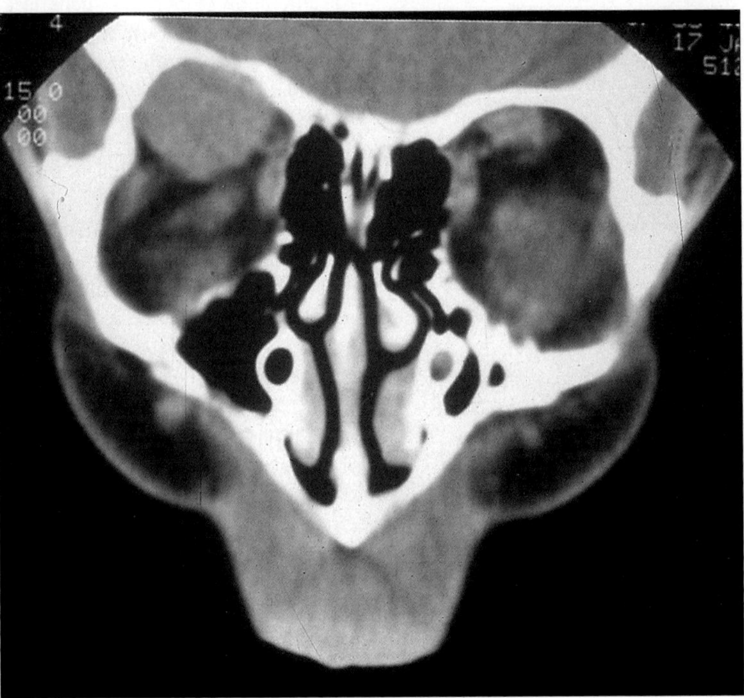

B

Figure 14-12 Schwannoma **A.** *and* **B.** *A 45-year-old female with gradual onset of right eye proptosis. CT scan shows a well-circumscribed mass in the superior orbit. There is some bony fossa formation. On excision, this was a schwannoma. Schwannomas are most commonly intraconal. (Continued.)*

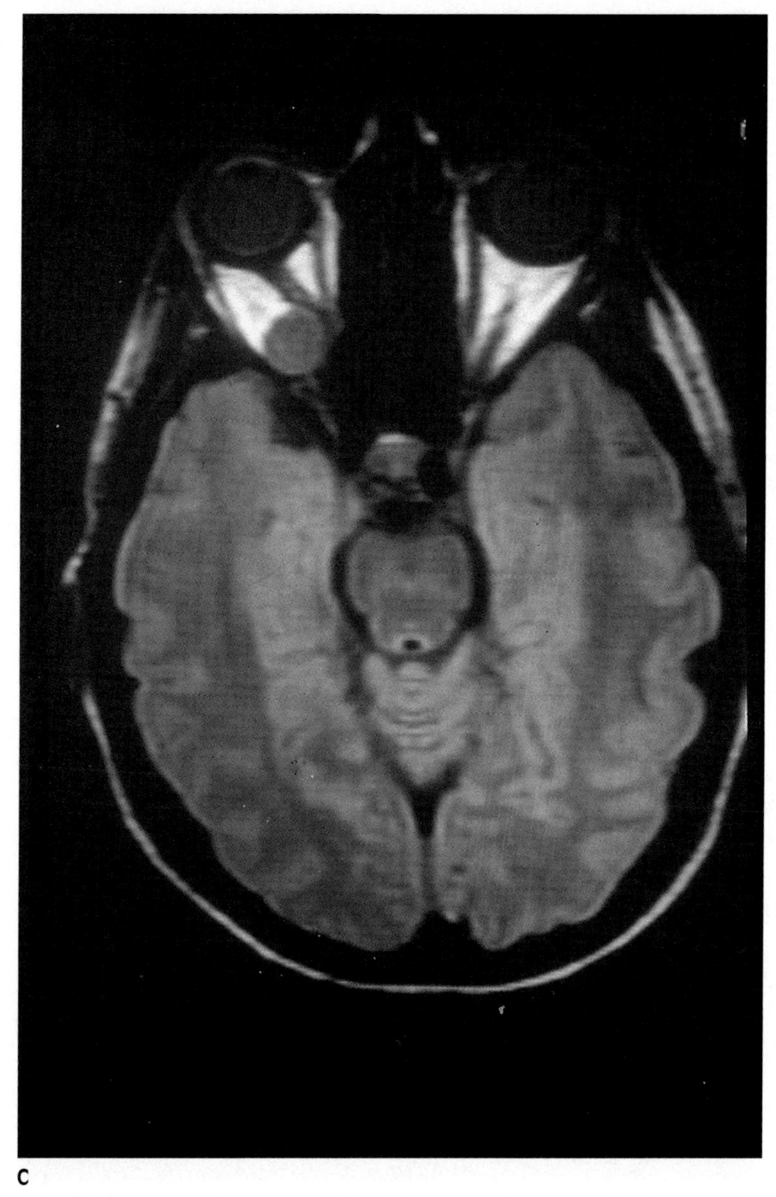
C

Figure 14-12 Schwannoma (cont.) **C.** *MRI shows a well-circumscribed lesion. The* T_1*-weighted image* **(C)** *shows the lesion isointense to muscle and hypointense to fat. (Continued.)*

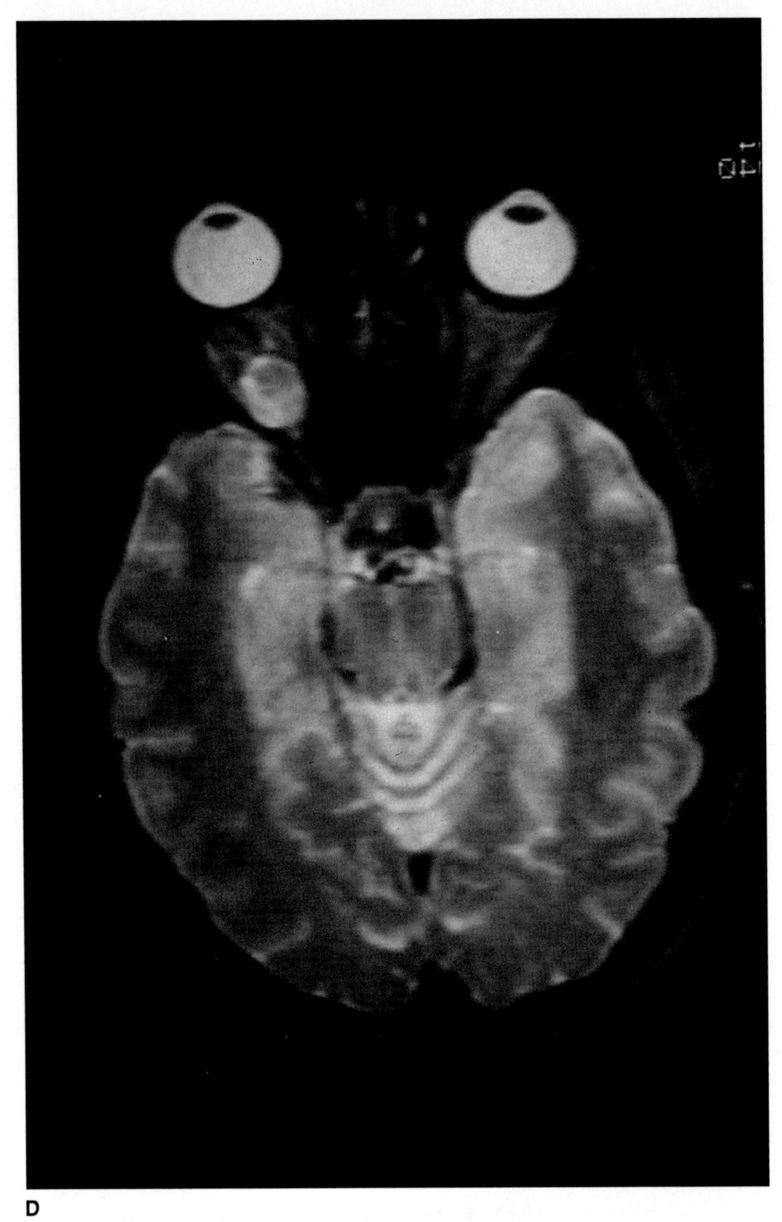

D

Figure 14-12 Schwannoma (cont.) **D.** *On the T_2-weighted image* (**D**)*, the lesion is hyperintense to fat and muscle.*

MESENCHYMAL TUMORS

RHABDOMYOSARCOMA

Rhabdomyosarcoma is the most common primary orbital malignancy of childhood. Classically, the child presents with sudden onset of proptosis over days to weeks with an orbital mass found on imaging. Once suspected, the lesion should be immediately biopsied so treatment can be started as quickly as possible.

Epidemiology and Etiology

Age Average age 7 to 8 years.

Gender Equal incidence in males and females.

Etiology Rhabdomyosarcomas develop from undifferentiated pluripotential mesenchymal cells.

History

Classically, rapid onset of unilateral proptosis is seen over days to a week but some patients may present less rapidly over many weeks.

Examination

Proptosis is seen with variable amounts of adenexal response, such as edema, erythema, and globe displacement, and sometimes a palpable mass. The superior nasal orbit is the most common location (Fig. 14-13).

Imaging

CT scan: homogenous mass that may have bony erosion.
MRI: hypointense on T_1 and hyperintense on T_2. Variable enhancement with gadolinium.

Special Considerations

Acute proptosis in a child is an emergency. Once a rhabdomyosarcoma is suspected, the lesion needs to be biopsied within 24 hours followed by prompt initiation of treatment.

Differential Diagnosis

- Capillary hemangioma
- Orbital pseudotumor
- Orbital cellulitis
- Ruptured dermoid cyst
- Metastatic tumor

Pathology

There are four distinct forms of rhabdomyosarcoma.

- Embryonic: poorly differentiated spindle cells
- Alveolar: shows rounded rhabdomyoblasts
- Pleomorphic: rounded or strap-like cells with cross-striations
- Botryoid: rare form with grape-like clusters

Treatment

Once suspected, a CT scan is done to identify the lesion. Urgent orbital biopsy with pathologic evaluation is then done to confirm the diagnosis and classify the type of rhabdomyosarcoma. Systemic evaluation by a pediatric oncologist is then done. Radiation and systemic chemotherapy are the mainstay of treatment.

Prognosis

Survival rates are 90 percent with this treatment.

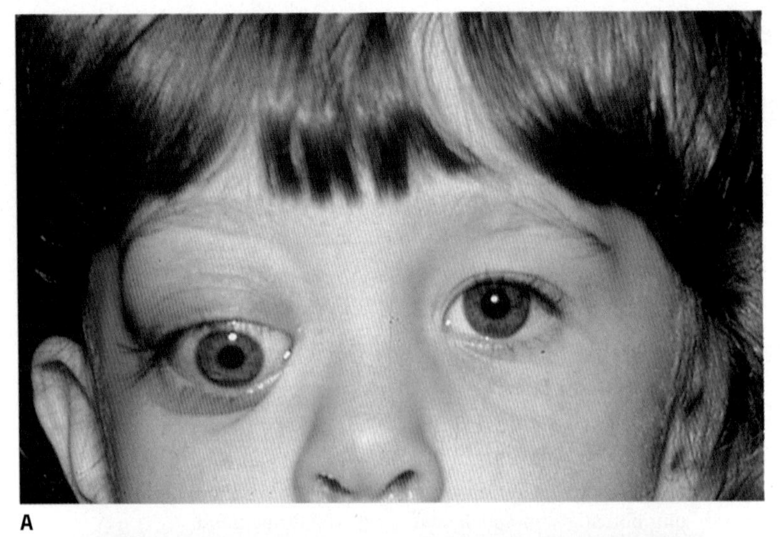

A

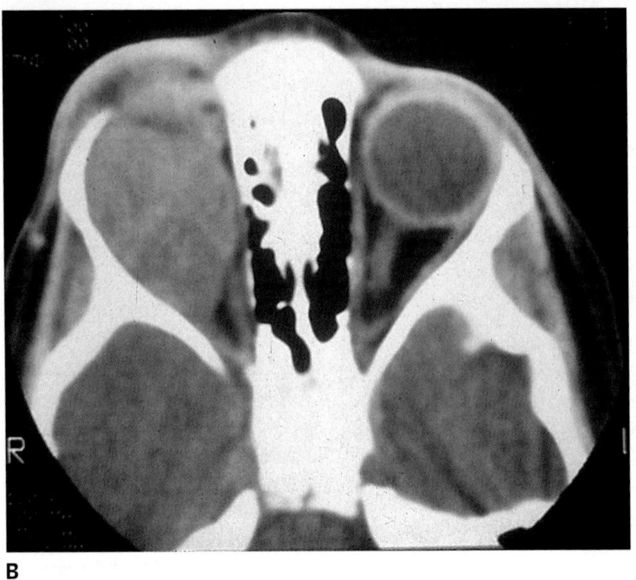

B

Figure 14-13 Rhabdomyosarcoma **A.** *An 8-year-old female with 3-week history of progressive swelling of the right eye.* **B.** *CT scan shows large mass of the orbit, which on biopsy was a rhabdomyosarcoma. (Continued.)*

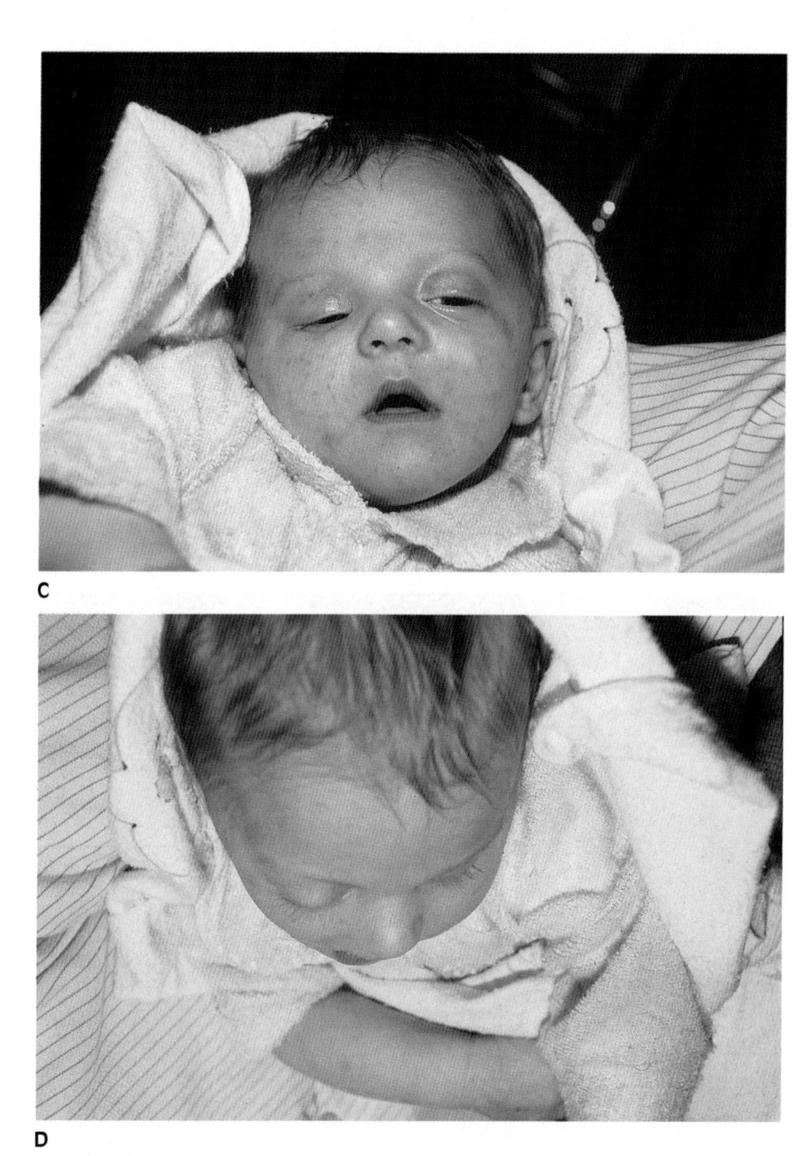

Figure 14-13 Rhabdomyosarcoma (cont.) **C.** *and* **D.** *A 3-month-old female with 1- to 2-week history of swelling of the right eye. (Continued.)*

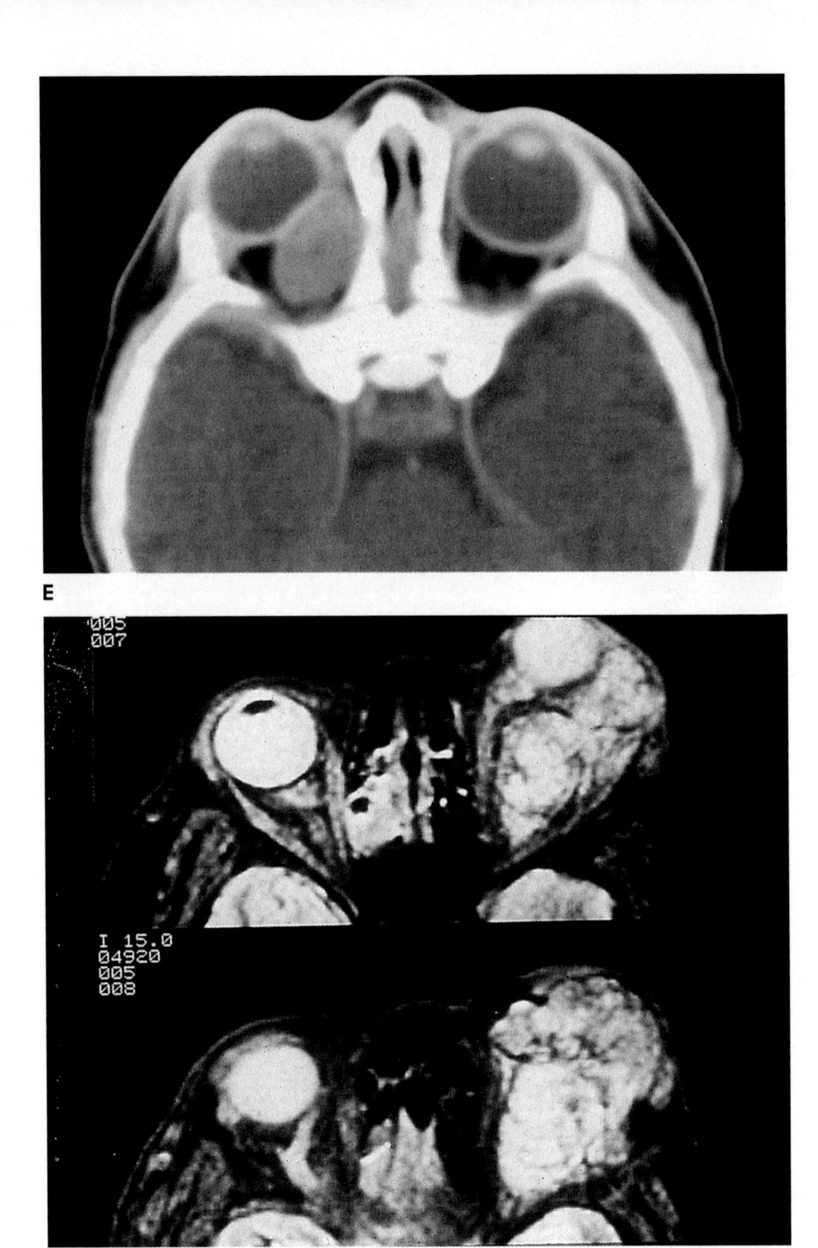

Figure 14-13 Rhabdomyosarcoma (cont.) **E.** *CT scan shows well-circumscribed mass with indentation of the globe. Biopsy of the mass revealed a rhabdomyosarcoma. The fact that this patient is younger than the typical rhabdomyosarcoma patient shows that rhabdomyosarcoma can present at various ages.* **F.** *MRI of a rhabdomyosarcoma. The T_2-weighted image shows the lesion is hyperintense to muscle and fat.*

FIBROUS HISTIOCYTOMA

Fibrous histiocytoma is a tumor that can be benign, locally aggressive, or malignant. If not completely excised, the benign forms can become malignant. The tumor is usually infiltrating and not encapsulated. It usually presents with proptosis and is often accompanied by various forms of orbital dysfunction depending on the tumor location.

Epidemiology and Etiology

Age Middle age.

Gender Equal occurrence in males and females.

Etiology Arises de novo from mesenchymal tissue. The tumor can be benign, intermediate, or malignant.

History

Usually slow onset of proptosis with no definitive onset in the least aggressive form. The malignant form can present more rapidly accompanied by diplopia, pain, swelling, and restricted eye movements.

Examination

Proptosis with few other orbital signs in the benign form. The more aggressive forms show signs of inflammation, restricted eye movements, chemosis, and swelling (Fig. 14-14).

Imaging

CT scan: well-circumscribed orbital mass but the intermediate and malignant forms can be more infiltrative.
MRI: isointense on T_1 and hyperintense on T_2. Enhances with gadolinium.

Special Considerations

Incomplete excision can lead to recurrence and the recurrence can be malignant. The malignant, most aggressive form can metastasize.

Differential Diagnosis

- Hemangiopericytoma
- Capillary hemangioma
- Schwannoma

Pathology

Fibrous appearing histiocytic cells that form a characteristic cartwheel or storiform pattern.

Treatment

Complete surgical excision. The histology will reveal the prognosis.

Prognosis

Depends on histologic type. If the benign or locally aggressive forms are completely excised, the prognosis is usually good.

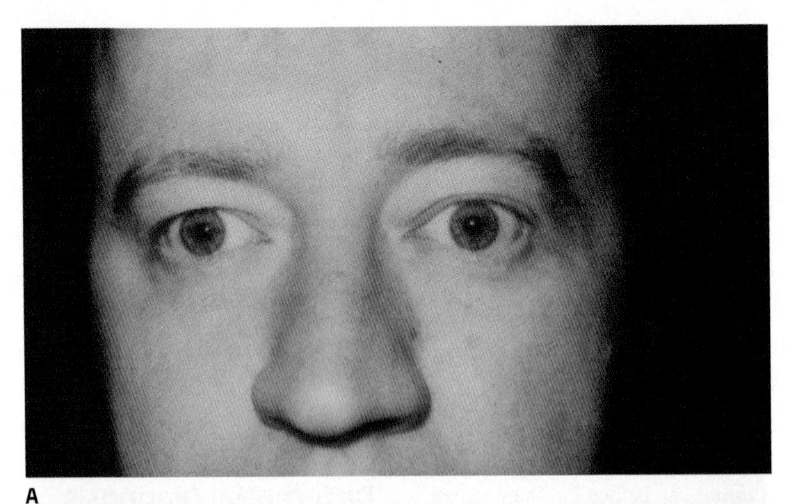

A

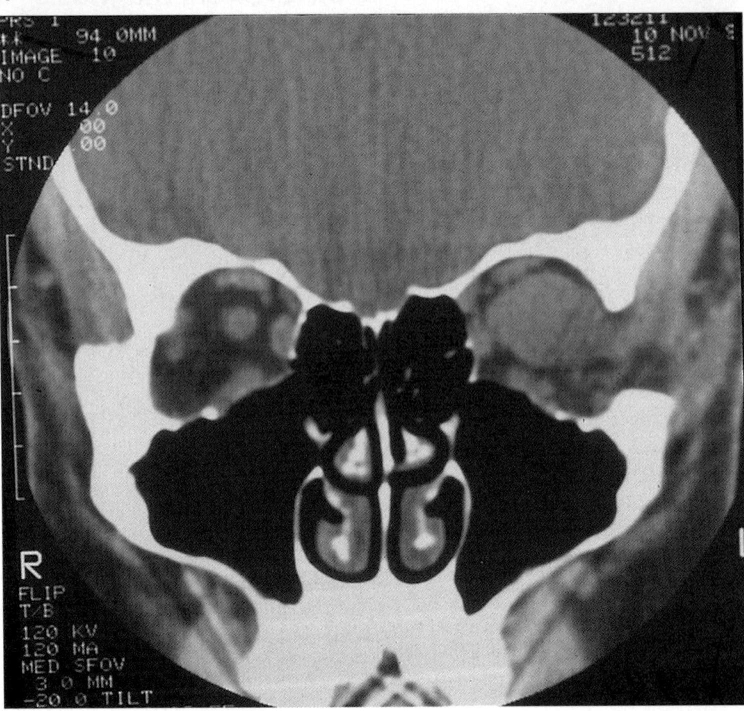

B

Figure 14-14 Fibrous histiocytoma **A.** *A 42-year-old male with progressive proptosis of the left eye over 2 to 3 months, increasing diplopia, and blurred vision.* **B.** *CT scan shows an intraconal mass with possible infiltration of the optic nerve. (Continued.)*

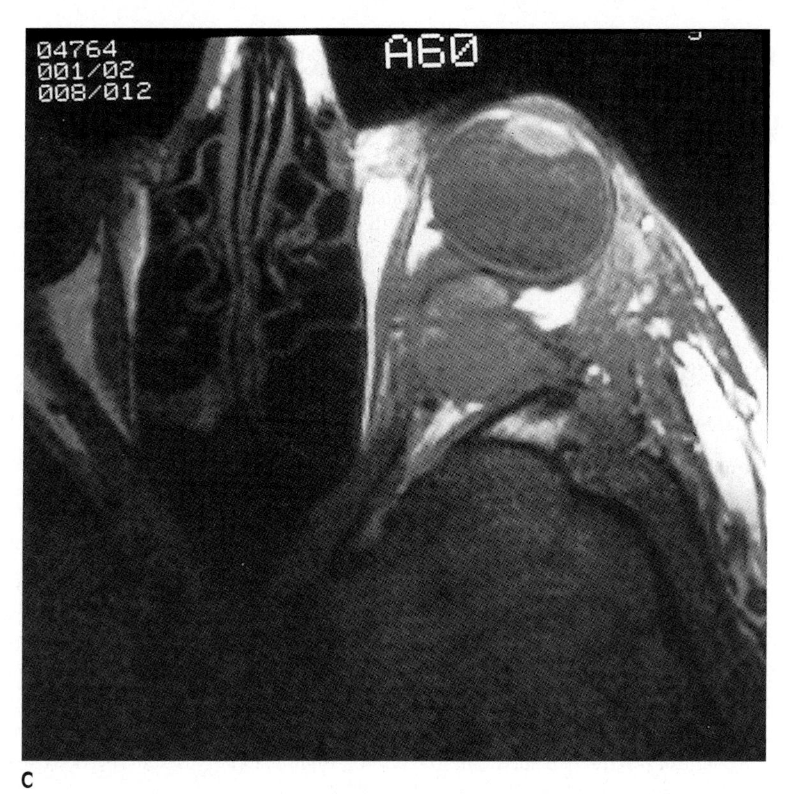

C

Figure 14-14 Fibrous histiocytoma (cont.) **C.** *On MRI, the mass abuts but does not infiltrate the optic nerve. The mass was removed and was a benign fibrous histiocytoma.*

LYMPHOPROLIFERATIVE TUMORS

LYMPHOID HYPERPLASIA AND LYMPHOMAS

Lymphoid lesions include a spectrum of lesions from benign to malignant. Presence of even the benign lymphoid hyperplasia implies a risk in the future for the development of a lymphoma somewhere in the body. These lesions can occur in the orbit or subconjunctival area and tend to mold around structures rather than displacing structures.

Epidemiology and Etiology

Age Older adults.

Gender Equal occurrence in males and females.

Etiology Clonal expansion of abnormal precursor cells. There is a continuum of disease from the benign, localized lymphoid hyperplasia through malignant lymphoma.

History

A history of a painless, progressive mass. The exact history depends on the location of the mass. Anteriorly, it can present as a visible, palpable mass. More posteriorly, the symptoms will be more of proptosis or globe displacement depending on the location.

Examination

Anteriorly, a visible, subconjunctival salmon-patch mass can be observed. A soft, diffuse mass can be palpated if the mass is in the anterior orbit but not visible. More posterior tumors will cause proptosis with symptoms depending on the tumor location. These tumors tend to mold around orbital structures and rarely displace or infiltrate structures so motility or visual disturbances are rare (Fig. 14-15A–D).

Imaging

CT scan: a mass that molds around orbital structures rather than displacing or infiltrating (Fig. 14-15E).

MRI: shows extent of tumor but does not differentiate orbital inflammation and cannot separate lymphoid hyperplasia from lymphoma (Fig. 14-15F).

Special Considerations

There are multiple ways to evaluate a lymphoid lesion to determine whether it is a benign or a malignant lesion. Not all lesions can be clearly determined to be benign or malignant. Even the patient with benign lymphoid hyperplasia must be observed systemically for the development of a lymphoma elsewhere in the body over future years.

Differential Diagnosis

- Orbital pseudotumor
- Metastatic orbital tumor
- Lymphangioma

Pathology

A collection of lymphocytes is seen, which identifies the lesion as lymphoid. Microscopic appearance will give some evidence of the lesion as benign or malignant. Fresh tissue is evaluated to identify cell surface markers. Polyclonal lymphocytic populations are less likely to develop systemic disease, monoclonal lesions are more likely to accompany lymphoma elsewhere in the body. The attempt to separate lymphoid lesions into benign and malignant is not exact and is both controversial and confusing; however, at this time, it is the best we have.

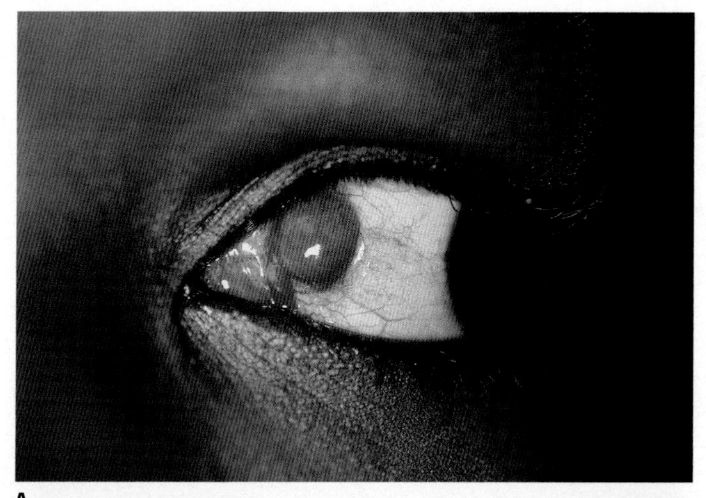
A

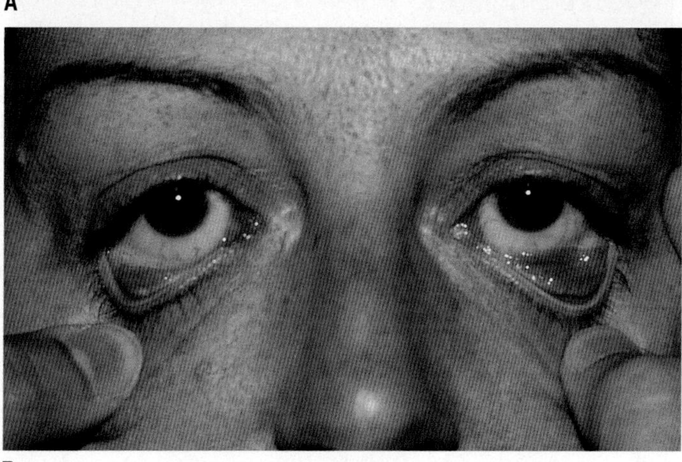
B

Figure 14-15 Lymphoid hyperplasia and lymphoma **A.** *and* **B.** *Both figures show subconjunctival lymphoid infiltrates. These may be isolated or there may be orbital extension. They may be a reactive process or a lymphoma. Where these lesions fall on the spectrum of benign versus malignant can only be differentiated on biopsy. Figure 14-15A was benign reactive lymphoid hyperplasia and Figure 14-15B was a low-grade lymphoma. (Continued.)*

Treatment

The lesions require biopsy to identify whether they are benign or malignant. A systemic work-up is done to look for evidence of lymphoid lesions elsewhere in the body. Treatment for localized benign orbital disease is low-dose radiation. More malignant lesions or systemic disease usually requires radiation and systemic chemotherapy.

Prognosis

The prognosis is dependent on the type of lymphoma. Many lymphomas are very responsive to treatment but a high-grade lymphoma can be rapidly fatal, even with treatment.

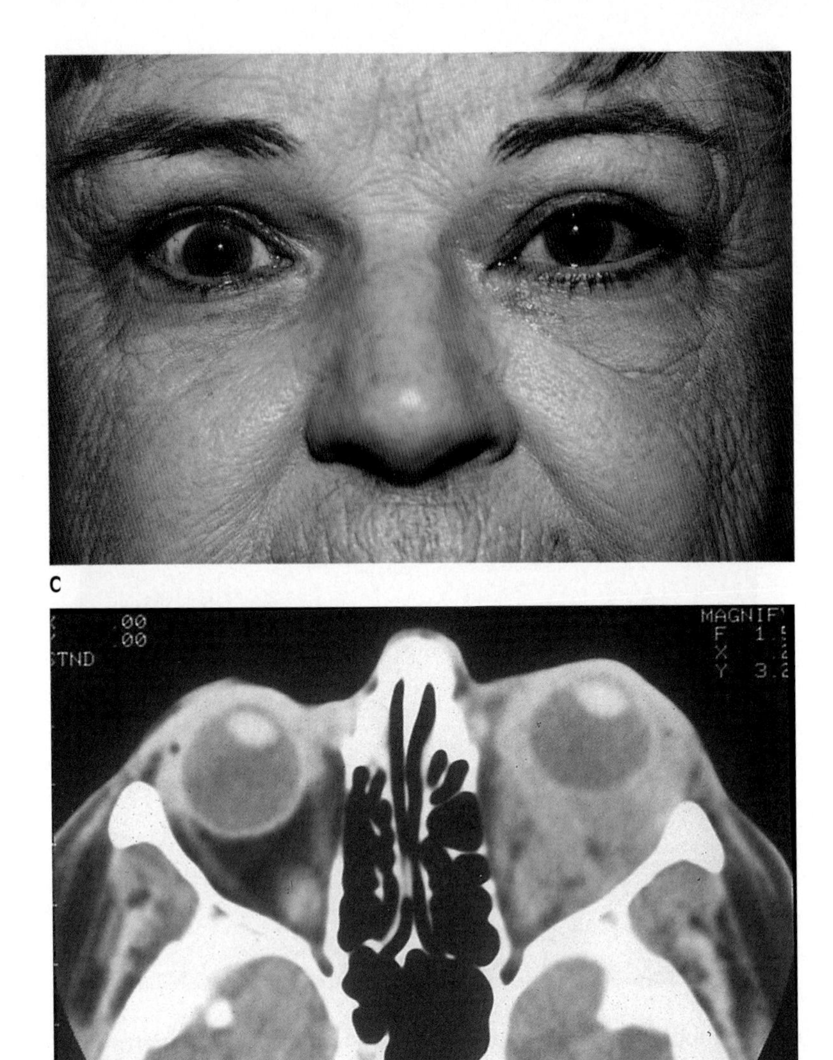

C

D

Figure 14-15 Lymphoma (cont.) **C.** *A 65-year-old female with swelling and redness of the left eye.* **D.** *CT scan shows a diffuse orbital process, which on biopsy was a lymphoma. Patient was treated with radiation and chemotherapy. (Continued.)*

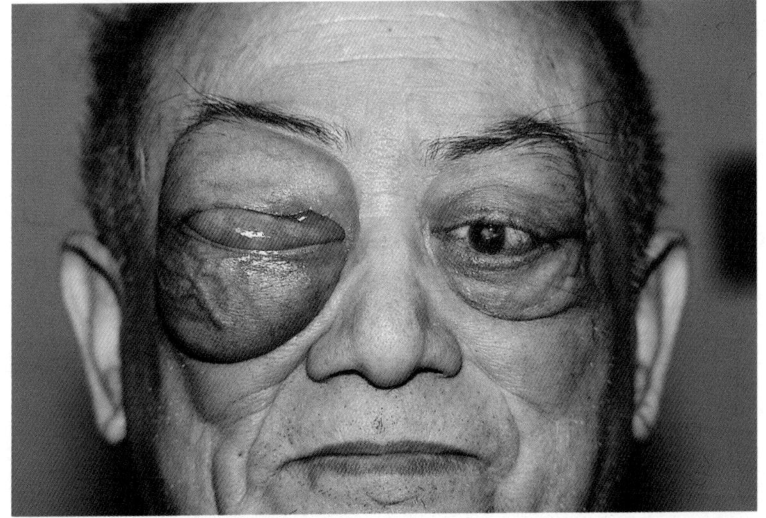

E

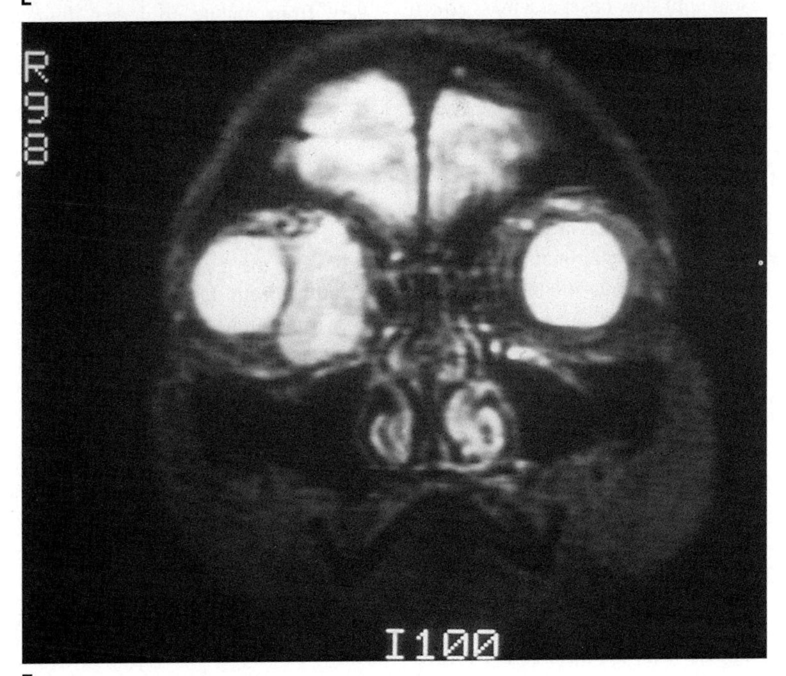

F

Figure 14-15 Lymphoma (cont.) **E.** *Massive lid and orbital infiltration by a lymphoma on the right.* **F.** *MRI of a lymphoma. The T_2-weighted image shows the lesion to be hyperintense to muscle and fat.*

PLASMACYTOMA

Plasmacytoma is an isolated mass of plasma cells that occurs in the bone. This lesion can extend from the bone into the orbital soft tissue. Progression to a systemic plasma cell tumor is termed multiple myeloma.

Epidemiology and Etiology

Age Sixth and seventh decades.

Gender Males more commonly affected.

Etiology Rare proliferation of plasma cells in soft tissues or bone of the orbit.

History

Patients present with slow onset of a mass effect with some inflammatory signs but very rarely pain. Symptoms depend on the location of the tumor.

Examination

If located anteriorly, there is a palpable mass over or adjacent to an orbital bone. There may be proptosis or globe displacement depending on the location (Fig. 14-16).

Imaging

CT scan shows a lesion in or adjacent to bone with bony destruction.

Special Considerations

Like lymphoma, plasma cell tumors can be benign or malignant. They are differentiated from multiple myeloma on the basis of systemic involvement in multiple myeloma.

Differential Diagnosis

- Multiple myeloma
- Metastatic disease
- Histiocytic disorders
- Malignant tumor of the sinus

Pathology

Classic plasma cells make up the tumor. These vary from mature to larger, immature cells depending on the tumor. Differentiation from multiple myeloma is on the basis of systemic work-up; multiple myeloma having other systemic manifestations.

Treatment

Biopsy of the lesion, and then a complete systemic work-up. If the lesion is isolated, higher dose irradiation is indicated. Chemotherapy may be indicated.

Prognosis

Variable depending on the aggressiveness of the tumor.

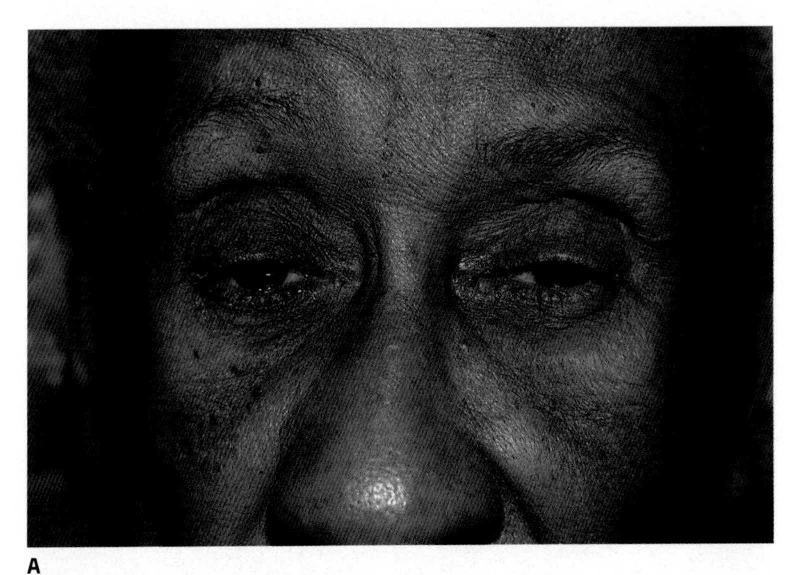

A

Figure 14-16 Plasma cell tumor **A.** *A 70-year-old female was noted to have swelling around the left eye. Examination shows proptosis with downward displacement of the left eye. (Continued.)*

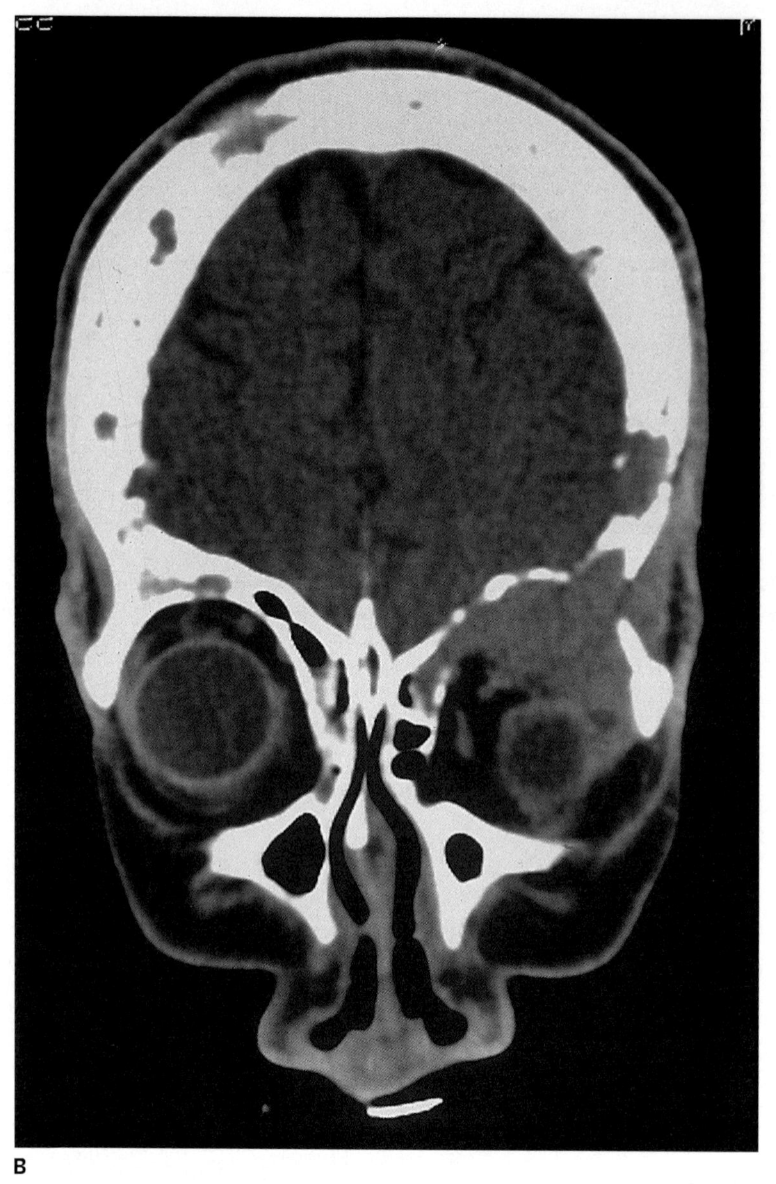

B

Figure 14-16 Plasma cell tumor (cont.) **B.** *and* **C.** *CT scan shows a superior temporal lesion that has eroded bone and may even be centered in bone. Biopsy revealed a plasmacytoma. (Continued.)*

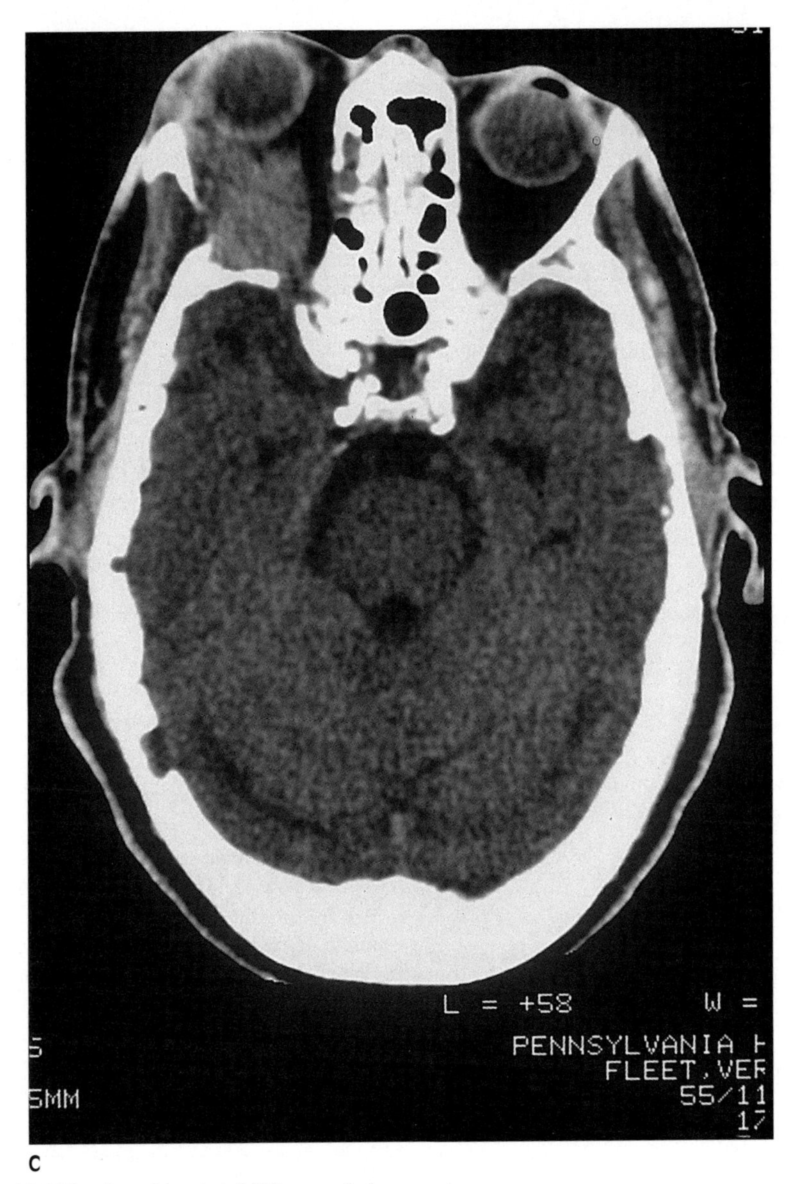

C

Figure 14-16C. (cont.) *Axial CT scan of plasmacytoma.*

HISTIOCYTIC DISORDERS

Histiocytic disorders are a rare group of abnormalities of the mononuclear phagocytic system. In the orbit, they most commonly present as a unifocal lesion of the superior bone of the orbit with secondary progressive proptosis.

Epidemiology and Etiology

Age Children. Children less than age 2 years are more likely to have systemic disease, which is up to 50 percent fatal. Over the age 2 years the disease involves the bone without systemic involvement but is often multifocal. The older the child, the more likely the disease will be unifocal and less severe.

Gender Males more commonly affected.

Etiology Abnormal immune regulation resulting in an accumulation of proliferating dendritic histiocytes.

History

Orbital swelling most commonly superiorly over days to weeks.

Examination

Superior orbital swelling with a variable amount of mass effect is the most common presentation. Younger children are more likely to have more swelling, multifocal bony involvement, and systemic involvement (Fig. 14-17).

Imaging

CT scan will show a lesion adjacent to bone with bone erosion. Most commonly in the superior, temporal orbit.

Special Considerations

The older term for these disorders was histiocytosis X with specific manifestations termed Letterer–Siwe disease, Hand–Schüller–Christian disease, and eosinophilic granuloma of bone. These terms are replaced by diffuse soft tissue histiocytosis, multiple eosinophilic granuloma of bone, and unifocal granuloma of bone.

Differential Diagnosis

- Cholesteatoma
- Reparative granuloma

Pathology

Proliferation of dendritic histiocytes along with granulocytes and lymphocytes.

Treatment

Bony lesions require a confirmatory biopsy and then debulking. This treatment is often curative but in younger children, evidence of systemic disease must be sought. Rarely, steroids or low-dose radiation is needed. Treatment for systemic disease in younger children may include steroids, irradiation, or cytotoxic agents. In some cases, the disease may not respond to anything.

Prognosis

Excellent in unifocal disease in older children. Very young children with systemic disease have a 50 percent mortality rate.

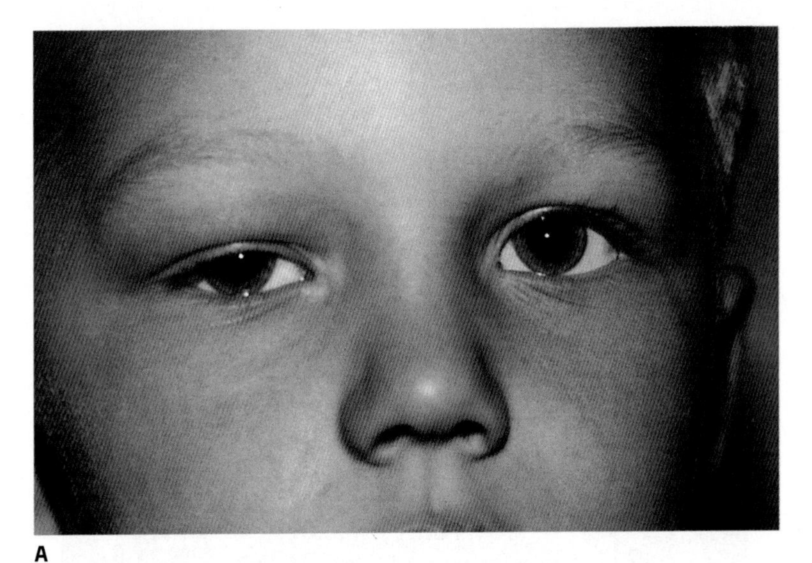

A

Figure 14-17 Histiocytic disorder **A.** *An 8-year-old male with a 1- to 2-week history of swelling of his right eye. Mild erythema and swelling superiorly and downward displacement of the globe on the right is shown. (Continued.)*

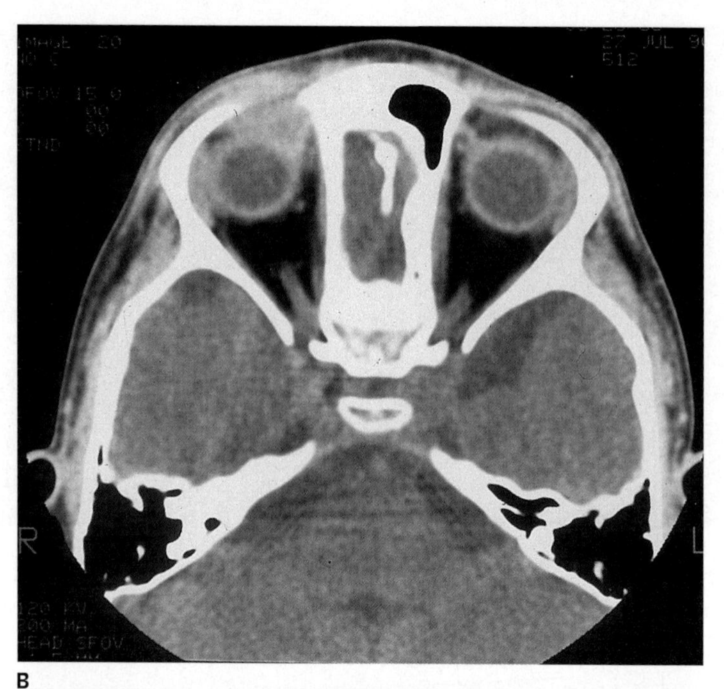

B

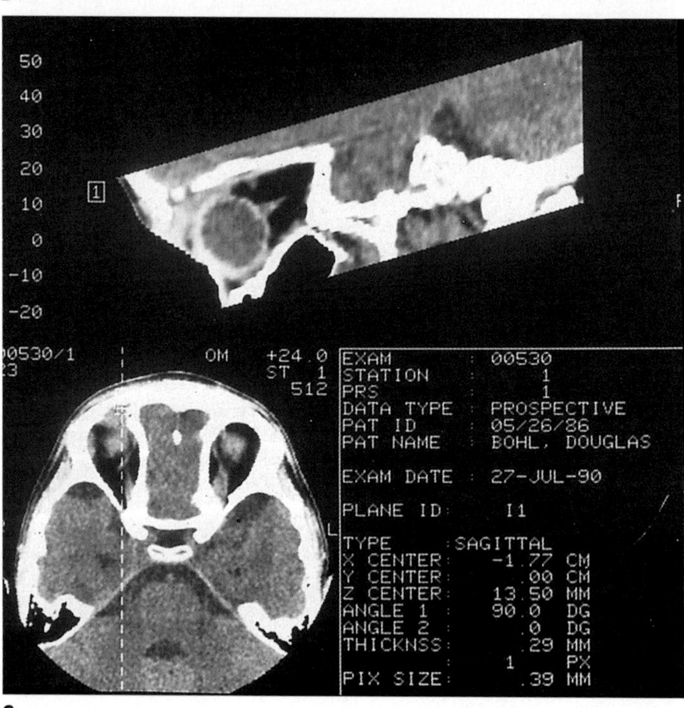

C

Figure 14-17 Histiocytic disorder (cont.) **B.** *and* **C.** *CT scan shows a superior infiltrate with bony erosion. Biopsy revealed a unifocal granuloma of bone, which was treated with curettage.*

LACRIMAL GLAND TUMORS

EPITHELIAL TUMORS OF THE LACRIMAL GLAND

The lacrimal gland can harbor multiple disease processes. The most common is inflammatory disease. Benign and malignant processes inherent to the lacrimal gland also occur. Biopsy is often required to identify these processes.

Epidemiology and Etiology

This group includes a number of entities that involve the lacrimal gland. This does not include idiopathic inflammation or lymphoid infiltration of the lacrimal gland.

Age Pleomorphic adenoma occurs in the fourth and fifth decades. Malignant mixed tumors occur at an older age. Adenoid cystic carcinoma has a peak incidence in the second and fourth decades.

Gender Equal male and female incidence.

Etiology Proliferation of epithelial cells.

History

Pleomorphic adenomas present with progressive, downward and inward displacement of the globe, sometimes with axial proptosis. The process is painless, unlike the malignant tumors of the lacrimal gland.

Malignant mixed tumors usually arise from existing pleomorphic adenomas. Adenoid cystic carcinoma will present with more rapid growth associated with significant pain. This pain is what easily separates many malignant lacrimal gland tumors from a benign pleomorphic adenoma.

Examination

Palpable mass in the superior, temporal quadrant with displacement of the globe down and in. The presence of inflammation and the amount of globe displacement is variable depending on the etiology of the lacrimal gland mass (Fig. 14-18).

Imaging

CT scan: pleomorphic adenomas show a globular, circumscribed mass. The mass flattens and deforms the globe. There can be pressure expansion of the lacrimal fossa but no erosion. Malignant lesions are not globular, are less well-defined, and may have bony erosions and calcifications.

MRI: valuable to define the extent of intracranial extension in aggressive, malignant tumors.

Special Considerations

Must completely excise a pleomorphic adenoma or it can recur as a malignant tumor.

Differential Diagnosis

- Idiopathic inflammation of the lacrimal gland
- Lymphoid infiltration of the lacrimal gland
- Sarcoidosis

Pathophysiology

Pleomorphic adenoma: proliferation of epithelial cells with ductal and secretory elements.

Adenoid cystic carcinoma: small, benign-appearing cells arranged in nests, tubules, or in a cribiform, Swiss-cheese pattern.

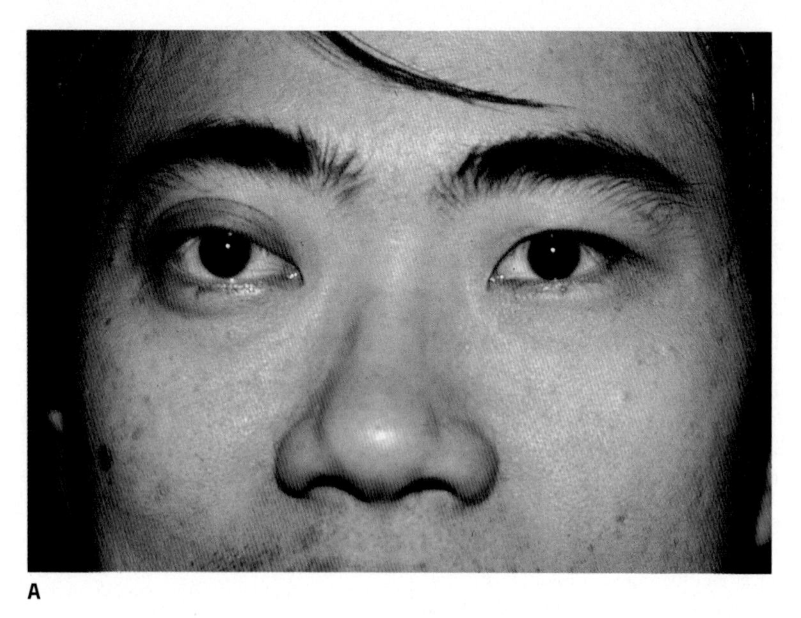

A

Figure 14-18 Lacrimal gland tumor **A.** *A 33-year-old male with slowly progressive, painless proptosis over a few years. (Continued.)*

Treatment

Pleomorphic adenoma: complete excision within the capsule.

Malignant tumors: individualize treatment. Generally extensive excision, especially with adenoid cystic carcinoma and high-dose radiation. Some tumors will require orbital exenteration.

Prognosis

Pleomorphic adenoma: excellent if completely excised.

Malignant tumors: high rate of recurrence over time.

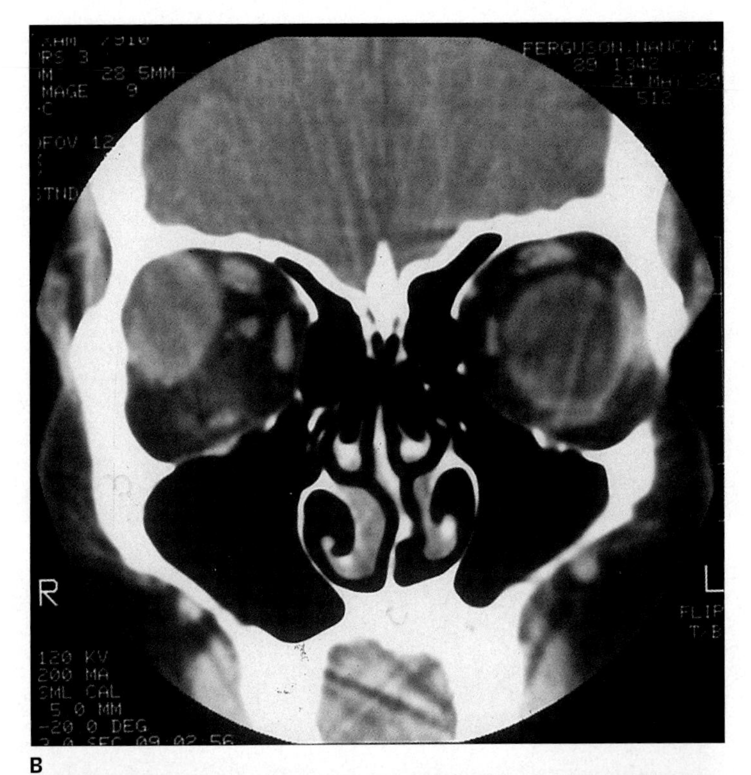

B

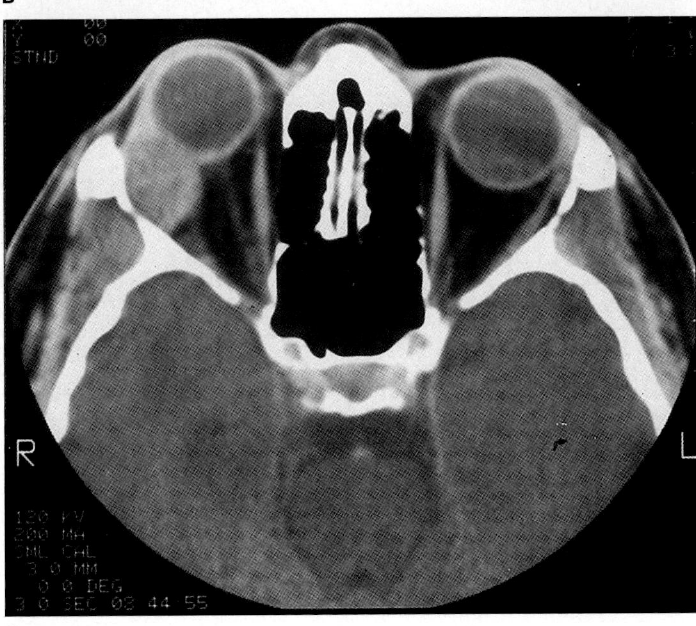

C

Figure 14-18 Lacrimal gland tumor (cont.) **B.** *and* **C.** *CT scan shows a round, well-circumscribed mass replacing the lacrimal gland. Complete excision showed a pleomorphic adenoma. (Continued.)*

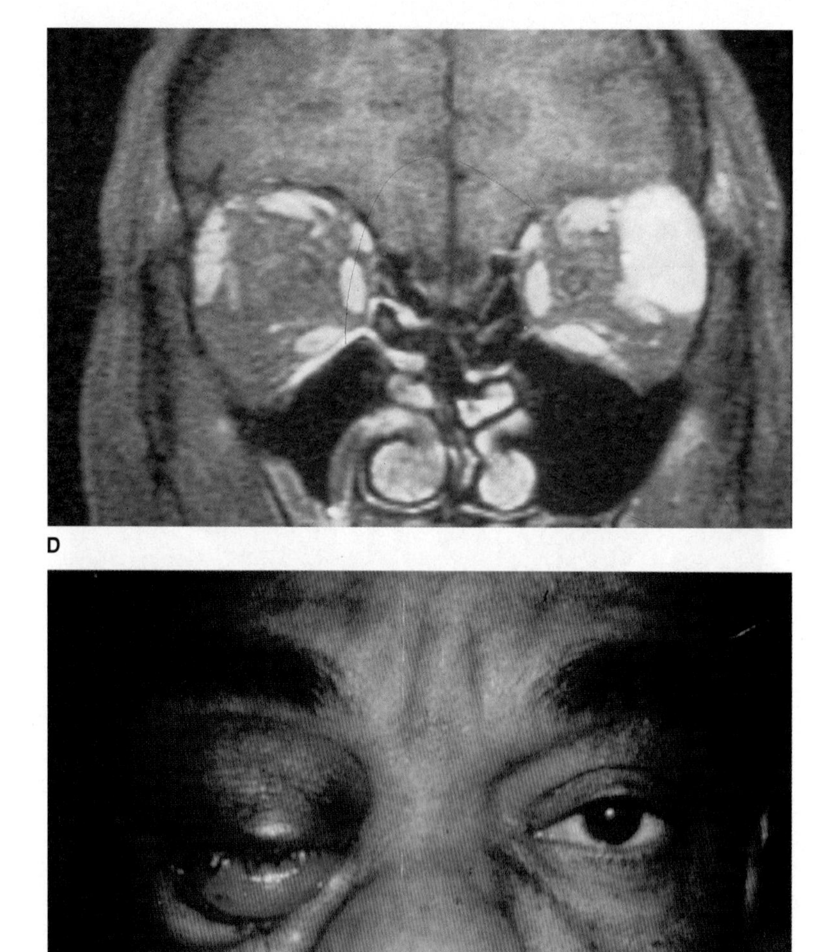

Figure 14-18 Lacrimal gland tumor (cont.) **D.** *MRI of a pleomorphic adenoma. The T_2-weighted image shows the lesion is hyperintense to fat and muscle.* **E.** *A 58-year-old male with 6-month history of swelling and pain around the left eye. Massive proptosis and swelling with downward displacement of the eye are seen. (Continued.)*

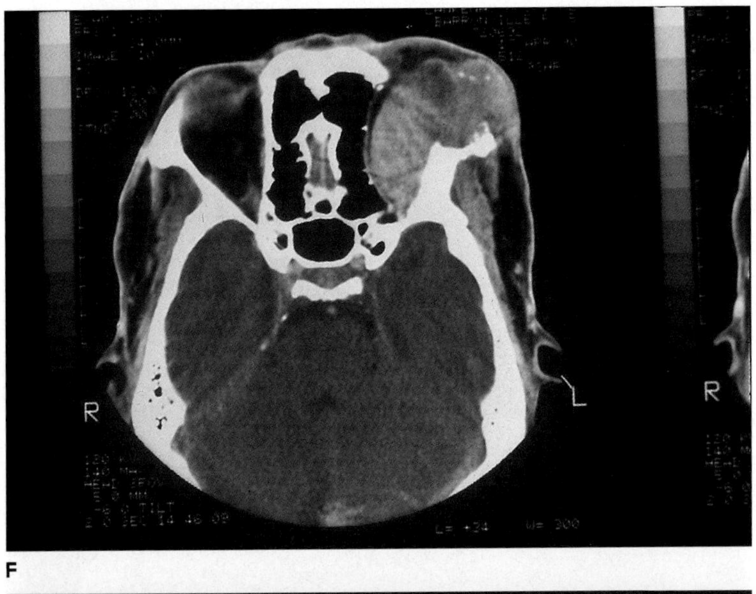

F

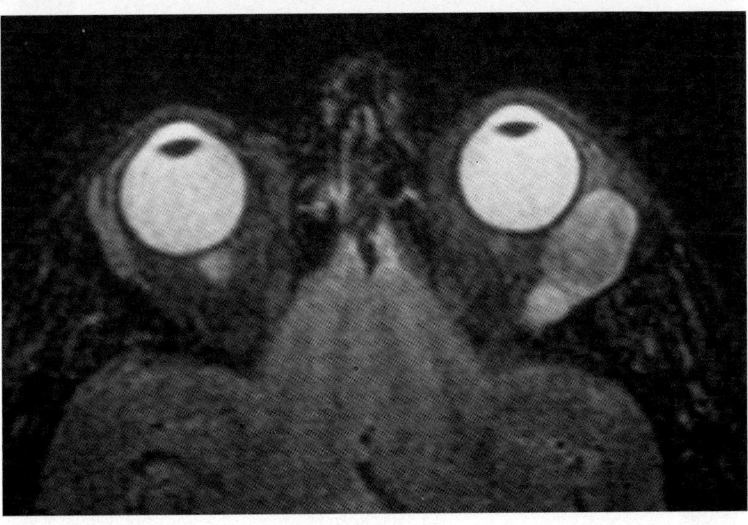

G

Figure 14-18 Lacrimal gland tumor (cont.) **F.** *CT scan shows a large mass in the lacrimal gland area with bony destruction. This was adenoid cystic carcinoma of the lacrimal gland.* **G.** *MRI of an adenoid cystic carcinoma. The T_2-weighted image shows the lesion is hyperintense to muscle and fat. (Continued.)*

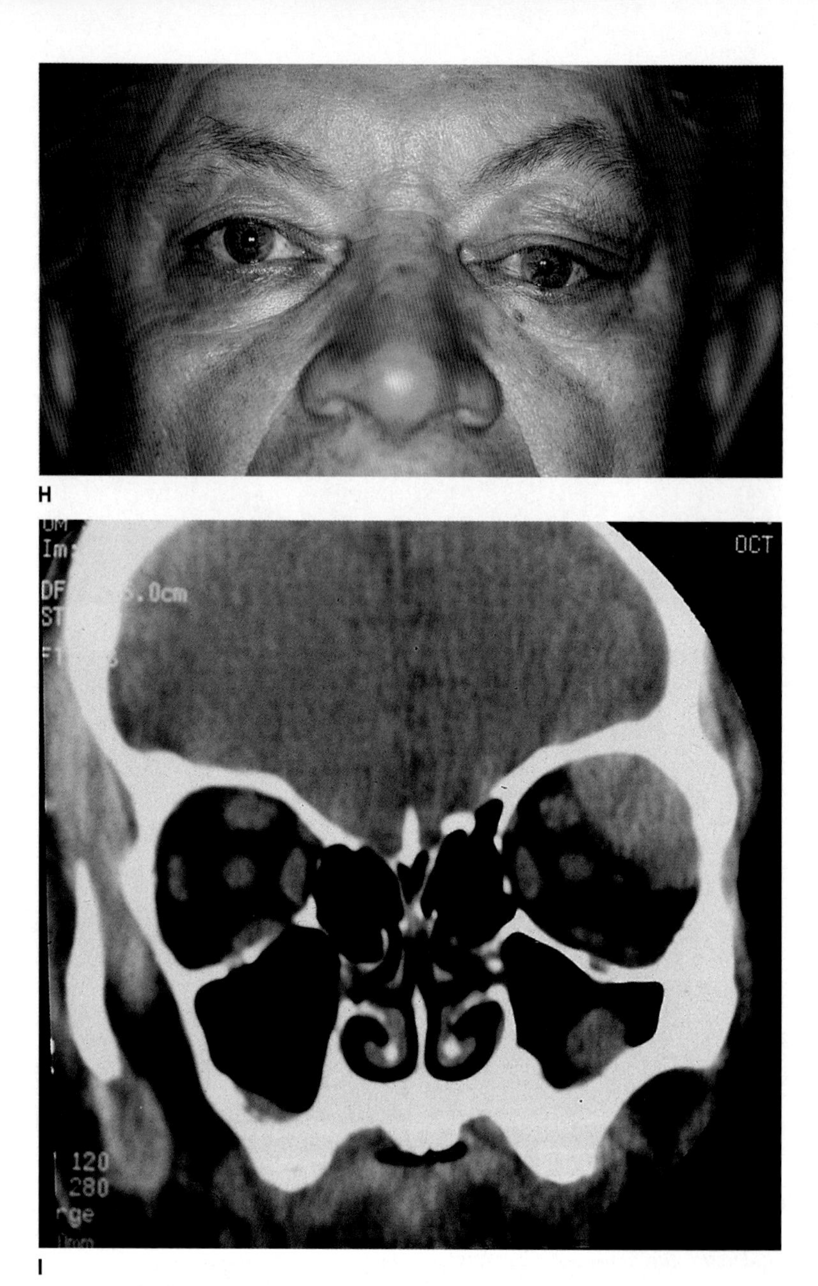

I

Figure 14-18 Lacrimal gland tumor (cont.) **H.** *and* **I.** *This 75-year-old male had swelling and downward displacement of the left eye for 2 to 3 months. CT scan shows an enlarged lacrimal gland, which was a lymphoma on biopsy. Contrast the shape of this mass with the very round contour in Figure 14-18B and C.*

MISCELLANEOUS ORBITAL TUMORS

SECONDARY ORBITAL TUMORS

Secondary orbital tumors are tumors that invade the orbit from adjacent structures including sinus tumors, eyelid tumors, and tumors that extend into the orbit from within the globe.

Epidemiology and Etiology

Etiology Includes tumors that invade the orbit from the sinus, eyelid, or globe. Sinus processes include mucoceles and squamous cell carcinoma. Eyelid tumors include basal cell carcinoma (Fig. 14-19A to C), sebaceous adenocarcinoma, and squamous cell carcinoma (Fig. 14-19E to G). Retinoblastoma and choroidal melanoma (Fig. 14-19D) can extend from the globe into the orbit.

Age and Gender Variable based on primary tumor.

History

Often, there is a history of either a neglected primary malignancy or a history of previous treatment of the primary malignancy. The time course of symptoms and growth is dependent on the primary malignancy.

Examination

There may be obvious external signs of the primary tumor such as in a neglected basal cell carcinoma. Likewise, intraocular tumors that extend outside the globe usually have external signs of inflammation. Sinus tumors that extend into the orbit may only show proptosis, often with some directional displacement of the globe.

Imaging

CT scan: dependent on the primary source. A tumor from the sinuses will show sinus changes. MRI: may help to define extraocular extension of a primary ocular tumor.

Differential Diagnosis

- If the primary tumor is known, the secondary process is easily suspected.

Pathology

The pathology is specific for each of the individual processes.

Treatment

Treatment is aimed at complete excision if possible. If the tumor is resectable and there is no evidence of distant metastasis then that is the treatment of choice. Depending on the tumor, irradiation after excision can be used. For those tumors unresectable, the use of irradiation and chemotherapy can be considered. Treatment must be individualized.

Prognosis

Generally poor. Even if the tumor is thought to be removed, there is often recurrence.

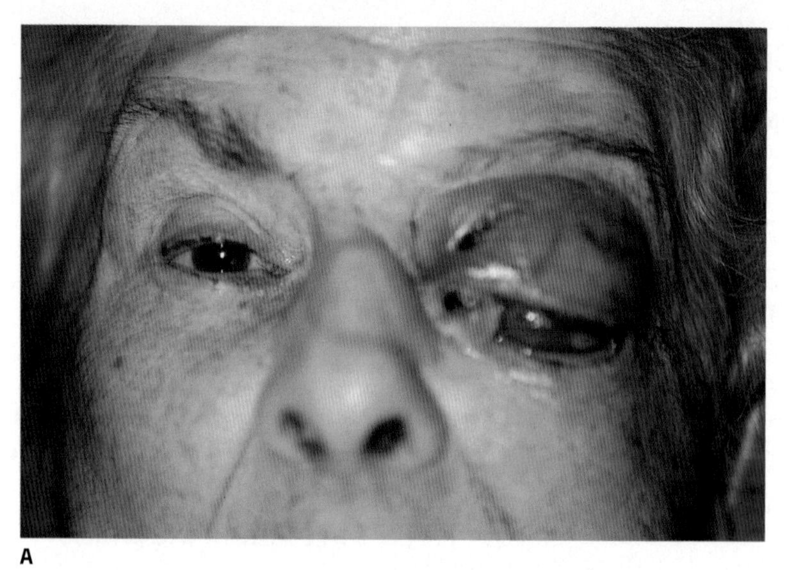

A

Figure 14-19 Basal cell carcinoma with orbital invasion **A.** *A patient with a neglected medial canthal basal cell carcinoma presents with proptosis. (Continued.)*

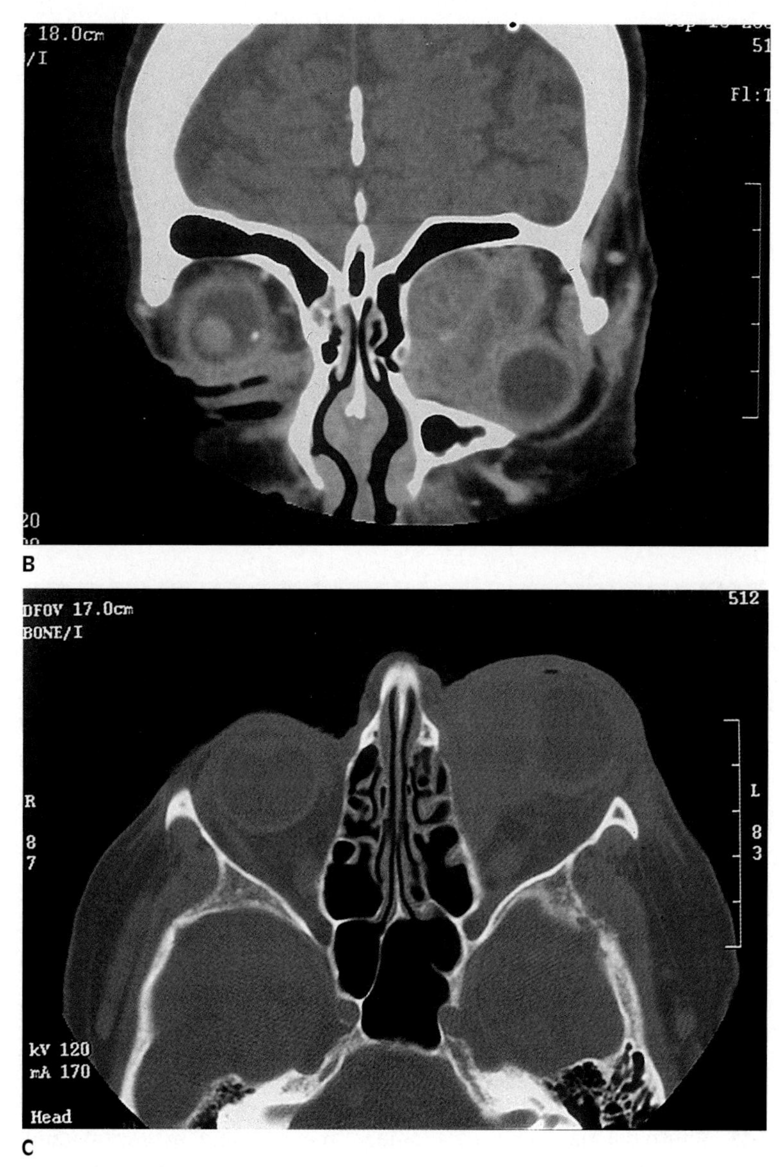

Figure 14-19 Basal cell carcinoma with orbital invasion (cont.) **B.** *and* **C.** *Axial and coronal CT scan shows a large medial orbital mass that was basal cell carcinoma on biopsy. The patient required an orbital exenteration. (Continued.)*

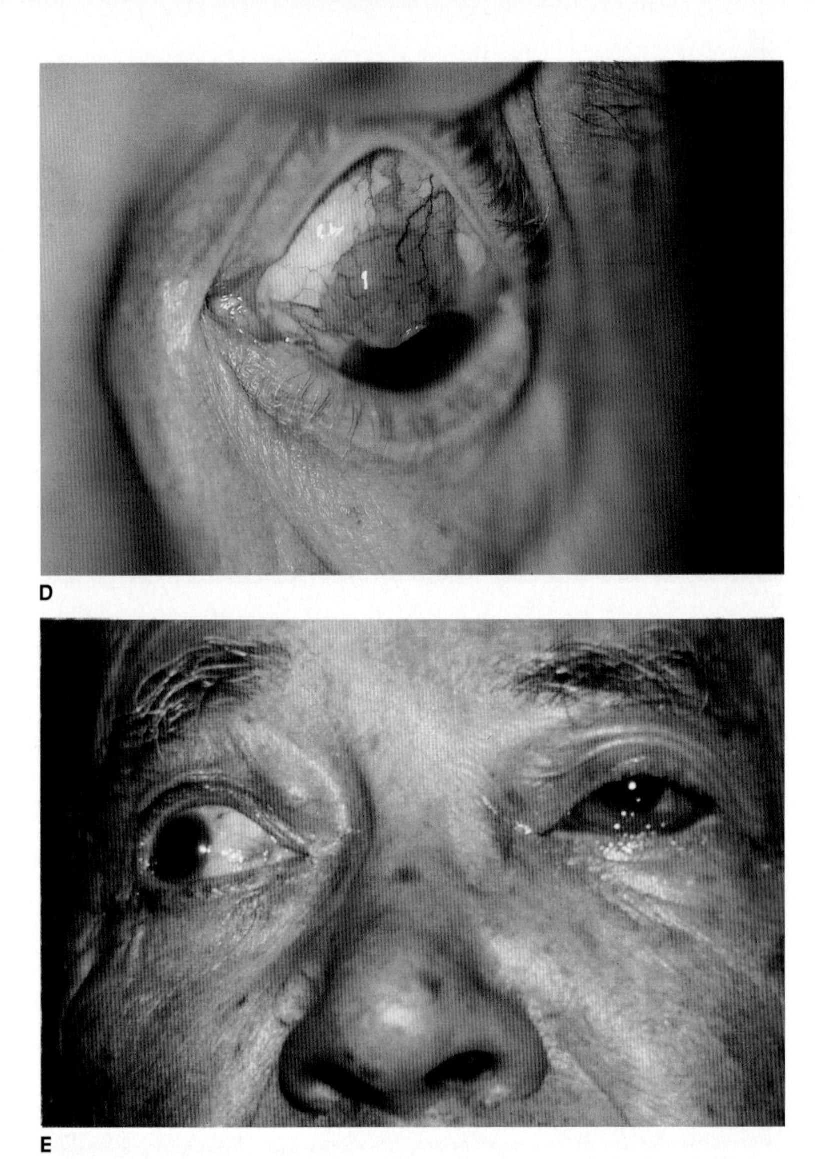

Figure 14-19 Choroidal malignant melanoma with extrascleral extension (cont.) **D.** *A patient with a large limbal mass. On fundus examination, there was a large choroidal melanoma that had extended extrasclerally.* **Squamous cell carcinoma with perineural spread** **E.** *A 77-year-old male with an orbital apex syndrome. (Continued.)*

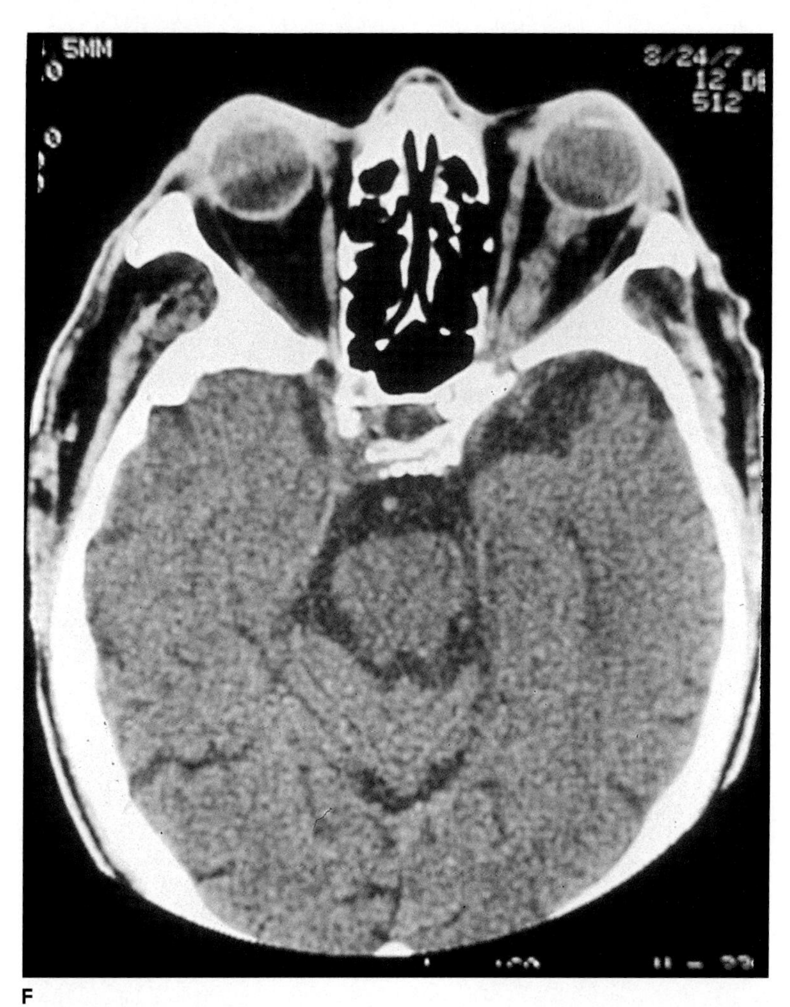

F

Figure 14-19 Squamous cell carcinoma with perineural spread (cont.) **F.** *and* **G.** *CT scan shows an infiltrating mass at the apex with thickening along the superior orbit. Biopsy showed squamous cell carcinoma that had spread into the apex along the frontal nerve. The patient had the history of a squamous cell carcinoma of the forehead excised 2 years prior. (Continued.)*

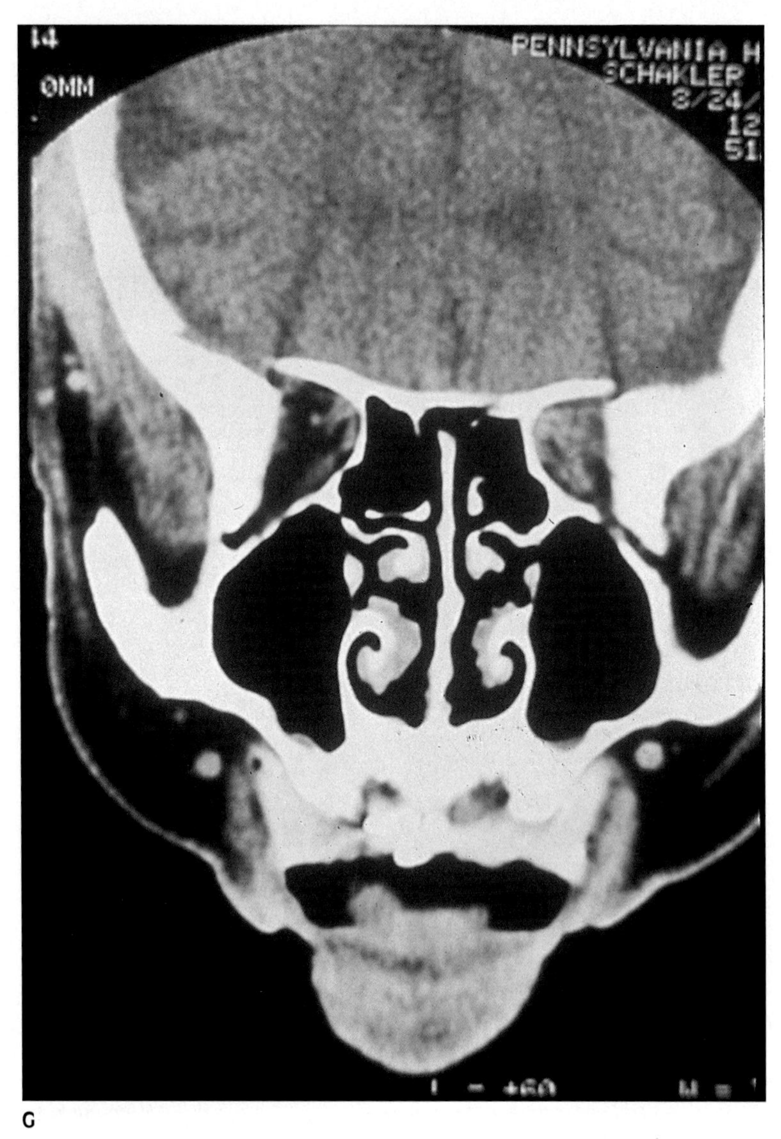

G

Figure 14-19 Squamous cell carcinoma with perineural spread (cont.) *Coronal CT showing lesion at apex.*

METASTATIC ORBITAL TUMORS

Metastatic orbital tumors usually present with orbital inflammation, pain, proptosis, and bony destruction. Most cases will have a known primary malignancy but in up to 25 percent, the primary site is unknown.

Epidemiology and Etiology

Age Most commonly in the fifth, sixth, and seventh decades.

Etiology and Gender Breast metastasis is the most common in women. Lung metastasis is the most common in men and second in women. Other etiologies include prostate in men, gastrointestinal, and many have an unknown primary site.

History

The majority of patients will have a known primary malignancy at the time of orbital occurrence. The onset of symptoms tends to be more rapid than in most orbital tumors and can be accompanied by pain.

Examination

Proptosis is the most common finding. This can be axial or displace the globe. A palpable mass may be present that is usually firm. Ptosis, motility disturbances, and decreased vision may be present because of the infiltrative nature of the metastasis (Fig. 14-20).

Imaging

CT scan: highly variable appearance of these lesions. May be discrete or invasive, cause bony erosion or hyperostosis (prostate), and may only show muscle enlargement.
MRI: not diagnostic and does not define bone well. May show extent into soft tissues.

Differential Diagnosis

- Lymphoma
- Wegener's granulomatosis
- Orbital pseudotumor

Pathology

Special stains and marker studies can help identify the tissue of origin in those cases that do not have a primary malignancy already identified.

Treatment

Biopsy to identify the tumor as metastatic. Systemic treatment of the carcinoma is then that of the primary malignancy. Orbital irradiation will often shrink the orbital tumor and diminish symptoms, either alone or in combination with chemotherapy.

Prognosis

The prognosis is that of the primary tumor with metastasis. In most cases, the prognosis is poor.

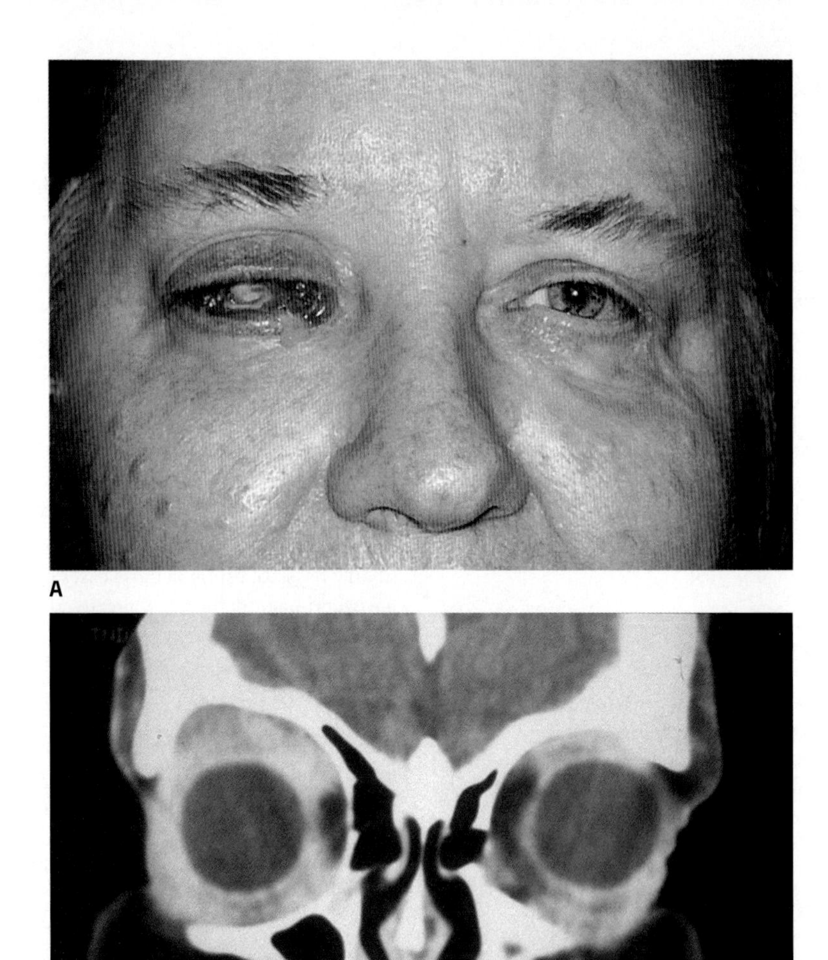

B

Figure 14-20 Metastatic breast carcinoma **A.** *and* **B.** *A 65-year-old female with known history of breast cancer presents with swollen, painful right eye. The patient has proptosis with a frozen globe and a corneal ulcer. CT scan shows diffuse infiltration of the orbit with metastatic breast carcinoma. Further work up revealed other areas of metastatic disease. (Continued.)*

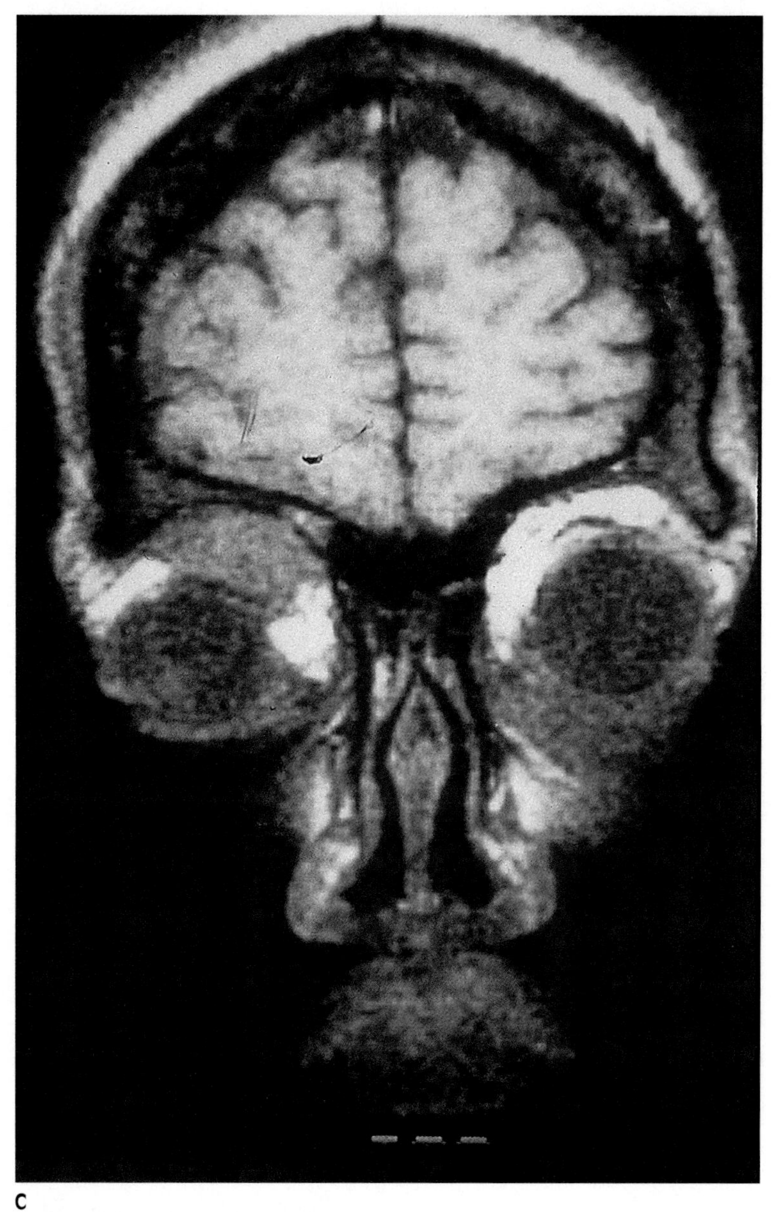

C

Figure 14-20 Metastatic breast carcinoma (cont.) **C.** *MRI T_1-weighted image shows the lesion hypointense to fat and muscle. (Continued.)*

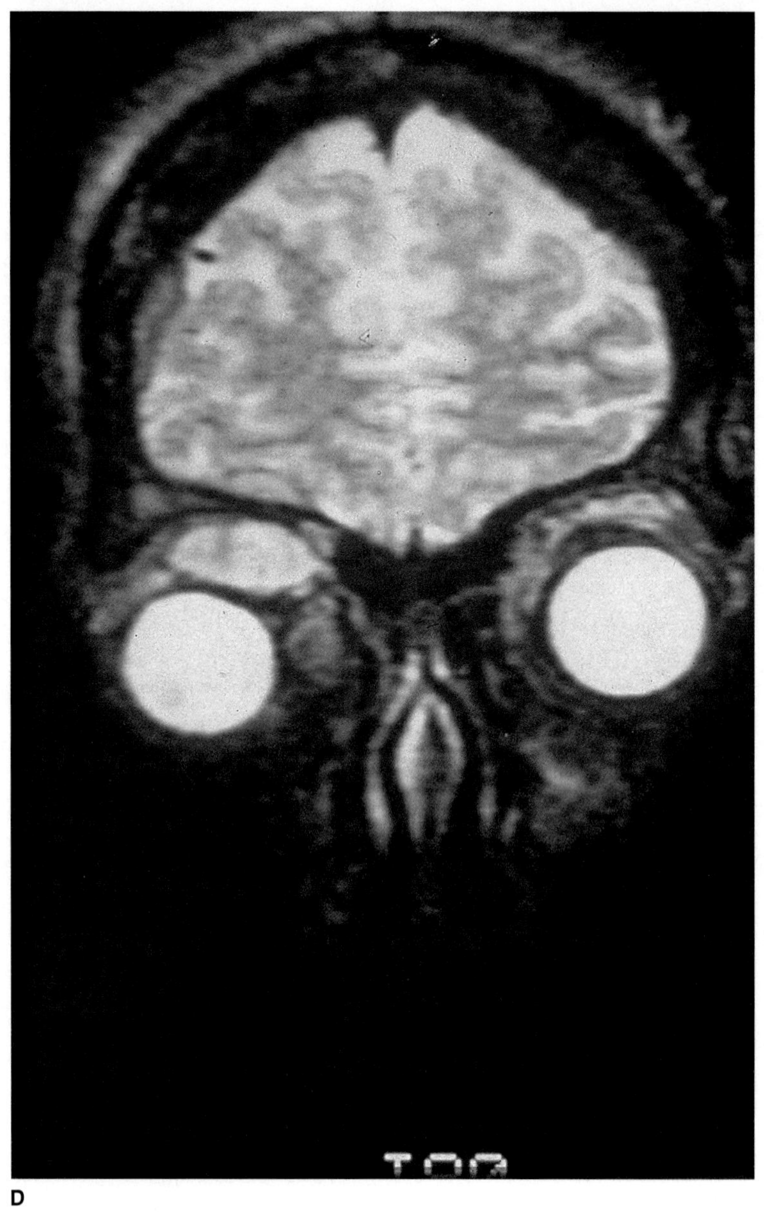

D

Figure 14-20 Metastatic breast carcinoma (cont.) **D.** *The T_2-weighted image shows the lesion hyperintense to fat and muscle. (Continued.)*

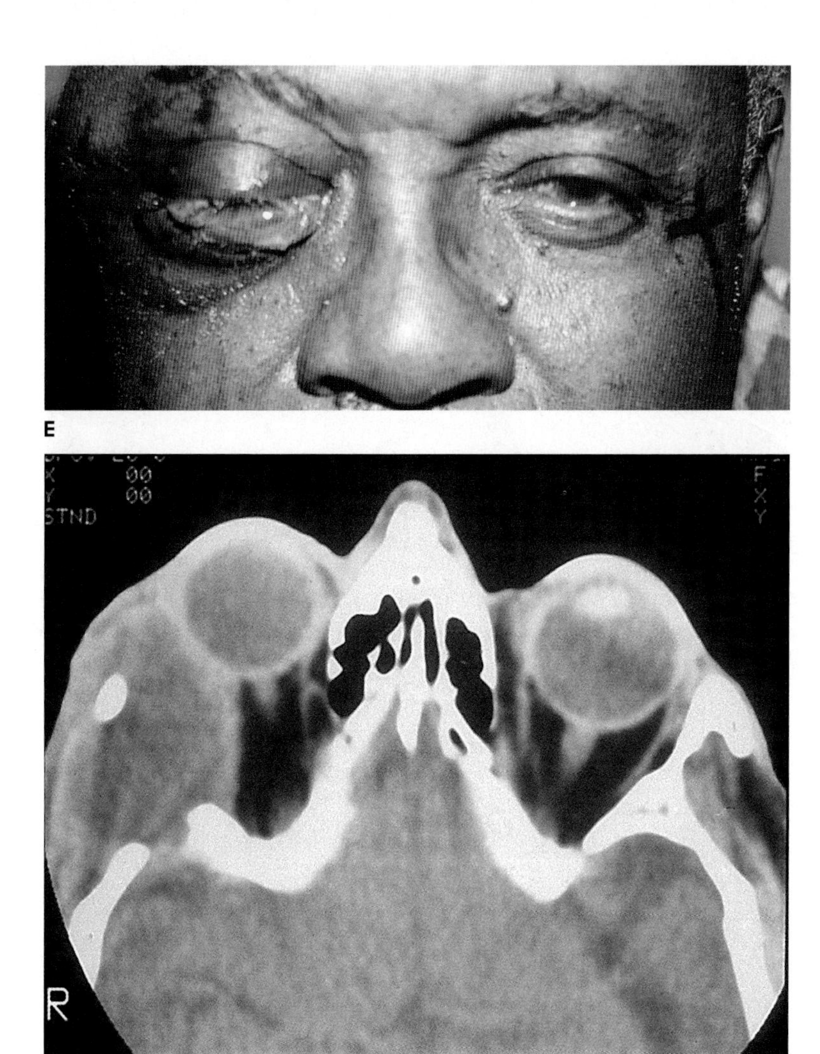

Figure 14-20 Metastatic lung carcinoma (cont.) **E.** *and* **F.** *A 68-year-old male with known metastatic lung adenocarcinoma presents with proptosis and pain. Note the lateral mass on the right. CT scan shows a lateral orbital mass with bone destruction. (Continued.)*

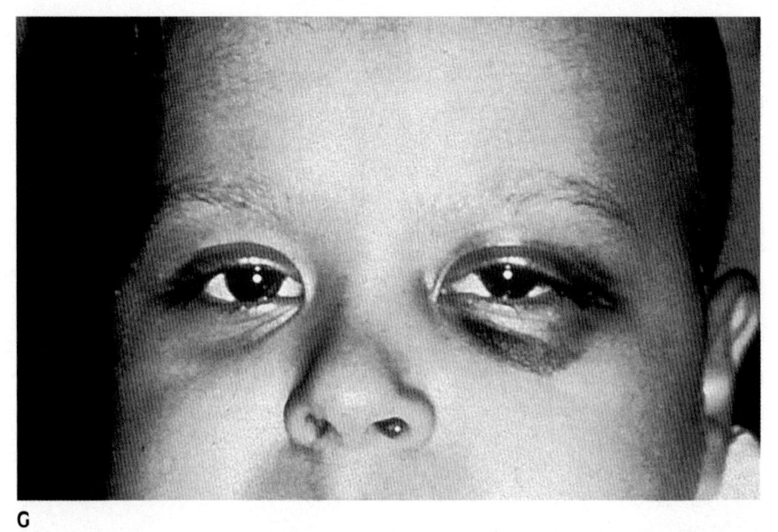

G

Figure 14-20 Metastatic neuroblastoma (cont.) **G.** *An 8-year-old child with known neuroblastoma with orbital metastasis. The photograph shows the classic orbital ecchymosis along with proptosis.*

Chapter 15

ORBITAL TRAUMA

ORBITAL FRACTURES

ORBITAL FLOOR FRACTURE

Orbital floor fractures are the most common type of orbital fracture. This is the result of a blow to the eye itself or to the bony rim. Many fractures only result in swelling and ecchymosis of the orbital tissues. Those with entrapped tissue and persistent diplopia, or with a large fracture and enophthalmos, will require repair.

Epidemiology and Etiology

Age Most common in second through fourth decades.

Gender More common in males.

Etiology Direct force to the inferior orbital rim with buckling and fracture of the floor is one mechanism. The second mechanism consists of forces which raise the intraorbital pressure and then "blow-out" the thin orbital floor.

History

Trauma such as fist, fingers, elbow, hit with a ball, and so forth. The patient will often have double vision after the injury. Less commonly, the patient may note orbital swelling after the trauma from orbital emphysema after blowing the nose.

Examination

Orbital swelling and ecchymosis is variable. Some fractures have very little. Infraorbital hypesthesia and restricted motility with diplopia are the most specific signs. As the orbital swelling decreases, large fractures will develop enophthalmos. Variable degrees of crepitance may be present as an indication of the fracture (Fig. 15-1).

Imaging

CT scanning shows a fracture of the orbital floor often with blood in the sinuses. A fracture that is very small is more likely to have entrapment of orbital tissue than a very large fracture. The inferior rectus is almost never in the fracture itself but tissues around the muscle are entrapped. MRI does not image bone well and should not be used initially after trauma.

Special Considerations

Children may sustain a fracture with no ecchymosis, but with severe entrapment of the inferior rectus muscle and associated nausea and vomiting. These patients are very uncomfortable and difficult to examine. The entrapment needs to be released within 24 to 48 hours, as the muscle will become ischemic if not released.

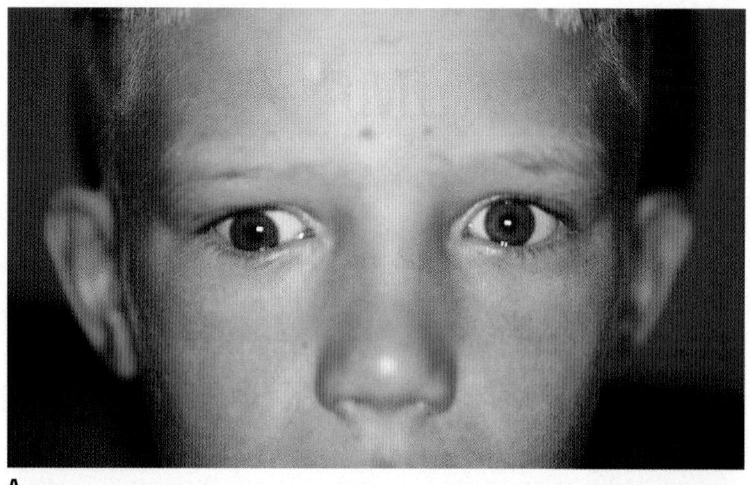

A

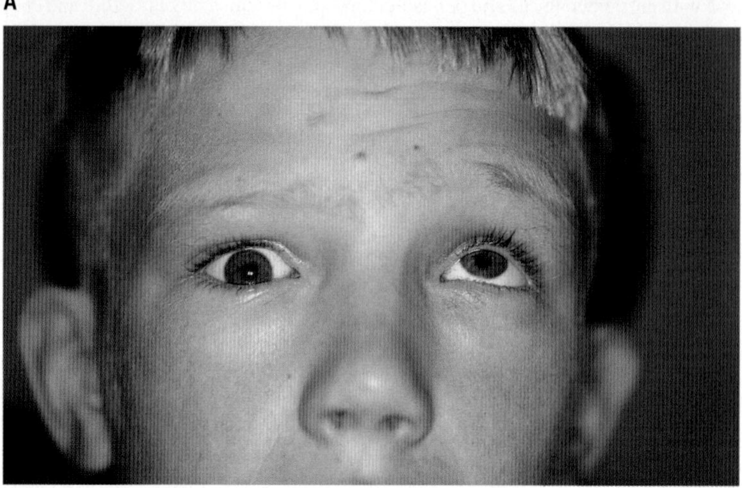

B

Figure 15-1 Orbital floor fracture **A.** *and* **B.** *A 9-year-old male with a history of being hit with an elbow 1 day prior. He has pain, worse with eye movement; double vision; and has had nausea and some vomiting. The photograph shows his lack of ecchymosis and swelling as well as severe restriction of upgaze. (Continued.)*

Treatment

Open repair is required for patients with functional diplopia that does not improve as the swelling resolves. Fractures involving more than 50 percent of the floor will result in significant enophthalmos and also should be considered for repair. Fractures should be repaired within 2 weeks of trauma. Most fractures that are repaired will require an implant of some type.

Prognosis

Good if repaired within 2 weeks. Some patients will have direct muscle or nerve injury and either will not improve or may take months to improve.

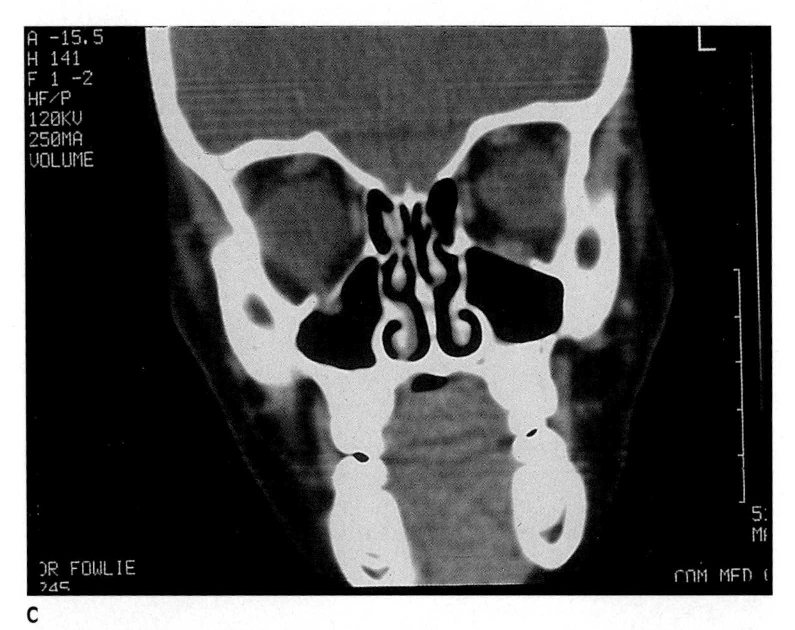

C

Figure 15-1 Orbital floor fracture (cont.) **C.** *CT scan shows a small trap-door floor fracture with tissue entrapment. This fracture needs to be repaired promptly as the entrapped muscle may become ischemic. (Continued.)*

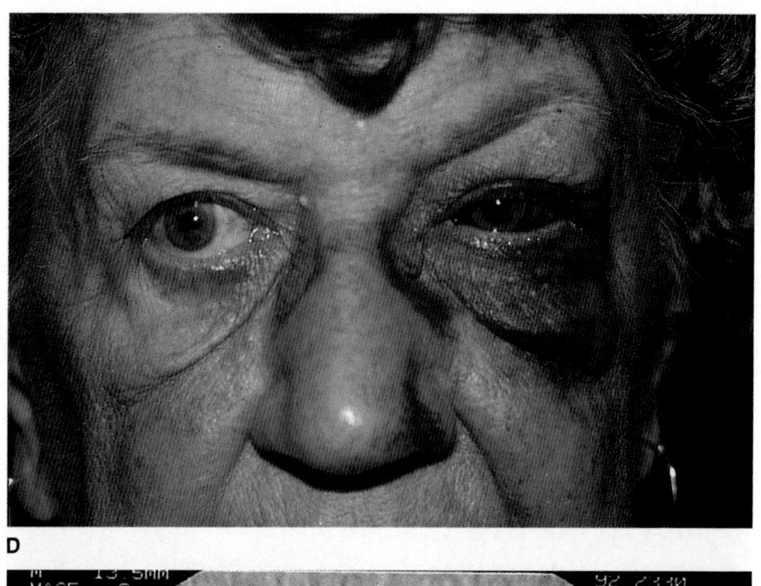

D

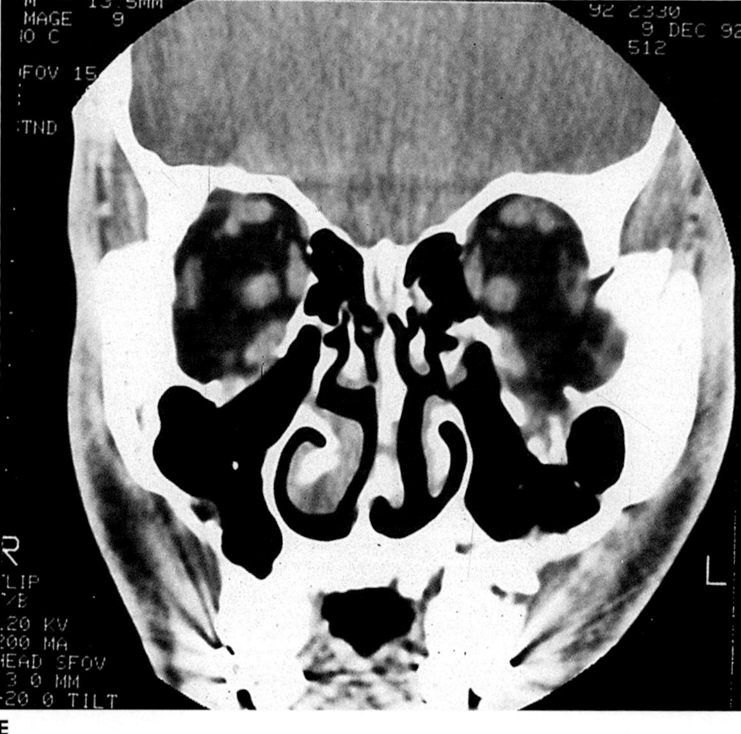

E

Figure 15-1 Orbital floor fracture (cont.) **D.** *and* **E.** *This 72-year-old female fell and hit her eye on her bedpost. She has full motility but significant swelling, ecchymosis, and infraorbital hypesthesia. CT scan shows a large orbital floor fracture. The patient is at risk for development of enophthalmos from the large fracture.*

MEDIAL WALL FRACTURE

Medial wall fractures can be isolated fractures of the medial wall only or they can be a part of larger fractures involving the nose and sinuses. Isolated fractures are treated much like orbital floor fractures. Larger fractures usually involve a multidiscipline approach to the repair of the fractures.

Epidemiology and Etiology

Age Most common in second through fourth decades.

Gender More common in males.

Etiology Direct fractures occur from striking a solid object. Indirect (blow-out) fractures occur in association with and by similar mechanisms as orbital floor fractures.

History

Trauma history is variable. Symptoms include diplopia and cosmetic deformities depending on the extent of the nasal fractures.

Examination

Medial rectus entrapment with diplopia and eventual enophthalmos are the two ocular manifestations that may occur. Direct fractures often have significant damage to the nasal bridge and medial orbit. The nasal bridge may be depressed with telecanthus. Other findings that can occur include epistaxis, orbital hematoma, cerebral spinal fluid rhinorrhea, and damage to the lacrimal drainage system (Fig. 15-2).

Imaging

CT scanning will show the extent of the fracture and assist with potential planning of the repair. MRI does not image bone well and should not be used initially after trauma.

Special Considerations

Medial wall fractures with entrapment of the medial rectus need to be repaired sooner than floor fractures (within 1 week) if possible.

Treatment

If isolated, medial wall fractures often do not need repair. Medial rectus entrapment with diplopia is one indication for repair. If the fracture is large, enophthalmos can develop and require surgery to build up the orbit. Implants are sometimes placed. Larger fractures involving the nasal bridge and medial orbit require repair and plating, usually in conjunction with an otolaryngology specialist.

Prognosis

Good. Larger fractures may require multiple surgeries and revisions.

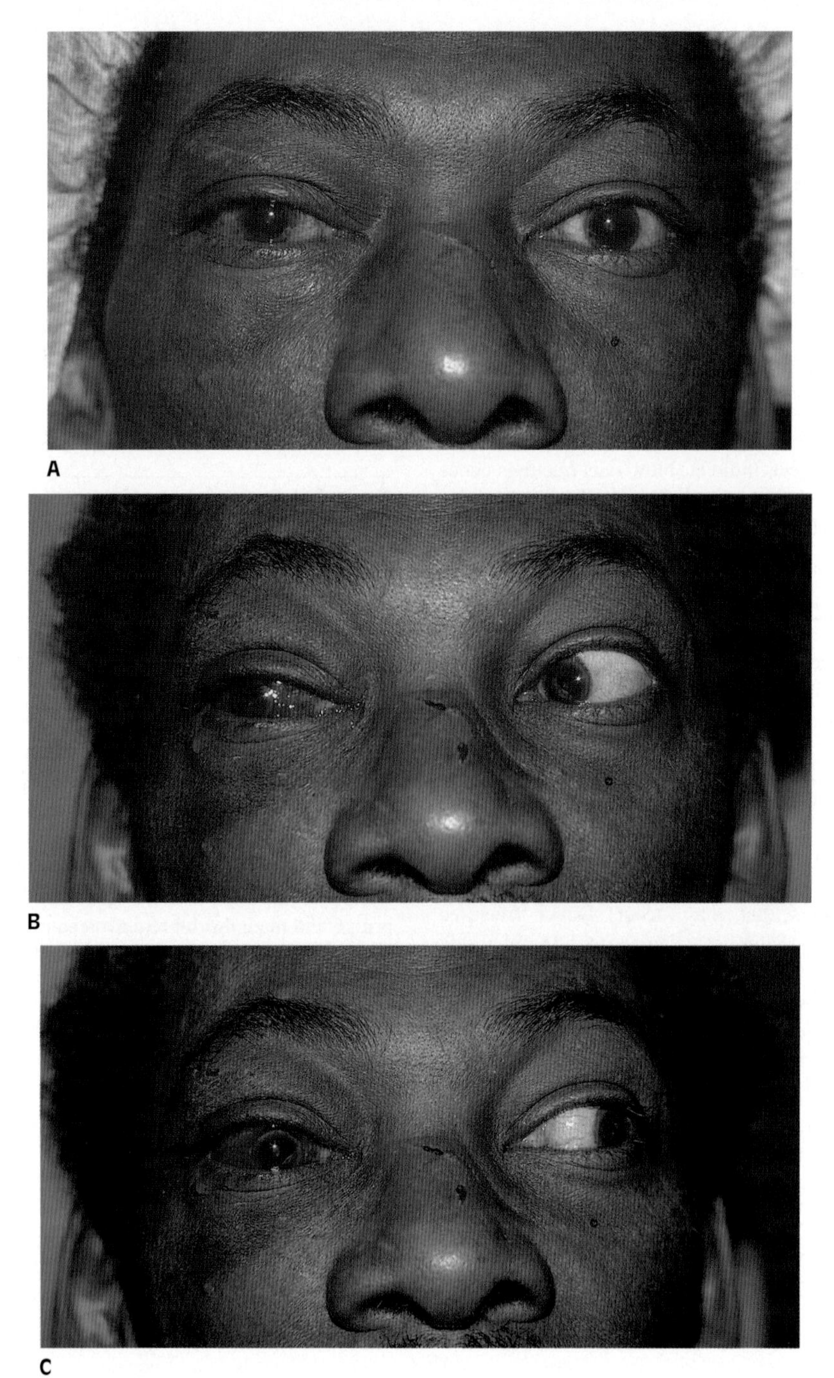

Figure 15-2 Medial wall fracture **A.** *through* **C.** *A 55-year-old male struck in the face with an unknown object presents with horizontal diplopia. Motility is restricted in the right eye in both adduction and abduction. (Continued.)*

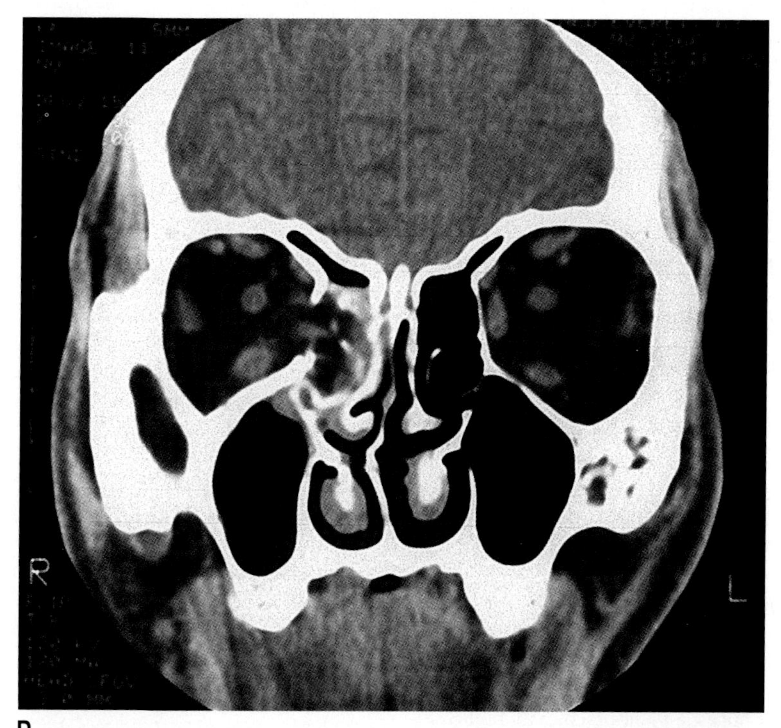

D

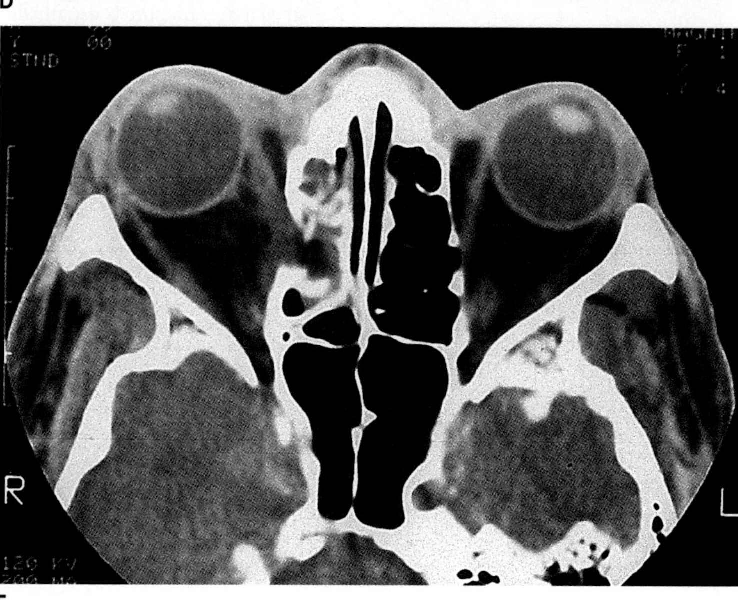

E

Figure 15-2 Medial wall fracture (cont.) **D.** *and* **E.** *CT scan shows a medial wall orbital fracture with the medial rectus muscle pulled into the fracture.*

ORBITAL ROOF FRACTURE

Orbital roof fractures are rare fractures that need to be recognized because of the potential for life-threatening neurologic sequelae. There may just be a small fracture with no neurologic problems or there may be significant intracranial air and bleeding. Treatment is in conjunction with neurosurgery.

Epidemiology and Etiology

Age Most common in second through fourth decades.

Gender More common in males.

Etiology Blunt trauma or direct injury by a thin object that goes above the globe under the superior orbital rim. An isolated roof fracture is rare.

History

Trauma history will often suggest high-energy forces that caused the injury. These include hydraulic air hoses, a blunt object with high velocity, and so forth.

Examination

Poor upgaze, supraorbital hypesthesia, and more swelling superiorly than inferiorly suggest an orbital roof fracture. Entrapment of the superior rectus muscle is extremely rare (Fig. 15-3).

Imaging

CT scanning will show the fracture usually just inside the orbital rim. MRI does not image bone well and should not be used initially after trauma. MRI can be of value to evaluate intracranial injury.

Special Considerations

Important to consult neurosurgery for the potential of CNS complications with a roof fracture.

Treatment

Repair of a roof fracture is usually done for neurologic reasons rather than ocular. Any plating and repair is done via craniotomy. Nondisplaced fractures do not require repair.

Prognosis

Variable depending on the extent of associated CNS injuries.

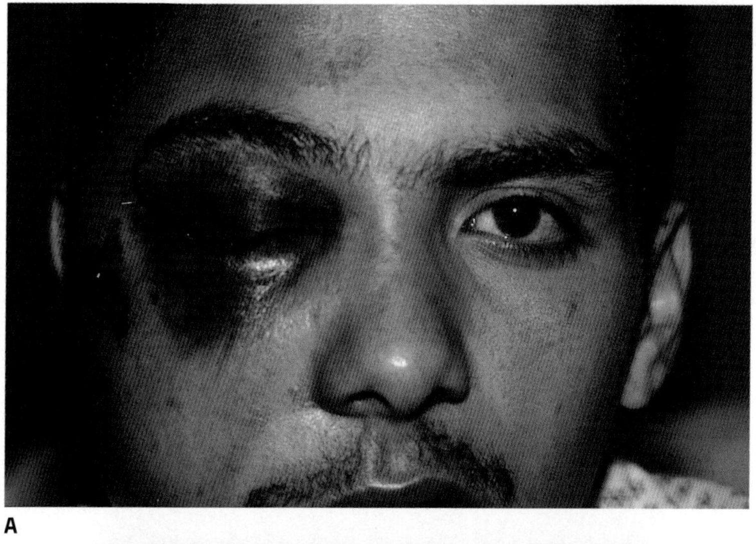

A

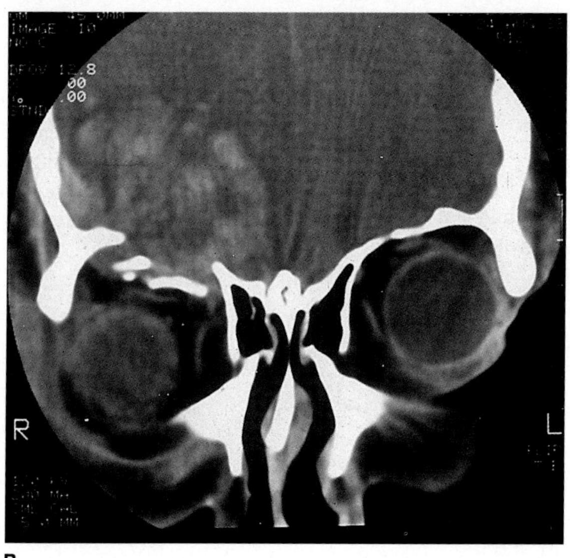

B

Figure 15-3 Orbital roof fracture **A.** *The patient was struck in the eye with a hydraulic air hose. Examination shows significant swelling, with decreased upgaze, and supraorbital hypesthesia.* **B.** *CT scan shows an orbital roof fracture with intracranial hemorrhage.*

ZYGOMATIC FRACTURE

Zygomatic fractures are the result of significant traumatic force to the zygomatic area. The result injury and symptom depend on the direction and amount of displacement of the bone. Repair should be done within the first week when needed.

Epidemiology and Etiology

Age Young adults.

Gender Males most common.

Etiology Trauma with force directed at the zygote.

History

Trauma with significant force. Patients often complain of pain and difficulty opening their mouth and chewing.

Examination

Initial findings may be minimal if there is significant swelling and ecchymosis of the orbit and cheek. Depressed cheek, orbital rim step off, and inability to open the mouth wide are common findings (Fig. 15-4A).

Imaging

CT scanning shows fracture of the zygomatic arch at the frontal-zygomatic suture and at the maxillary–zygomatic suture. The zygomatic arch is displaced in various directions depending on the direction of trauma. There is usually an associated orbital floor fracture (Fig. 15-4B to E). MRI does not image bone well and should not be used initially after trauma.

Treatment

Repair is required for most fractures with any significant displacement. This should be done as soon as the swelling has lessened. This is done with open reduction and plating as needed. Nondisplaced fractures do not require repair.

Prognosis

Excellent if repaired promptly.

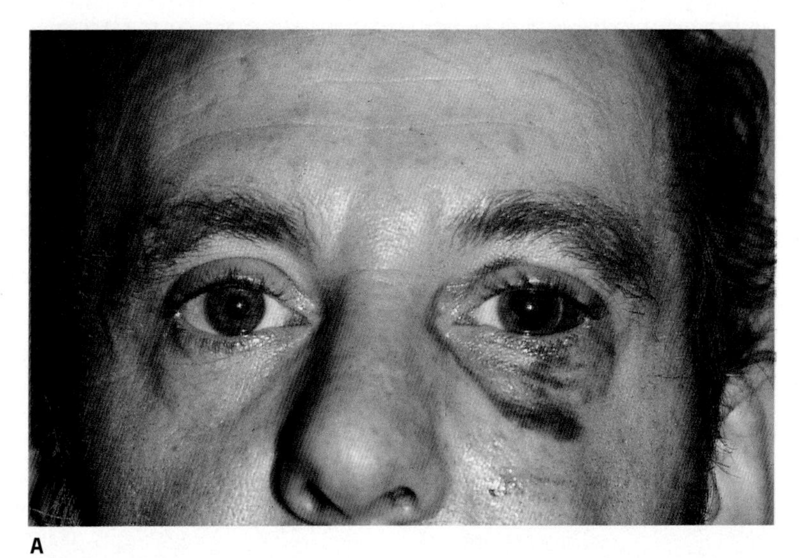

A

Figure 15-4 Zygomatic fracture **A.** *A 43-year-old male struck on the right cheek and eye with a bat. There is flattening of the cheek with trismus. (Continued.)*

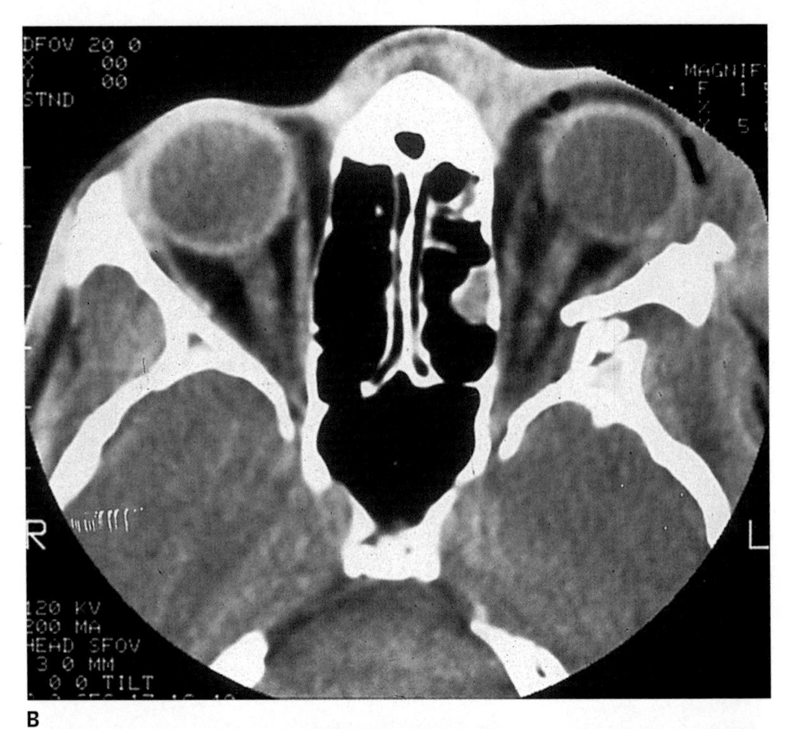

B

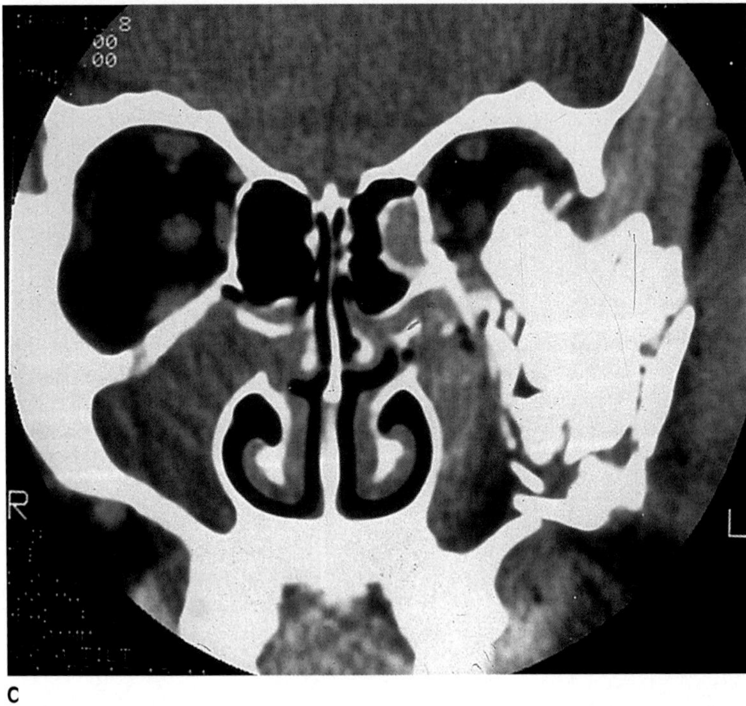

C

Figure 15-4 Zygomatic fracture (cont.) **B.** *and* **C.** *CT scan shows a zygomatic fracture. (Continued.)*

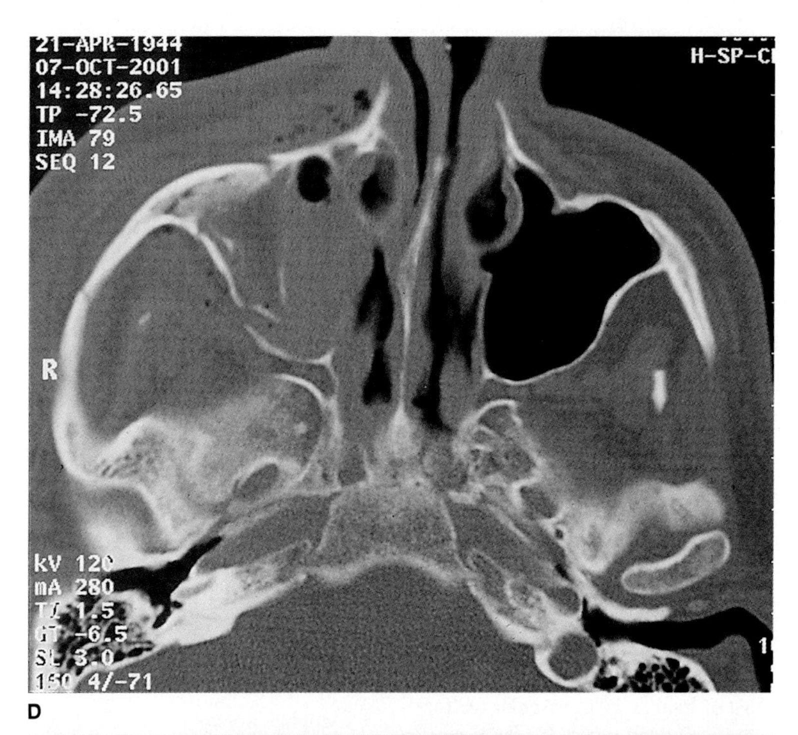

D

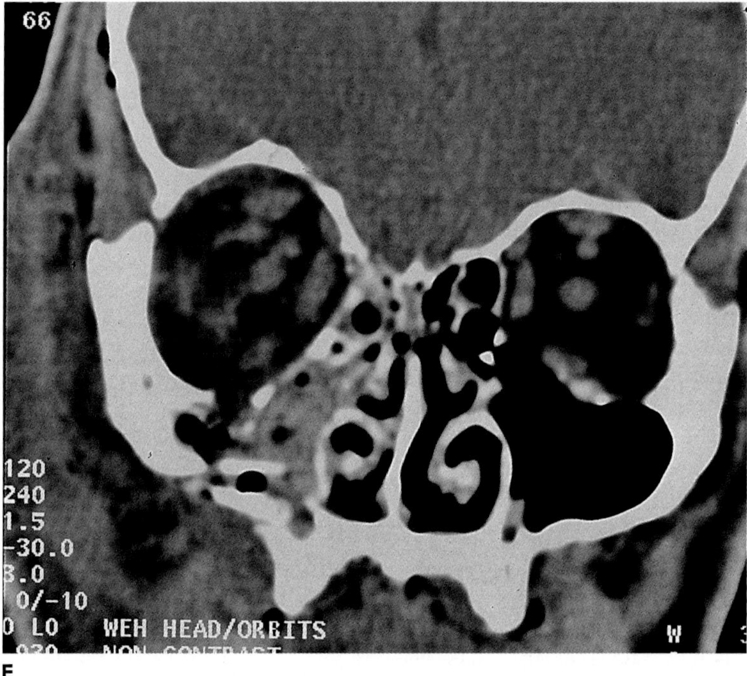

E

Figure 15-4 Zygomatic fracture (cont.) **D.** *and* **E.** *CT scan shows a smaller minimally displaced zygomatic fracture with associated orbital floor fracture.*

MISCELLANEOUS TRAUMA

ORBITAL HEMORRHAGE

Orbital hemorrhage as the result of orbital trauma is common and rarely requires any specific treatment. Spontaneous orbital hemorrhage is rare and requires evaluation of the orbit for a source of bleeding, although none may be found. The need to drain an orbital bleed is very rare.

Epidemiology and Etiology

Age Any.

Gender Males more common because of the higher incidence of trauma.

Etiology Trauma or orbital vascular lesion such as lymphangioma or vascular malformation.

History

History is that of trauma. With vascular malformations, there is sudden onset of orbital pain, pressure, proptosis, and sometimes ecchymosis.

Examination

Examination reveals proptosis with variable symptoms depending on the severity of the hemorrhage. There can be other ocular and orbital injuries if the cause is trauma. Mild hemorrhage may only reveal proptosis. Severe hemorrhage can result in no light perception vision, with severe proptosis, corneal exposure, frozen globe, elevated intraocular pressure, and inability to close the eye because of the severe proptosis (Fig. 15-5).

Imaging

CT scan: may show a discrete mass or more infiltrative lesion.
MRI: acute hemorrhage is hypointense on T_1 and hyperintense in T_2. When blood is more than 7 days old, it will become hyperintense on T_1 and variable on T_2.

Special Considerations

In spontaneous hemorrhage, an orbital vascular malformation needs to be looked for. If nothing is seen on imaging after the acute hemorrhage, a follow up MRI with gadolinium may identify a lesion.

Differential Diagnosis

Spontaneous hemorrhage (no trauma) includes the following.

- Lymphangioma
- Venous malformation and varix
- Arteriovenous malformation

Treatment

Observation, unless there is visual loss. Mild visual loss needs monitoring with intravenous steroids, acetazolamide, and possible lateral canthotomy. If visual loss is more severe, immediate lateral cantholysis is indicated along with high-dose intravenous steroids. Orbital imaging is done to look for loculated blood. The blood is usually within the orbital tissues and orbital drainage or even decompression is rarely of value. The exception would be a loculated hemorrhage such as in a lymphangioma.

Prognosis

Chance of permanent visual loss is present with severe hemorrhage. Less severe hemorrhages resolve without sequelae.

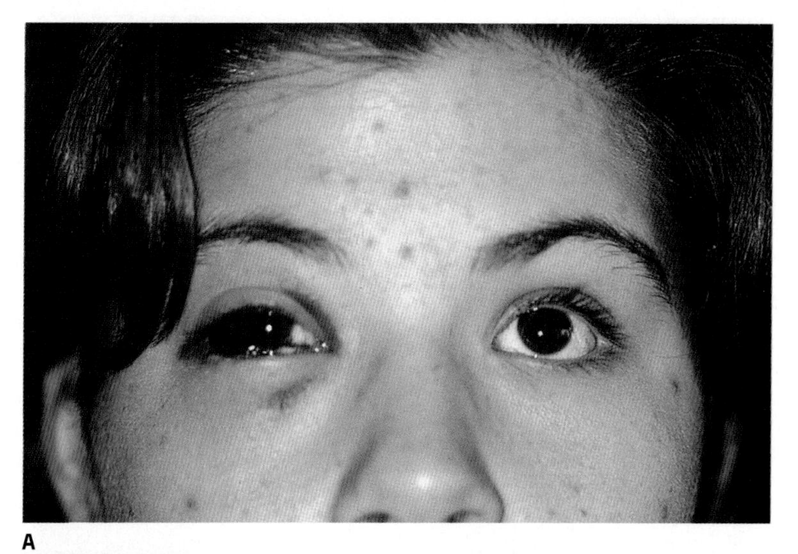

A

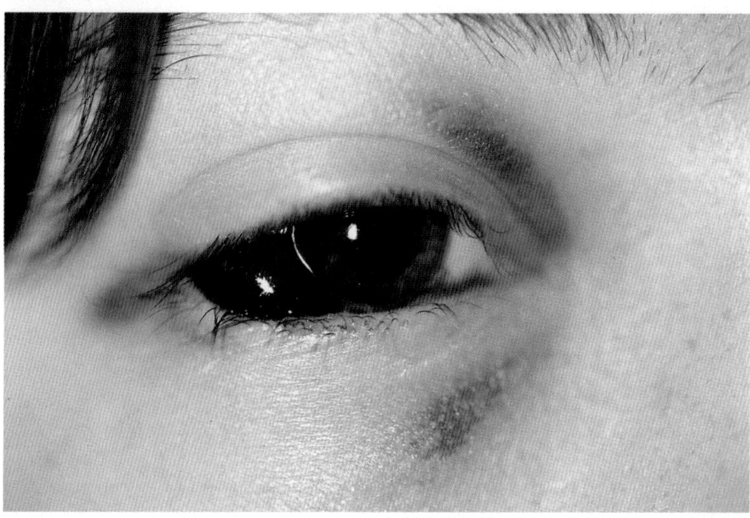

B

Figure 15-5 Orbital hemorrhage **A.** *A 17-year-old female with orbital hemorrhage after being poked in the eye with a field hockey stick. There was no other injury noted on CT scan. Vision was normal but the orbit was moderately tight. She was observed for progressive hemorrhage but the fullness of the orbit resolved overnight.* **B.** *There was a small corneal delle that resolved with lubrication and resolution of the hemorrhage. (Continued.)*

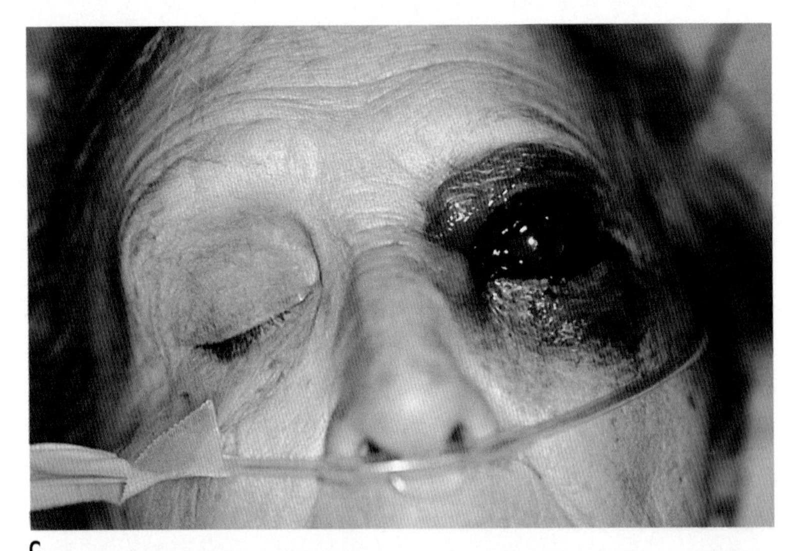

C

D

Figure 15-5 Orbital hemorrhage (cont.) **C.** *Severe orbital hemorrhage after retrobulbar injection in patient on coumadin.* **D.** *CT scan shows diffuse hemorrhage within the tissue and no loculated blood. Note the stretching and straightening of the optic nerve. (Continued.)*

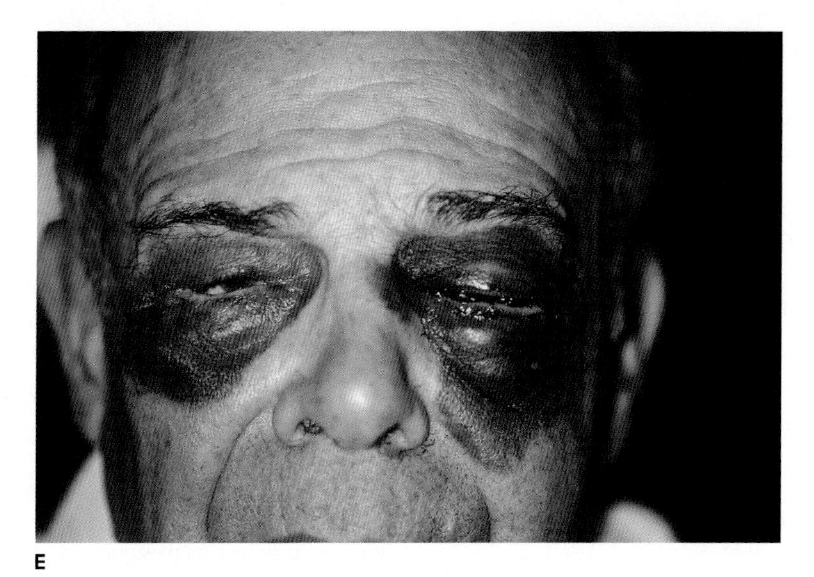

E

Figure 15-5 Orbital hemorrhage (cont.) **E.** *Bilateral orbital hemorrhage after blepharoplasty.*

ORBITAL FOREIGN BODIES

Orbital foreign bodies must always be suspected in any kind of orbital trauma. Most foreign bodies are removed surgically with the exception of certain inert materials that are deep in the orbit.

Epidemiology and Etiology

Age Any age.

Gender More common in males.

Etiology Foreign bodies can enter the orbit between the globe and the orbital wall or by double perforation of the globe.

History

The history may be of a specific foreign body entering the orbit. The more difficult situation is where there is trauma with a poor history but with wounds that could suggest a foreign body.

Examination

If the foreign body is anterior, it may be palpable or even visible. If it is deeper, there may very few signs except an entrance wound, or there may be significant hemorrhage and swelling (Fig. 15-6).

Imaging

Imaging is key to identifying and localizing an orbital foreign body and CT scanning is the imaging modality of choice. MRI should never be done after trauma unless a metallic foreign body has been ruled out. Glass, plastic, and organic foreign bodies may not show up well with CT scanning. These can be better visualized with MRI scanning but even MRI may not show these foreign bodies.

Treatment

Orbital foreign bodies should be removed if they are organic, cause symptoms, or if they have sharp edges so that migration could cause damage. The position of the foreign body can affect the decision to remove a foreign body. The more posterior it is, the more difficult it will be to remove it. Any foreign body left in place requires counseling of the patient about the potential for future extrusion or infection. If a foreign body is suspected, explanation is required even if imaging is negative.

Prognosis

Good. Organic foreign bodies can sometimes be retained and lead to chronic inflammation or infection.

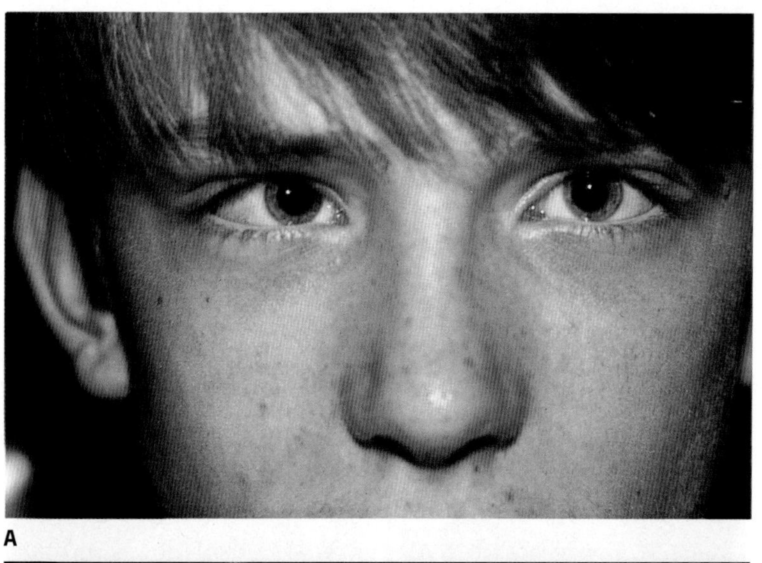

A

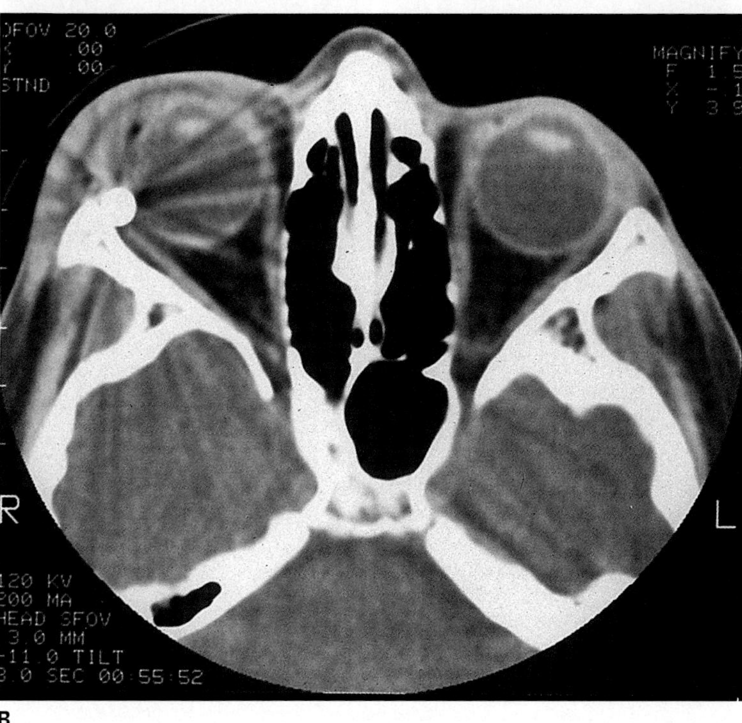

B

Figure 15-6 Orbital foreign body **A.** *A 12-year-old shot with a BB gun 2 weeks prior. The child has a long-standing esotropia. Note the mild erythema of the lateral right globe.* **B.** *CT scan shows the BB in the anterior lateral orbit. BBs can be left in the orbit without a problem. In this case, because of the anterior location and relative ease of removal, the BB was removed. (Continued.)*

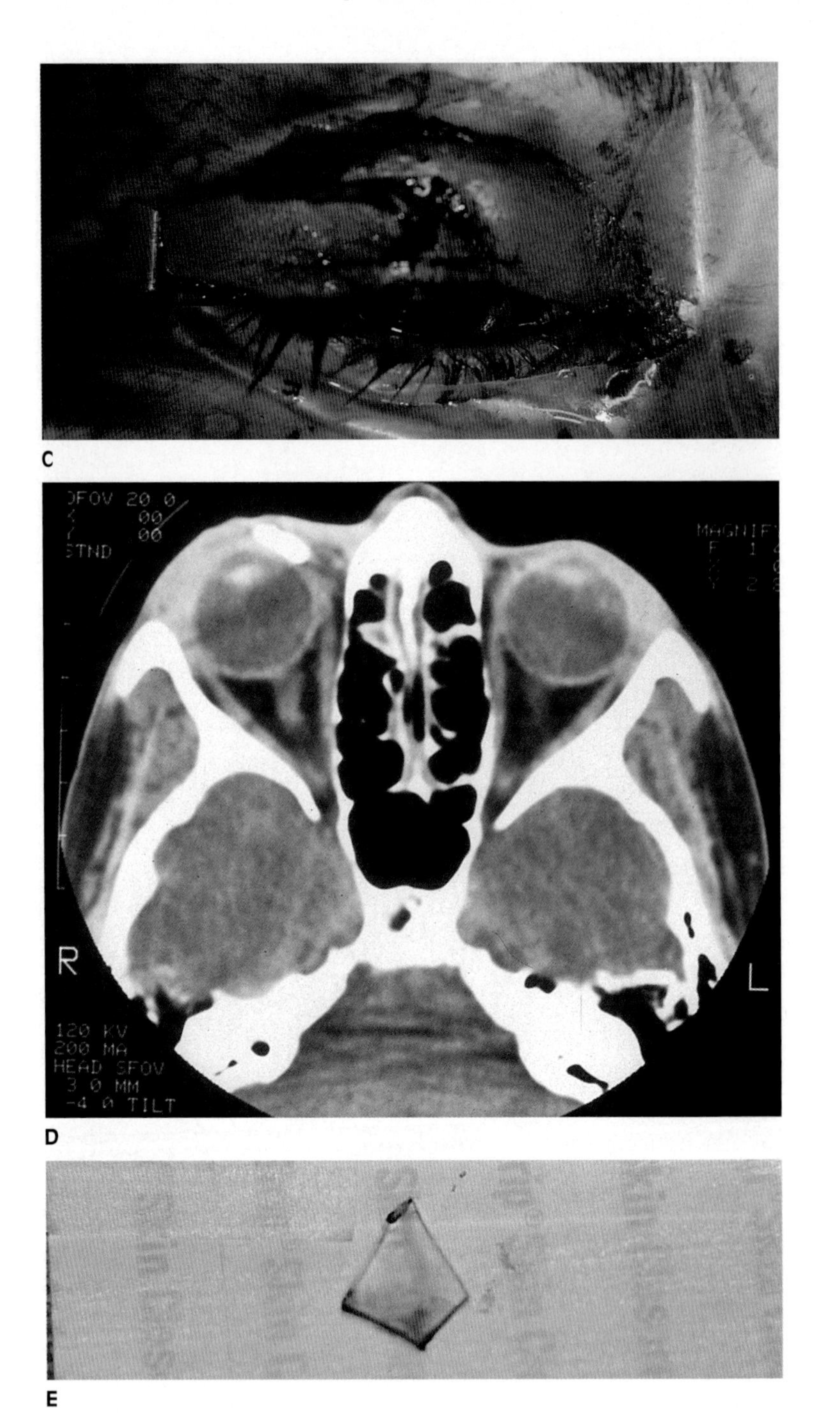

Figure 15-6 Orbital foreign body (cont.) **C.** *and* **D.** *Multiple eyelid lacerations from being struck with a wineglass that broke. A retained foreign body must always be suspected with broken glass. On CT scan, a foreign body is noted.* **E.** *The glass foreign body that was removed. The wineglass was leaded crystal, which is why it showed up so well on CT scan. (Continued.)*

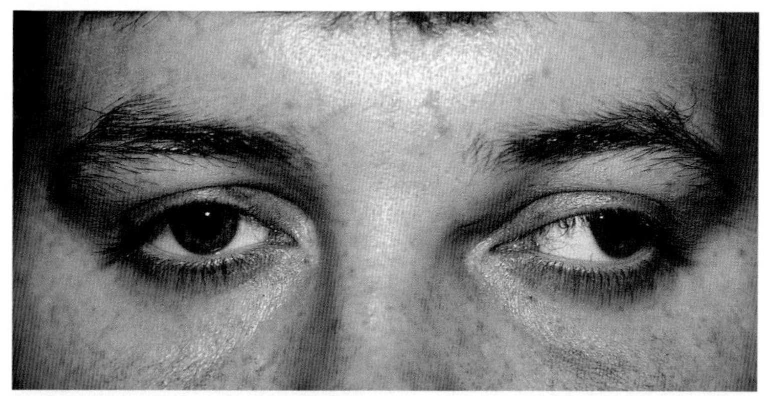

F

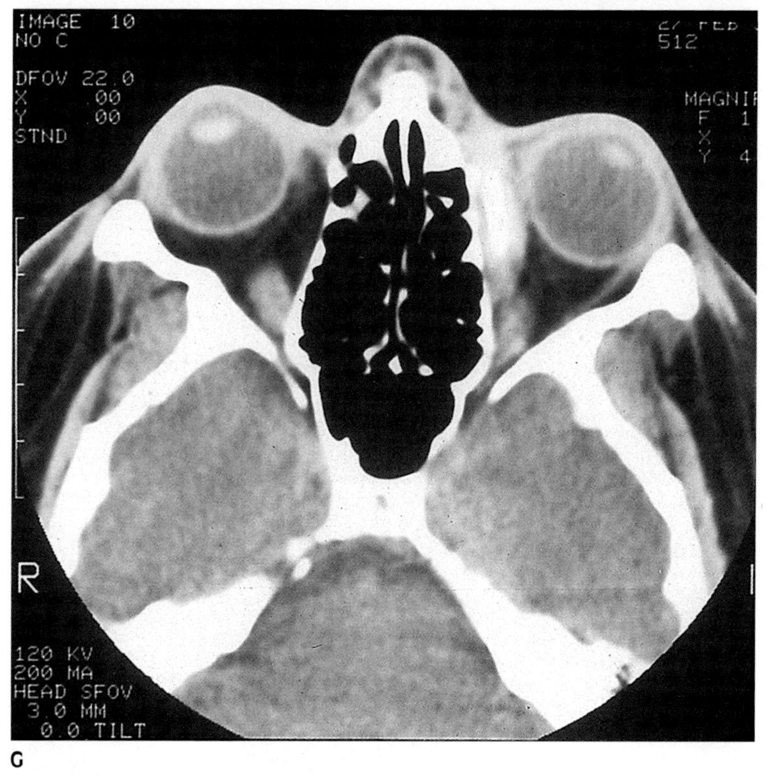

G

Figure 15-6 Orbital foreign body (cont.) **F.** *The patient was struck in the eye with a pencil 4 months prior. He presented with mild irritation of the left orbit. Note the lump in the left medial canthus.* **G.** *CT scan shows a medial orbital opacity. (Continued.)*

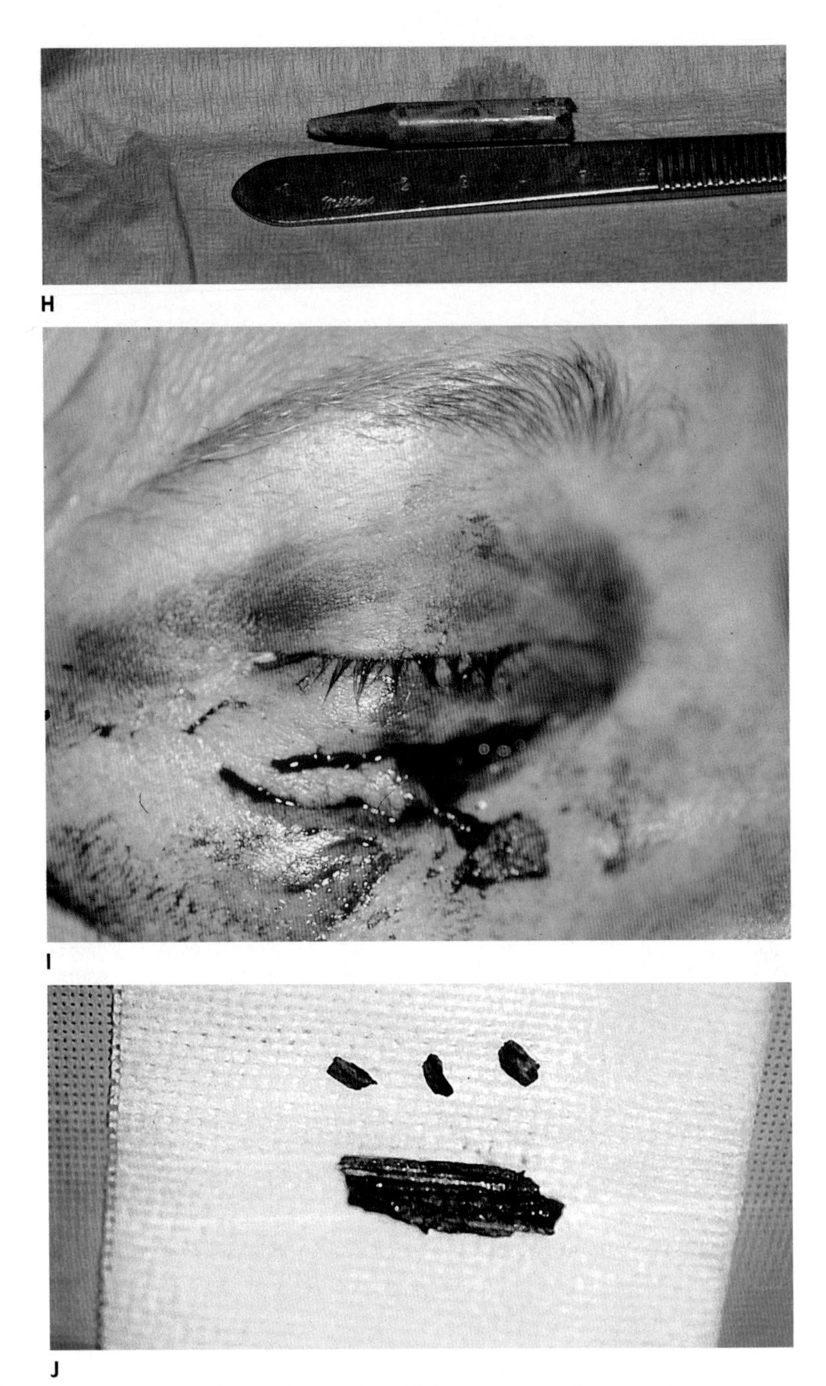

Figure 15-6 Orbital foreign body (cont.) **H.** *The medical orbital opacity turned out to be part of a pencil.* **I.** *and* **J.** *The patient ran into a bush and an eyelid laceration was revealed on examination. CT scan showed no foreign body. Exploration showed multiple wood fragments* (**J**).

MUCOCELE

Destruction of the sinus ostium from trauma or sinus disease can result in a mucous-filled sinus that can then expand into the orbit. Symptoms depend on the location of the mucocele. Treatment is usually aimed at excision of the cyst and obliteration of the sinus.

Epidemiology and Etiology

Age Any age but most common age is 40 to 70 years.

Gender More common in males.

Etiology Blockage of the sinus ostium results in a mucous-filled cyst that can expand with time.

History

There is usually a history of trauma to the sinuses or a long history of sinus disease. The orbital process shows very slow insidious onset of proptosis or globe displacement. More posterior mucoceles can present with slow visual loss. Rarely, if the mucocele becomes infected, the symptoms can have a rapid progression.

Examination

Findings will depend on the location of the mucocele. The mass expands slowly and will displace the globe, cause proptosis, and, if posterior, may cause optic nerve compression and/or an orbital apex syndrome (Fig. 15-7).

Special Considerations

Frontal and ethmoidal sinus mucoceles are the most common, with sphenoid sinus mucoceles being less common.

Differential Diagnosis

- Orbital abscess
- Primary sinus tumor with orbital extension

Treatment

Surgical excision with obliteration of the affected sinus.

Prognosis

There can be recurrences. Most mucoceles are easily treated surgically unless extremely large.

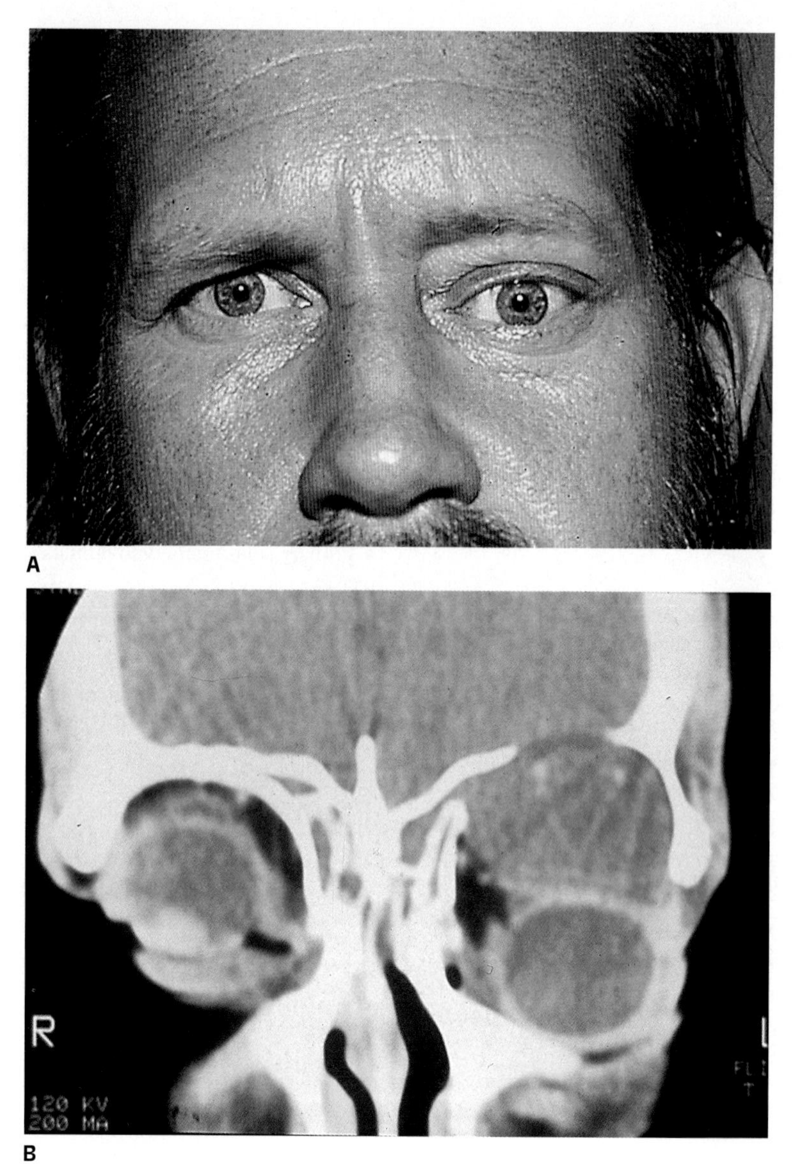

Figure 15-7 Orbital mucocele **A.** *A patient with a history of prior facial fractures presents with the complaint that his left eye is "out of place." The duration of this condition is unknown.* **B.** *CT scan shows a large frontal sinus mucocele displacing the globe downward.*

INDEX

Page numbers followed by f *indicate figures.*

F

G

O

P

R

S

T

V

W

X

Z